Progress in
CARDIOLOGY

Progress in CARDIOLOGY

Editor
Suman Bhandari MD DM FCSI FACC FSCAI FESC
Director, Interventional Cardiology
Department of Cardiology
Fortis Escorts Heart Institute
New Delhi, India

Forewords
Dhiman Kahali
Sanjay Tyagi

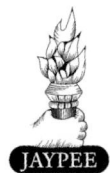

JAYPEE BROTHERS MEDICAL PUBLISHERS
The Health Sciences Publisher
New Delhi | London

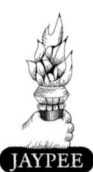# Jaypee Brothers Medical Publishers (P) Ltd

Headquarters
EMCA House, 23/23-B
Ansari Road, Daryaganj
New Delhi 110 002, India
Landline: +91-11-23272143, +91-11-23272703
+91-11-23282021, +91-11-23245672
e-mail: jaypee@jaypeebrothers.com

Corporate Office
4838/24, Ansari Road, Daryaganj
New Delhi 110 002, India
Phone: +91-11-43574357
Fax: +91-11-43574314
e-mail: jaypee@jaypeebrothers.com

Overseas Office
JP Medical Ltd.
83, Victoria Street, London
SW1H 0HW (UK)
Phone: +44-20 3170 8910
e-mail: info@jpmedpub.com

EU GPSR Authorised Representative
Logos Europe, 9 rue Nicolas Poussin
17000, La Rochelle, France
Phone: +33 (0) 6 67 93 73 78
e-mail: contact@logoseurope.eu

Website: www.jaypeebrothers.com
Website: www.jaypeedigital.com

© 2026, Jaypee Brothers Medical Publishers

The views and opinions expressed in this book are solely those of the original contributor(s)/author(s) and do not necessarily represent those of editor(s) or publisher of the book.

All rights reserved. No part of this publication may be reproduced, stored or transmitted in any form or by any means, electronic, mechanical, photocopying, recording or otherwise, without the prior permission in writing of the publishers.

All brand names and product names used in this book are trade names, service marks, trademarks or registered trademarks of their respective owners. The publisher is not associated with any product or vendor mentioned in this book.

Medical knowledge and practice change constantly. This book is designed to provide accurate, authoritative information about the subject matter in question. However, readers are advised to check the most current information available on procedures included and check information from the manufacturer of each product to be administered, to verify the recommended dose, formula, method and duration of administration, adverse effects and contraindications. It is the responsibility of the practitioner to take all appropriate safety precautions. Neither the publisher nor the author(s)/editor(s) assume any liability for any injury and/or damage to persons or property arising from or related to use of material in this book.

This book is sold on the understanding that the publisher is not engaged in providing professional medical services. If such advice or services are required, the services of a competent medical professional should be sought.

Every effort has been made where necessary to contact holders of copyright to obtain permission to reproduce copyright material. If any have been inadvertently overlooked, the publisher will be pleased to make the necessary arrangements at the first opportunity.

Inquiries for bulk sales may be solicited at: jaypee@jaypeebrothers.com

Progress in Cardiology

First Edition: **2026**

ISBN: 978-93-7202-079-3

Printed at: Samrat Offset Pvt. Ltd.

Dedication

Dedicated to my cheerleaders and support:
My wife and daughter who have been with my "ups and downs"
with exemplary equanimity
My late parents for the values they taught me
My teachers and my mentors who have had my back for such a long while
My patients who have had faith and trust in me and for teaching me the value of renewal of skills and knowledge—keeping me going in this complex life and helping me be of value.

Contributors

Abhishek Kumar Tiwari MD DM (Cardiology)
Associate Consultant
Department of Cardiology
Medanta—The Medicity
Gurugram, Haryana, India

Ajeet Bana MS MCh
Chair
Department of Cardiothoracic and Vascular Surgery
Eternal Heart Care Centre and Research Centre
Jaipur, Rajasthan, India

Akhilendra Bhushan Gupta MTech PhD
Head
Department of Civil Engineering
Malviya National Institute of Engineering
Jaipur, Rajasthan, India

Akhilesh Kumar MD (Medicine) DrNB (Cardiology)
Associate Consultant
Department of Cardiology
Fortis Escort Heart Institute
New Delhi, India

Anil Yadav MD (General Medicine) DM (Cardiology)
Associate Consultant
Department of Cardiology
Max Hospital
New Delhi, India

Anindita Das MSc (Clinical Nutrition)
Honorary Pediatric Dietitian
Department of Clinical Dietetic
NHS Greater Glasgow and Clyde
Glasgow, Scotland

Ankit Kumar Sahu MD DM
Assistant Professor
Department of Cardiology
Sanjay Gandhi Postgraduate Institute of Medical Sciences
Lucknow, Uttar Pradesh, India

Anupam Goel MD DM (Cardiology)
Director Intervention Cardiology
Department of Cardiology
Max Superspeciality Hospital
New Delhi, India

Aparajita Kumar PGDCC PCAC AMCD
Associate Consultant
Department of Clinical and
Preventive Cardiology
Medanta—The Medicity
Gurugram, Haryana, India

Ashutosh Marwah MD (Pediatrics)
Director
Department of Pediatric Cardiology
Fortis Escorts Heart Institute
New Delhi, India

Atul Kaushik MD (Medicine) DrNB
3rd-year DrNB Cardiology Resident
Department of Cardiology
Fortis Escorts Heart Institute
New Delhi, India

B Hilbert Sahoo MD
Senior Resident
Department of Cardiology
Sanjay Gandhi Postgraduate Institute of Medical Sciences
Lucknow, Uttar Pradesh, India

Babu Ezhumalai
MD DM FNB FACC FESC FSCAI FAPSIC FHFA FCSI FICC FISE
Senior Consultant and
Interventional Cardiologist
Department of Cardiology
MGM Healthcare
Chennai, Tamil Nadu, India

Balakrishnan KR MBBS MS MCh
Head and Director (Cardiac Surgery)
Department of Mechanical Circulatory Support and Heart/Lung Transplant
Institute of Heart/Lung and Mechanical Circulatory Support
Chennai, Tamil Nadu, India

Bhavana Mastebhakti MD (Medicine) DrNB (Cardiology)
Associate Consultant
Department of Cardiology
Fortis Escorts Heart Institute
New Delhi, India

Chhavi Agrawal DM (Endocrinology) MD
Consultant
Department of Endocrinology
Fortis Escorts Heart Institute
Gurugram, Haryana, India

Chris Alvis Shaji MD (Medicine)
Senior Resident
Department of Clinical and Preventive Cardiology
Medanta—The Medicity
Gurugram, Haryana, India

Deepak Reddy MD DM
Interventional Cardiologist
Department of Cardiology
Apollo Speciality Hospitals
Chennai, Tamil Nadu, India

Deepti Yadav MD DM
Consultant and Interventional Cardiologist
Department of Cardiology
Medanta—The Medicity
Gurugram, Haryana, India

GC Khilnani MD FCCP (USA) FAMS FICCM FICP FNCCP FISDA
Chairman
Department of Pulmonary, Critical Care, and Sleep Medicine
Pushpawati Singhania Research Institute
New Delhi, India

Ishi Khosla MSc (Clinical Nutrition)
Clinical Nutritionist
Celiac Society of India
New Delhi, India

Jagadish A MD DM FTEE FIECMO
Associate Consultant (Cardiac Anesthesia)
Department of Mechanical Circulatory Support and Heart/Lung Transplant
Institute of Heart/Lung and Mechanical Circulatory Support
Chennai, Tamil Nadu, India

Karthikeyan B MD DM
Consultant Cardiologist
Department of Cardiology
Hindu Mission Hospital
Chennai, Tamil Nadu, India

Leon M Ptaszek MD PhD FACC FHRS
Assistant Professor
Department of Medicine
Harvard Medical School
Associate Physician
Department of Medicine
Massachusetts General Hospital and Harvard Medical School
Boston, MA, USA

Madhu Agarwal MTech PhD
Associate Professor
Department of Chemical Engineering
Malviya National Institute of Technology
Jaipur, Rajasthan, India

Mitendra Singh Yadav MD DNB (Cardiology) FESC
Senior Consultant and Interventional Cardiologist
Department of Cardiology
Max Hospital
New Delhi, India

Mohd Akram DNB (General Medicine) DrNB (Cardiology)
3rd-year DrNB Cardiology Trainee
Department of Interventional Cardiology
Fortis Escorts Heart Institute
New Delhi, India

Mrinal Kanti Das MD (Medicine) DM (Cardiology)
Senior Consultant and Interventional Cardiologist
Department of Cardiology
CK Birla Hospitals (BMB/CMRI)
Kolkata, West Bengal, India

Nagendra Chouhan MD DM
Director
Department of Cardiology
Medanta—The Medicity
Gurugram, Haryana, India

Nilashish Dey MBBS DNB
DrNB (Resident)
Department of Cardiology
Fortis Escorts Heart Institute
New Delhi, India

Palanivel Rajan MD DM
Consultant Cardiologist
Department of Cardiology
Apollo Hospitals
Chennai, Tamil Nadu, India

Praveen Chandra MD DM
Chairman, Institute of Cardiac Science
Department of Cardiology
Medanta—The Medicity
Gurugram, Haryana, India

Pravin K Goel MD DM FACC FSCAI FICC MAMS
Director, Interventional Cardiology
Department of Cardiology
Medanta Heart Institute
Lucknow, Uttar Pradesh, India

Rajeev Gupta MD PhD
Chair
Department of Preventive Cardiology and Medicine
Eternal Heart Care Centre and Research Centre
Jaipur, Rajasthan, India

Rajiv Parakh FRCS MS (Surgery)
Chairman
Department of Peripheral Vascular and Endovascular Sciences
Medanta—The Medicity
Gurugram, Haryana, India

Salil K Midha MD FACC
Chief of Cardiology
Department of Medicine
Melrose-Wakefield Hospital
Melrose, MA, USA

Sangeeta Dhir MDS (Periodontology) Fellow (Implantology)
Consultant Dentistry and Clinical Research
Department of Cardiology
Max Hospital
New Delhi, India

Sanjay Mittal MD DM (Cardiology)
Vice Chairman
Department of Clinical and Preventive Cardiology
Medanta—The Medicity
Gurugram, Haryana, India

Satyavir Yadav MD DM
Associate Professor
Department of Cardiology
All India Institute of Medical Sciences
New Delhi, India

Sebastian E Beyer MD MPH
Clinical and Research Fellow in Medicine
Department of Medicine
Massachusetts General Hospital and
Harvard Medical School
Boston MA, USA

Shiv Kumar Goel DM (Endocrinology) MD
Consultant
Department of Cardiology
Sarvottam Superspeciality Clinic
Gurugram, Haryana, India

Siddarth Varshney MD DM
Consultant Interventional Cardiologist
Department of Cardiology
Medanta—The Medicity
Gurugram, Haryana, India

Siddhartha Paturi
DrNB (Vascular Surgery) MS (Surgery)
Senior Resident
Department of Peripheral Vascular and
Endovascular Sciences
Medanta—The Medicity
Gurugram, Haryana, India

Smit Shrivastava
MD DM PGDHHM FACC FICP FISE FIMSA FIACM FSCAI FICN FCSI
Professor and Head
Department of Cardiology
Advanced Cardiac Institute
Pt. JNM Medical College Raipur (Cg)
Raipur, Chhattisgarh, India

Sonali Bansal MD DrNB
Associate Director
Department of Critical Care
Park Hospital
Gurugram, Haryana, India

Suman Banerjee MBBS EDIC
Consultant Critical Care Medicine
Department of Pulmonology, Sleep Medicine, and
Critical Care Medicine
Pushpawati Singhania Research Institute
New Delhi, India

Suman Bhandari MD DM FCSI FACC FSCAI FESC
Director, Interventional Cardiology
Department of Cardiology
Fortis Escorts Heart Institute
New Delhi, India

Surendra Singh MD
Head
Department of Pathology
Eternal Heart Care Centre and Research Centre
Jaipur, Rajasthan, India

Suresh Rao KG MD MBA
Head and Co-Director (Cardiac Anesthesia)
Department of Mechanical Circulatory Support and
Heart/Lung Transplant
Institute of Heart/Lung and Mechanical Circulatory
Support
Chennai, Tamil Nadu, India

Tanu Chaudhary MD DrNB
Consultant Interventional Cardiologist
Department of Cardiology
Medanta—The Medicity
Gurugram, Haryana, India

Vaibhav Bandil MD (Medicine) DrNB (Cardiology)
Senior Interventional Cardiologist
Department of Cardiology
Arogy Adham Hospital and Research Centre
Gwalior, Madhya Pradesh, India

Vibhav Sharma MD (Medicine, PGI Chandigarh) DM (Cardiology, AIIMS, New Delhi)
Assistant Professor
Department of Cardiology
Amrita institute of Medical Sciences
Faridabad, Haryana, India

Vijayakumar S MD DM FNB
Senior Consultant and Cardiologist
Department of Cardiology
Apollo Hospitals
Chennai, Tamil Nadu, India

Viveka Kumar
MD DM FSCAI FACC FECS FAPSIC FRCP (Edin)
Principal Director and Chief, Cath Labs (Pan Max)–
Cardiac Sciences
Max Super Speciality Hospital
New Delhi, India

Foreword

I am very impressed with *Progress in Cardiology*. The selection of topics is contemporary and has advanced my current knowledge in the broad field of cardiology. Key topics on preventive, clinical, and intervention, as well as burnout—which is quite common among cardiologists, are very apt and informative. Such books help busy cardiologists keep pace with this rapidly moving specialty. We definitely need such wide selections of key reviews of current cardiology topics, especially with an Indian context. I hope and believe that Dr Suman Bhandari will make this a regular feature and involve other key opinion leaders from neighboring countries and expand it to a global and regional yearly series of *Progress in Cardiology*.

The contributors have done a marvelous job and I would like to congratulate them too for helping bring out the best current reviews.

I would definitely recommend it as a must-read for all levels of cardiologists to keep themselves updated and remain on top of the field.

Dhiman Kahali
MD DM
Director of Interventional Cardiology
Department of Interventional Cardiology
BM Birla, Heart Research Centre
President-Elect, CSI 2025

Foreword

It is an honor and a pleasure to write the foreword for the book *Progress in Cardiology* edited by Dr Suman Bhandari. It is an excellent book with 28 chapters that cover the current landscape of cardiology, covering preventive, clinical, and interventional cardiology, including recent key trials.

I found this a must-read and would recommend it to all cardiologists at whatever stage they may be, to get up to date with the rapid paced progress in cardiology. It is a great initiative from India and Southeast Asia. I hope that as it broadens, it will have a far widespread authorship and readers.

Once again, I congratulate Dr Suman Bhandari for this initiative and wish him all success in further *Progress in Cardiology* series. I will surely reserve my copy of this and all further issues.

Sanjay Tyagi
MD DM FAMS FESC
BC Roy Awardee
Clinical Director
Department of Cardiology
Apollo Group Hospitals
New Delhi, India
President, CSI 2025

Preface

Progress in Cardiology is the first of its kind in Southeast Asia (India). This is a contemporary review of the topics in the field of cardiology by key opinion leaders from India and overseas and will serve to provide early leaners in the field with "cutting-edge" topics and also help those established in this field with an update of the current understanding and new paradigms in this fast-paced field.

Thanks are due to M/s Jaypee Brothers Medical Publishers (P) Ltd, New Delhi, India for envisioning this need and for inviting me to serve as the editor and curator of this new important venture.

The authors deserve my sincerest gratitude for helping to bring out an excellent review of the current landscape of cardiology, despite their hectic schedule and engagements. Their love for this educational venture is highly applauded by all stakeholders.

The readers have 28 contemporary subjects updated for the assimilation and enhancement of their zeal in the field of cardiology, which continues to evolve at an exciting pace. Hopefully, such updates (*Progress in Cardiology*) will make this journey more informative and rewarding.

Suman Bhandari

Acknowledgments

I would like to acknowledge the team at M/s Jaypee Brothers Medical Publishers (P) Ltd, New Delhi, India especially Mr Ankit Vij (Managing Director), Mr Sabyasachi Hazra (Director, PG and PNR), and Ms Kajal Keshri (Development Editor), for being pillars of help, support, and understanding during the editing of the book *Progress in Cardiology*. They had the vision and deep knowledge of their field which helped me proceed with the processes as the end was quite visible and clear.

Thanks are due to the authors who despite a busy clinical schedule found some time to bring out their assignment with the excellence that you will surely relish. Their enthusiasm and discipline are really what give this volume its character.

I am also thankful to my Secretary, Mr Sourabh for helping me with many revisions and keeping me on track.

I am grateful to my family and my wife, Nita who have always backed my academic engagement and helped serve as a mirror to my life with encouragement and keen observations to put me back on path.

Thanks are due to my daughter, Sonakshi who has always been engaged with my life enthusiastically (daughters are precious and full of love) and her husband, Prashant for being truly understanding and positive.

I would like to mention my 5-year-old granddaughter, Alayna, who is full of fun and has the eagerness to live life to the fullest. This too has helped me see each day through her lens—in a very different, curious, and playful perspective.

Finally, the readers need their acknowledgment for it is with them in mind that one prepares the pudding that they would relish and ask for more.

Contents

1. **Cardiovascular–Kidney–Metabolic Syndrome: A New Actionable Cause** 1
   Babu Ezhumalai, Deepak Reddy

2. **Nanoplastics in Coronary Artery Disease** 12
   *Rajeev Gupta, Surendra Singh, Madhu Agarwal,
   Ajeet Bana, Akhilendra Bhushan Gupta*

3. **The Lancet Commission: Relooking at Coronary Heart Disease in 2025** 24
   Rajeev Gupta

4. **Are SGLT2 Inhibitors New Wonder Drugs? Effects Beyond Their Task** 41
   Mohd Akram, Suman Bhandari

5. **Atherosclerosis: Newer Concepts** 52
   Akhilesh Kumar, Suman Bhandari

6. **Late Myocardial Infarction Presentation: Current Strategy for Best Practices 2025** 65
   Atul Kaushik, Suman Bhandari

7. **Vericiguat—The Fifth Pillar or Default Early Start in Heart Failure: Indian Data** 69
   Sanjay Mittal, Abhishek Kumar Tiwari, Aparajita Kumar, Chris Alvis Shaji

8. **Antihypertensive Management in 2025: Moving Toward a Single Pill (Triple/Quadruple)** 83
   Suman Bhandari, Bhavana Mastebhakti

9. **Cuffless Blood Pressure Measurement Devices: How Accurate and Feasible?** 91
   Akhilesh Kumar, Suman Bhandari

10. **Dual Antiplatelet Therapy: Newer Direction in 2025** 98
    Mrinal Kanti Das

11. **High Bleeding Risk: Making Antiplatelet Safe** 107
    Vaibhav Bandil, Suman Bhandari

12. **Infective Endocarditis: What is the Management in 2025?** 121
    Vibhav Sharma, Satyavir Yadav

13. **Advances in Atrial Fibrillation Ablation: Technology and Technique** 141
    Sebastian E Beyer, Salil K Midha, Leon M Ptaszek

14. **Microvascular Angina: How to Diagnose and Manage It** 149
    Viveka Kumar, Anil Yadav, Sangeeta Dhir, Mitendra Singh Yadav, Anupam Goel

15. **Myocardial Bridging: Current Perspectives** 157
    Suman Bhandari, Atul Kaushik

16. **Imaging as Class I Indication: Current Value of ICI and Strategies for Achieving Better Penetration in India** 161
    Palanivel Rajan, Karthikeyan B, Vijayakumar S

17. **Cardiogenic Shock: Diagnosis and Early Management—Status 2025** 180
    Siddarth Varshney, Deepti Yadav, Sonali Bansal, Praveen Chandra

18. **Coronary LASER—Light at the End of the Tunnel: Expanding Indications** 188
    Smit Shrivastava

19. **Indian Perspective in Chronic Total Occlusion Management and Algorithmic Approach** 201
    Pravin K Goel, Ankit Kumar Sahu, B Hilbert Sahoo

20. **Drug-eluting Balloon: Coming of Age** 209
    Siddarth Varshney, Deepti Yadav, Tanu Chaudhary, Praveen Chandra

21. **A Primary Approach Moving Toward Early Catheter Directed Interventions in Acute Pulmonary Embolism** 217
    Rajiv Parakh, Siddhartha Paturi

22. **Heart Transplant and Left Ventricular Assist Device: Chennai Experience** 231
    Jagadish A, Suresh Rao KG, Balakrishnan KR

23. **Step-by-Step Coiling in Coronary Tree: Why and How** 246
    Atul Kaushik, Ashutosh Marwah

24. **Clipping Valves for Regurgitation in 2025** 250
    Deepti Yadav, Siddarth Varshney, Nagendra Chouhan, Praveen Chandra

25. **Weight Reduction by Novel Drugs: What is Their Effect on Cardiovascular Events and Which One to Choose?** 262
    Chhavi Agrawal, Shiv Kumar Goel

26. **Vegetarian Diet versus Mediterranean Diet: What to Follow? Indian Mediterranean Diet?** 268
    Ishi Khosla, Anindita Das

27. **Recent Trials with Clinical Impact: A 360° View** 275
    Suman Bhandari, Nilashish Dey

28. **Burnout: Understanding and Managing it in 2025** 292
    Suman Banerjee, GC Khilnani

Index *297*

CHAPTER 1

Cardiovascular–Kidney–Metabolic Syndrome: A New Actionable Cause

Babu Ezhumalai, Deepak Reddy

INTRODUCTION

Cardiovascular–kidney–metabolic (CKM) syndrome is a disorder with interconnected pathogenesis involving metabolic risk factors (such as obesity and diabetes), chronic kidney disease (CKD), and cardiovascular disease (CVD) **(Fig. 1)**. In CKM syndrome, dysfunction in one system (metabolic, renal, or CV) can initiate or exacerbate dysfunction in the others, thereby creating a vicious cycle. This concept extends beyond earlier notions, such as cardiorenal syndrome, by incorporating metabolic dysfunction as a fundamental contributor to cardiac and renal disease.[1,2] In 2023, the American Heart Association (AHA) formally introduced the term CKM syndrome to promote integrated strategies for risk reduction. The presidential advisory of AHA highlighted that poor CKM health has a profound impact on CVD incidence and mortality, and it emphasized the need for unified definitions, staging, and management algorithms for CKM syndrome.[1] This new framework has garnered broad attention in the medical community, signifying a paradigm shift toward treating the "whole patient" rather than individual diseases.[3,4]

EPIDEMIOLOGY AND BURDEN

Globally, over 500 million people are living with diabetes, approximately 64 million with heart failure (HF), and nearly 700 million with CKD. These conditions frequently overlap; for instance, patients with HF have about a fourfold higher prevalence of type 2 diabetes (T2D) compared to those without HF (20% vs. 5%). Conversely, T2D confers a two to fourfold increased risk of developing CVD (including coronary disease and stroke), and 40% of individuals with T2D have concomitant CKD.[5] Likewise, about half of patients with HF show evidence of CKD, and CVD is far more common in CKD patients than in the general population, with prevalence rising as glomerular filtration rate (GFR) declines. In the United States, an analysis of National Health and Nutrition Examination Survey data (1999–2020) found that 24% of adults had at least one cardiac, renal, or metabolic condition, and approximately 15% had coexisting conditions across these domains. Overall, an estimated 25–30% of adults worldwide may have some form of CKM multimorbidity, underscoring the widespread nature of the syndrome. The co-occurrence of these diseases exponentially worsens outcomes. These data illustrate that CKM syndrome is not

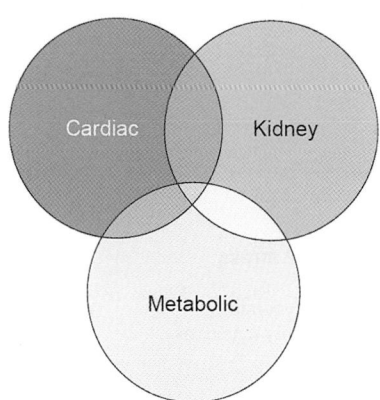

Fig. 1: Cardio-kidney-metabolic syndrome in a nutshell.

only highly prevalent but also confers a synergistic burden on morbidity and mortality.[6] Social determinants of health—such as food insecurity, poor access to healthcare, and environmental factors—drive risk factor clustering (obesity, hypertension, and diabetes) and poorer outcomes in CKM syndrome.[7]

PATHOPHYSIOLOGY

The pathophysiology of CKM syndrome is complex, involving shared pathways that link the heart, kidneys, and metabolic system. The primary underlying mechanism is chronic systemic inflammation, which is both a cause and consequence of the metabolic, renal, and CV abnormalities. Adiposity and insulin resistance in T2D promote a proinflammatory state, characterized by elevated cytokines (e.g., interleukin-6) and acute-phase reactants (such as high-sensitivity C-reactive protein), leading to endothelial dysfunction and atherosclerosis. Inflammatory mediators and oxidative stress not only damage blood vessels, accelerating coronary disease and stroke, but also impair pancreatic beta-cell function and insulin signaling, thereby worsening glycemic control **(Fig. 2)**.[8,9]

Hemodynamic and Neurohormonal Mechanisms

Cardiovascular-kidney-metabolic syndrome is further driven by neurohormonal activation, which is common to HF, CKD, and metabolic syndrome.[8,9] Activation of the renin–angiotensin–aldosterone system (RAAS) and sympathetic nervous system leads to vasoconstriction, sodium retention, and hypertension, placing strain on both the heart and kidneys. RAAS activation also promotes maladaptive cardiac remodeling (fibrosis and hypertrophy) and glomerular hypertension, while contributing to insulin resistance and lipid abnormalities through complex molecular crosstalk. In CKD, reduced renal clearance of sodium and water exacerbates volume overload and hypertension, further stressing the CV system.

Endothelial Dysfunction and Oxidative Stress

Endothelial dysfunction is a key mediator across the CKM spectrum. Hyperglycemia and proinflammatory cytokines reduce nitric oxide bioavailability, increasing oxidative stress in the endothelium and impairing vasodilation, which

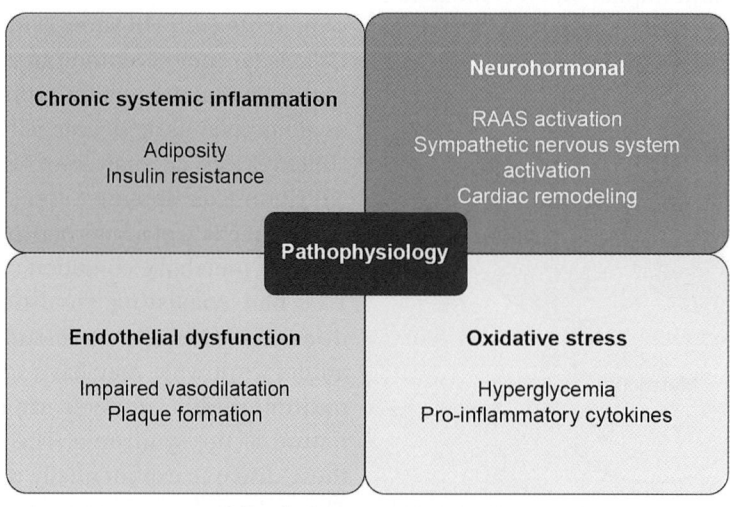

Fig. 2: Pathophysiology of CKM.

can trigger plaque formation in arteries. In the kidneys, endothelial injury in glomeruli leads to albuminuria and progressive nephron loss, while in the heart, it contributes to microvascular dysfunction and ischemia. These interrelated mechanisms underscore that CKM syndrome is not a linear sequence of events but rather a multidirectional network of pathophysiological processes.[8,9] Importantly, the progression of CKM syndrome is often gradual and subclinical in early stages. Initial insults such as obesity or prediabetes begin the cascade with relatively subtle effects (e.g., mild hypertension and microalbuminuria) that may go unnoticed. Without intervention, these changes progress to more significant organ damage, for instance, from microalbuminuria to overt CKD, or from left ventricular diastolic dysfunction to symptomatic HF, eventually culminating in advanced, irreversible end-organ failure. Hence, it reinforces the need for early, aggressive therapy targeting common pathways (such as inflammation and RAAS activation) to disrupt the cycle before it reaches a point of no return.[8,9]

DIAGNOSIS AND RISK STRATIFICATION

Early identification of CKM syndrome is critical, since patients have subclinical organ damage before manifesting obvious clinical disease. A comprehensive diagnostic approach involves screening for risk factors, laboratory biomarkers, and imaging for evidence of organ dysfunction across all three domains (cardio, renal, and metabolic).

Routine Risk Factor Screening

Adults with any component of CKM should undergo periodic assessment involving measuring blood pressure, fasting glucose or HbA1c, lipid profile, body mass index (BMI), estimated GFR (eGFR), and urine albumin-to-creatinine ratio (UACR). The AHA advisory recommends life-course screening for CKM risk factors (obesity, dyslipidemia, hypertension, and hyperglycemia) to facilitate timely prevention efforts.[1]

Laboratory Biomarkers

Certain biomarkers can detect organ stress before clinical symptoms develop. Albuminuria is a key early marker of kidney damage, even minimal persistent albuminuria (microalbuminuria) in a diabetic or hypertensive patient signals endothelial injury and heightened renal (and CV) risk. Patients with moderate eGFR reduction and albuminuria can be identified as high risk and targeted for intervention.[10] Natriuretic peptides (BNP or NT-proBNP), typically used to diagnose HF, also serve as sensitive indicators of subclinical cardiac strain. Even in patients without clinical HF, elevated BNP/NT-proBNP levels are associated with a higher risk of developing HF and adverse CV events.[11] Similarly, high-sensitivity cardiac troponin can detect minor myocardial injury (for example, from silent ischemia or microinfarctions) in stable patients; chronically elevated troponin T levels have been linked to higher long-term CV mortality. Incorporating these biomarkers into diabetes care may help unmask incipient cardiomyopathy or ischemic heart disease in the CKM population.

Imaging and Clinical Tests

Targeted use of imaging can reveal organ damage early. Echocardiography is recommended in asymptomatic diabetic patients with elevated BNP to evaluate for left ventricular hypertrophy or diastolic dysfunction. The presence of moderate diastolic dysfunction or a reduced ejection fraction (<50%) in such a patient would signal Stage 3 CKM (subclinical CVD) under the AHA scheme. Coronary artery calcium scoring or carotid ultrasound for plaque can detect subclinical atherosclerosis, which, if present in a CKD or diabetic patient, portends high CV risk (risk equivalent status). Renal ultrasound may be used to identify structural kidney disease that could expedite referral. Overall, the diagnostic strategy involves proactive surveillance, which involves detecting early warning signs of each organ's involvement in at-risk patients, thereby allowing for timely, multipronged interventions.[12]

Risk Stratification Tools

In diabetes care, investigators have advocated for incorporating biomarkers into risk models: For instance, adding high-sensitivity troponin and BNP significantly improved the prediction of HF and CV events in patients with T2D (as shown in the ARIC study). While no single unified "CKM risk score" is yet universally adopted, clinicians are encouraged to use a multifactorial risk assessment evaluating glycemic control (HbA1c), blood pressure, LDL cholesterol, eGFR, UACR, and perhaps BNP or troponin to categorize CKM patients as low, moderate, or high risk for progression to CV events or kidney failure. Such stratification can then guide the intensity of interventions (for example, aggressive risk factor modification and specialist referral for those in the highest risk categories).[13]

STAGING OF CARDIOVASCULAR–KIDNEY–METABOLIC SYNDROME

To facilitate clinical decision-making and research, staging systems for CKM syndrome have been proposed.[1] The AHA's 2023 advisory introduced a five-stage CKM classification (Stage 0–4) based on the presence and severity of risk factors and end-organ disease **(Fig. 3)**.

- *Stage 0:* (No CKM risk factors or disease): The individual has optimal metabolic health, normal kidney function, and no clinical CVD.[1] This stage, essentially a healthy state, underscores the importance of primordial prevention by maintaining a healthy lifestyle.
- *Stage 1:* [Presence of excess or dysfunctional adiposity (overweight/obesity) without established metabolic or organ damage]: The AHA defined Stage 1 primarily by adiposity.[1] Some experts, especially internationally, broaden this to include early metabolic risk factors such as hypertension, impaired glucose tolerance, or mild dyslipidemia

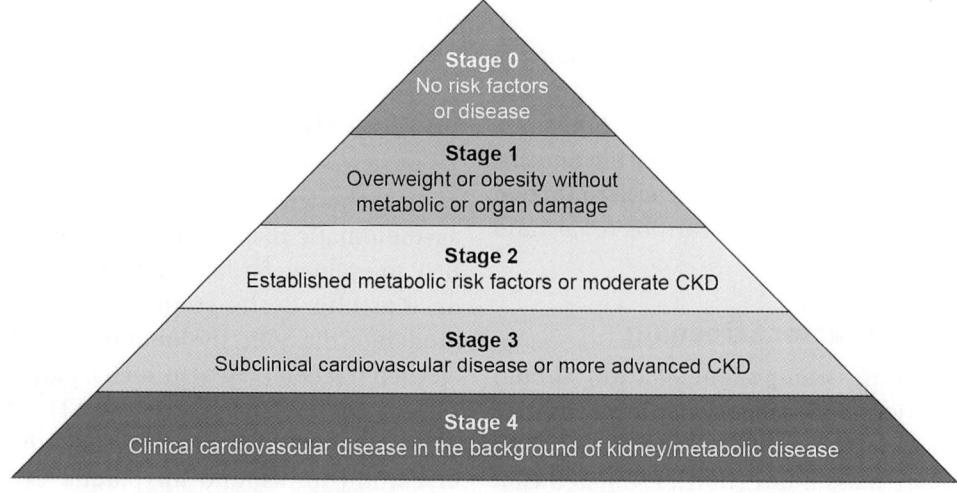

Fig. 3: Stages of CKM spectrum.

alongside adiposity. In any case, Stage 1 identifies those at risk due to lifestyle and anthropometric factors. Interventions focus on weight management, diet, physical activity, and addressing any emerging risk factor (e.g., prediabetes or prehypertension) to halt progression.

- *Stage 2:* (Presence of established metabolic risk factors or moderate CKD): This includes individuals with metabolic syndrome, T2D, or hypertension, and/or those with CKD defined as eGFR 45–59 mL/min/1.73 m² or evidence of kidney damage (e.g., persistent albuminuria) in the absence of clinical CVD.[1] Essentially, stage 2 encompasses patients who have significant risk factors that strongly predispose them to CVD, as well as those with early CKD that heightens CV risk (example includes middle-aged patient with T2D and microalbuminuria would be Stage 2 CKM). Management at this stage intensifies risk factor control, including strict glycemic control, blood pressure <130/80 mm Hg (often requiring multiple agents), statin therapy for dyslipidemia, and angiotensin-converting enzyme inhibitor (ACEi), or angiotensin receptor blocker (ARB) for kidney protection by reducing albuminuria, among other measures. The goal is to minimize risk to prevent progression to organ damage stages aggressively.

- *Stage 3:* (Presence of subclinical CVD or high predicted risk, or more advanced CKD, in the setting of the CKM syndrome): Subclinical CVD refers to objective evidence of cardiac or vascular target-organ damage without overt clinical events [examples include coronary artery calcification, left ventricular hypertrophy, or a reduced ejection fraction (<50%) on imaging, elevated cardiac biomarkers (BNP/troponin), or carotid plaque]. This stage also includes those with a high calculated 10-year CVD risk (based on risk scores) or very high-risk CKD (e.g., eGFR 30–44 mL/min or heavy proteinuria), even if no symptomatic CVD has yet occurred.[1] Recognition of Stage 3 is crucial as it signals the need for multidisciplinary care and possibly pre-emptive therapies (for instance, considering SGLT2 inhibitors or GLP-1 agonists if not already on board, tighter risk factor targets, and evaluation for silent ischemia or cardiomyopathy). It is at this juncture that a "CKM patient" may benefit from a combined cardiology-nephrology-diabetology evaluation.

- *Stage 4:* (Overt clinical CVD in the context of CKM syndrome): Established CV events or HF on top of underlying metabolic and kidney disease.[1] This includes patients who have had myocardial infarction, stroke, revascularization, acute coronary syndrome, decompensated HF, or other major CV events, and who also have diabetes, obesity, or CKD as part of their profile. Often by Stage 4, CKD may have progressed to late Stage 3 or Stage 4 CKD (eGFR <30, or even end-stage renal disease) due to the long-standing disease processes. Stage 4 represents advanced disease on all fronts, and these patients have the highest morbidity and mortality. Management is complex and requires shared care by cardiologists and nephrologists, as treating one aspect in isolation is insufficient.

The AHA staging system thus provides a scaffold to stage the continuum of CKM syndrome from at-risk to advanced disease.[1] However, some experts have argued for simplification to enhance clinical utility. An Italian expert panel proposed consolidating the AHA's multiple stages into two broader categories: "Early-stage CKM" (covering Stages 0–2, where risk factors and mild organ changes are present but no overt CVD) and "advanced-stage CKM" (covering

Stages 3–4, where significant organ dysfunction or clinical CVD has occurred). CKM syndrome is progressive, and each stage (or category) should trigger appropriate preventive or therapeutic actions to avert further deterioration.

THERAPEUTIC APPROACHES

Managing CKM syndrome requires an integrated approach targeting lifestyle, metabolic control, CV health, and organ-specific care **(Fig. 4)**. Combining lifestyle changes with evidence-based medications and novel agents helps slow disease progression, reduce complications, and improve overall outcomes.

Lifestyle Modification

Lifestyle interventions form the cornerstone at all stages of CKM. Dietary changes (such as a Mediterranean or DASH-style diet, reduced sodium intake, and avoidance of ultraprocessed foods) can favorably impact weight, blood pressure, and glycemic control, benefitting all three organ systems. A 5–10% weight reduction in an obese patient with diabetes can improve insulin sensitivity, lower blood pressure, and reduce albuminuria. Regular physical activity (at least 150 minutes of moderate exercise per week) improves cardiorespiratory fitness, assists with glycemic control, and may slow CKD. Smoking cessation is critical, as tobacco use exacerbates atherosclerosis and kidney function decline. Notably, intensive lifestyle intervention in diabetics has shown reductions in CV risk factors, though comprehensive risk reduction often requires adjunct pharmacotherapy. In CKD patients, lifestyle therapy must be tailored (for example, adjusting fluid intake and protein diet in advanced CKD, or avoiding strenuous exercise in unstable HF); however, it should be pursued whenever feasible.[14]

Glycemic Control

Tight glycemic control (target HbA1c individualized to ~7% or lower for many nonelderly adults) is fundamental to prevent microvascular complications in diabetes and has macrovascular benefits over the long term. In CKM syndrome, certain glucose-lowering medications have been shown to have cardiorenal protective effects beyond their glucose-lowering effects. SGLT2 inhibitors, such as empagliflozin and dapagliflozin, initially developed to treat hyperglycemia by inducing glycosuria, have shown remarkable outcomes in CV and renal trials. In the EMPA-REG OUTCOME trial, empagliflozin reduced the risk of major CV events and significantly lowered the risk of hospitalization for HF in patients with T2D and CVD.[15] Subsequent HF trials (e.g., EMPEROR-Reduced and EMPEROR-Preserved) confirmed that empagliflozin improves outcomes in patients with HFrEF and HFpEF, respectively, even in those without diabetes.[16,17] Equally important, SGLT2 inhibitors slow CKD progression by reducing albuminuria and attenuating eGFR decline, as evidenced by trials such as CREDENCE

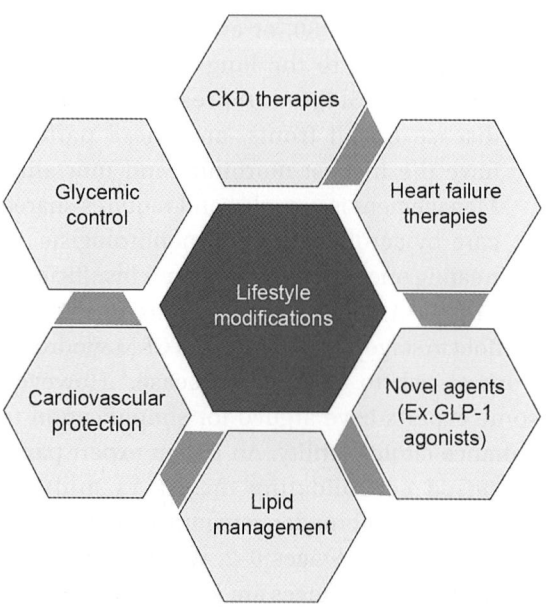

Fig. 4: Treatment of CKM syndrome.

and DAPA-CKD, as well as the kidney outcomes in EMPA-REG, where empagliflozin lowered the incidence of significant renal function loss.[15,18,19] Current guidelines strongly recommend SGLT2 inhibitors for patients with T2D who have CKD or HF, and even for nondiabetic CKD or HF patients, to reduce progression and events.

Cardiovascular Protection

All CKM patients with hypertension should be on optimized antihypertensive therapy, often with ACEi or ARB, which not only lowers blood pressure but also reduces intraglomerular pressure and proteinuria and has proven mortality benefits in systolic HF. In patients with CKM Stage 3 or 4 (clinical CVD), evidence-based therapies for heart disease are indicated, including beta-blockers and mineralocorticoid receptor antagonists (MRAs) in HFrEF, high-intensity statins for those with atherosclerotic CVD, and antiplatelet therapy (such as aspirin) for the secondary prevention of CV events. One emerging therapy bridging cardio-renal-metabolic benefits is finerenone, a nonsteroidal MRA. In clinical trials (FIDELIO-DKD and FIGARO-DKD), finerenone significantly reduced albuminuria and slowed CKD progression in T2D patients, while also reducing the incidence of CV outcomes like HF hospitalization.[20,21] A recent update on MRAs notes that finerenone provides added renal benefit over ACE/ARB in diabetic kidney disease, with a lower risk of hyperkalemia compared to traditional MRAs. Thus, finerenone is becoming part of the armamentarium for CKM patients with diabetic CKD and could be considered an organ-protective agent across the cardiorenal continuum.

Lipid Management

Management of dyslipidemia is critical for reducing atherosclerotic events in CKM.[1] As per guidelines, intensive statin therapy is indicated in virtually all CKM patients with diabetes or CKD, to achieve LDL-C targets (e.g., <70 mg/dL for high-risk individuals). CKD patients derive CV mortality reduction from statins, though in end-stage renal disease (dialysis), the benefit is less clear. Addition of ezetimibe or proprotein convertase subtilisin/kexin type 9 (PCSK9) inhibitors is considered for very high-risk patients who do not reach lipid goals.

Novel Antidiabetic Agents with Cardiorenal Benefits

Beyond SGLT2 inhibitors, GLP-1 receptor agonists have demonstrated significant CV benefits in individuals with diabetes.[22,23] Agents like liraglutide and semaglutide have demonstrated reduced rates of major adverse cardiovascular events (MACE) in T2D patients at high CV risk. Liraglutide was also associated with a slower progression of albuminuria and a lower incidence of new macroalbuminuria, suggesting renal benefit. GLP-1 RAs promote weight loss and lower blood pressure, which contribute to their cardiometabolic benefits. They are recommended for T2D patients with established CVD or CKD to reduce future events, independent of glucose control considerations. Moreover, their weight loss effect can be particularly valuable in Stage 1–2 CKM patients (those who are obese/overweight with risk factors) to help reverse the course of the disease. Metformin remains a foundational therapy for T2D and is generally safe in CKD until advanced stages; it has mild CV benefits (possibly via weight and slight lipid improvements) and should be used if no contraindications.

Heart Failure and Chronic Kidney Disease-specific Therapies

Cardiovascular-kidney-metabolic patients who progress to HF with reduced EF should receive the full suite of guideline-directed medical therapy (GDMT), now often summarized as quadruple therapy: An ACEi/ARB or angiotensin receptor-neprilysin inhibitor (ARNI), a beta-blocker, an MRA, and an SGLT2 inhibitor.[24,25] This combination has synergistic effects on reducing mortality and hospitalizations. In HFpEF, treatments are more limited, but SGLT2 inhibitors have demonstrated a reduction in HF hospitalization even in preserved EF, and MRAs may help a subset of patients. For CKD, especially diabetic CKD, ACEi or ARB is disease-modifying, reducing proteinuria and slowing GFR decline. These medications should be titrated to the maximum tolerated dose. Renal replacement therapy initiation in Stage 4 CKM should be planned collaboratively, considering CV stability and diabetic care during dialysis. Some CKM patients may even be candidates for combined kidney–heart transplantation in extreme cases.

▪ INTEGRATED CARE MODELS

An integrated, multidisciplinary care model **(Fig. 5)** aims to bring together cardiology, nephrology, endocrinology/diabetology, primary care, and other professionals (such as nutritionists and pharmacists) to develop and implement a unified care plan.[26] Primary care providers (PCPs) play a pivotal role in performing early CKM risk screening (checking blood pressure, HbA1c, eGFR, etc., during routine visits) and in initiating first-line therapies for risk factors. Once risk factors are identified, timely referrals to specialists are made. Under an integrated model, these referrals involve dynamic consultations where the specialist evaluates and provides recommendations. At the same time, the PCP continues to manage the overall care and implement suggestions, thereby maintaining continuity.

Multidisciplinary Clinics

One successful model is the establishment of cardio-renal-metabolic clinics, where a team of specialists can see patients in a single, coordinated visit or series of visits. A report from a UK tertiary center described a novel multidisciplinary cardiometabolic clinic, which led to high rates of therapeutic optimization and risk factor control in patients with combined diabetes, CKD, and CVD.[27] Pharmacists in such teams can assist with medication reconciliation and titration, while dietitians or diabetes educators can provide focused education.

Telemedicine and Remote Monitoring

Telemedicine has emerged as a powerful tool in CKM care.[28,29] Virtual consultations enable patients in rural areas to receive expert input without travelling long distances, which can improve concordance of advice. Remote patient monitoring is another component that allows patients to transmit blood pressure readings, weight, or blood glucose logs electronically to their care team. A systematic review found that clinicians perceived remote monitoring as beneficial for timely intervention.

Unified Guidelines and Protocols

Diabetes-Cardiorenal-Metabolic (DCRM) multi-disciplinary recommendations 2.0 consensus in

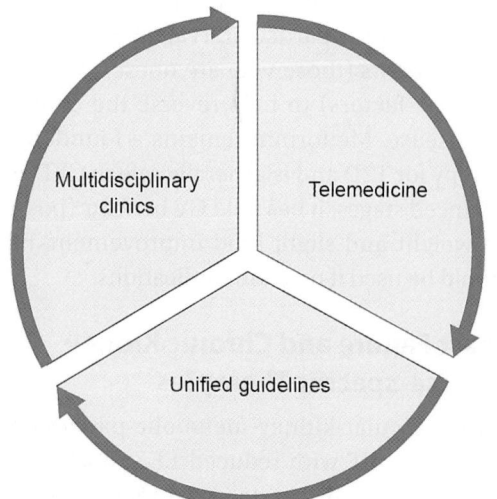

Fig. 5: Integrated care models.

2024 provided practice recommendations that span across diseases (recommending an SGLT2 inhibitor for any patient with diabetes and either CVD or CKD and detailing how to monitor and adjust therapy in the presence of multiple comorbidities).[30] By implementing unified protocols in clinics, care providers can work more easily in sync. Early evidence suggests that these models can improve risk factor control and reduce hospitalization. For instance, a virtual integrated care program in Australia (I-CONNECT CKD) for patients with CKD, hypertension, and diabetes resulted in better blood pressure and glucose management, as well as high patient satisfaction.[31] As CKM syndrome becomes a more recognized entity, healthcare systems will increasingly invest in such collaborative approaches.

EMERGING TRENDS AND FUTURE DIRECTIONS

The recognition of CKM syndrome as an actionable clinical entity is relatively recent, and ongoing developments promise to refine the prevention and treatment of this condition in the years to come in the ways described here.

Refinement of Cardiovascular–Kidney–Metabolic Definition and Risk Prediction

The evolving definition of CKM syndrome requires standardization to ensure consistent diagnosis and management. Future directions focus on integrating multiorgan risk into unified prediction tools that go beyond traditional CV or renal calculators. Advances in biomarkers (e.g., genomics, proteomics, and metabolomics), imaging modalities, and machine learning promise earlier and more accurate risk detection. By combining clinical, molecular, and social determinants of health, these approaches aim to enable personalized, equitable risk assessment and proactive intervention across diverse populations.[32]

Novel Therapeutics

Building on the success of SGLT2 inhibitors and GLP-1 agonists, new drug classes are under investigation. Dual- or triple-agonist drugs (for instance, combined GLP-1/GIP agonists or GLP-1/GIP/glucagon agonists) are being tested for obesity and diabetes and show even greater weight loss and metabolic improvements than current GLP-1 RAs. There is also interest in anti-inflammatory therapies, such as IL-6 or IL-1 inhibitors (tested in CVD trials, like CANTOS),[33] or novel agents targeting inflammation in diabetes (e.g., CCR2/CCR5 inhibitors). Lipid-lowering innovations [like RNA silencing therapies against PCSK9 or apolipoprotein(a)] can drastically lower atherogenic particles and may benefit CKM patients at high risk of atherosclerosis.

Digital Health and Remote Care

Remote monitoring programs designed explicitly for CKM patients utilize integrated apps/devices that enable patients to track their health data at home, with the data then flowing to their providers.[34] Emerging devices could include wearable sensors that continuously monitor heart rate and rhythm (detecting arrhythmias like atrial fibrillation, which is common in CKM), or patches that measure glucose without a fingerstick. These technologies, combined with AI-driven analytics, could alert care teams to warning signs, enabling proactive outreach to adjust treatment.

CONCLUSION

Cardiovascular-kidney-metabolic syndrome encapsulates the interconnected epidemics of obesity, diabetes, kidney disease, and CVD, where dysfunction in one system accelerates decline in the others. Recognizing CKM as a unified syndrome shifts care from organ-specific treatment to integrated, patient-centered strategies. With effective therapies, lifestyle interventions, and multidisciplinary models, CKM offers a pathway to earlier prevention, better treatment, and more patient-centered care. As evidence grows, CKM may serve as a model for managing other overlapping chronic diseases through holistic, collaborative approaches.

■ REFERENCES

1. Ndumele CE, Rangaswami J, Chow SL, et al. Cardiovascular-kidney-metabolic health: a presidential advisory from the American Heart Association. Circulation. 2023;148:1606-35.
2. Iacoviello M, Gori M, Grandaliano G, et al. A holistic approach to managing cardio-kidney metabolic syndrome: insights and recommendations from the Italian perspective. Front Cardiovasc Med. 2025;12:1583702.
3. Zoccali C, Zannad F. Refocusing cardio-renal problems: the cardiovascular-kidney-metabolic syndrome and the chronic cardiovascular-kidney disorder. Nephrol Dial Transplant. 2024;39:1378-80.
4. Kittelson KS, Junior AG, Fillmore N, et al. Cardiovascular-kidney-metabolic syndrome – an integrative review. Prog Cardiovasc Dis. 2024; 87:26-36.
5. Powell-Wiley TM, Poirier P, Burke LE, et al. Obesity and cardiovascular disease: a scientific statement from the American Heart Association. Circulation. 2021;143:e984-e1010.
6. Ostrominski JW, Arnold SV, Butler J, et al. Prevalence and overlap of cardiac, renal, and metabolic conditions in US adults, 1999–2020. JAMA Cardiol. 2023;8:1050-60.
7. Marassi M, Fadini GP. The cardio-renal-metabolic connection: a review of the evidence. Cardiovasc Diabetol. 2023;22:195.
8. Abreu AP, Drager LF, Almeida MQ, et al. Cardiovascular-kidney-metabolic Syndrome: a current and urgent concept. J Bras Nefrol. 2025; 47(2):e20240277.
9. Sebastian SA, Padda I, Johal G. Cardiovascular-Kidney-Metabolic (CKM) syndrome: A state-of-the-art review. Curr Probl Cardiol. 2024; 49(2):102344.
10. Grams ME, Coresh J, Matsushita K, et al. Estimated glomerular filtration rate, albuminuria, and adverse outcomes: an individual-participant data meta-analysis. JAMA. 2023;330:1266-77.
11. Jehn S, Mahabadi AA, Pfohl C, et al. BNP and NT-proBNP thresholds for the assessment of prognosis in patients without heart failure. JACC Adv. 2023;2:100688.
12. Mutruc V, Bologa C, Șorodoc V, et al. Cardiovascular-Kidney-Metabolic Syndrome: A New Paradigm in Clinical Medicine or Going Back to Basics?. J Clin Med. 2025;14(8):2833.
13. Zhao Y, Zhou P, Fan F, et al. A simple score, CKM2S2-BAG, to predict cardiovascular risk with cardiovascular-kidney-metabolic health metrics. iScience. 2025;28(7):112780.
14. Shahid NN, Clark D, Dave SA, et al. Lifestyle interventions in cardiovascular-kidney-metabolic syndrome. JACC Adv. 2025;4(6P2):101788.
15. Wanner C, Inzucchi SE, Lachin JM, et al. Empagliflozin and progression of kidney disease in type 2 diabetes. N Engl J Med. 2016;375:323-34.
16. Packer M, Anker SD, Butler J, et al. Cardiovascular and renal outcomes with empagliflozin in heart failure. N Engl J Med. 2020;383:1413-24.
17. Anker SD, Butler J, Filippatos G, et al. Empagliflozin in heart failure with a preserved ejection fraction. N Engl J Med. 2021;385:1451-61.
18. Perkovic V, Jardine MJ, Neal B, et al.; CREDENCE Trial Investigators. Canagliflozin and Renal Outcomes in Type 2 Diabetes and Nephropathy. N Engl J Med. 2019;380(24):2295-306.
19. Heerspink HJL, Stefánsson BV, Correa-Rotter R, et al.; DAPA-CKD Trial Committees and Investigators. Dapagliflozin in Patients with Chronic Kidney Disease. N Engl J Med. 2020; 383(15):1436-46.
20. Bakris GL, Agarwal R, Anker SD, et al.; FIDELIO-DKD Investigators. Effect of finerenone on chronic kidney disease outcomes in type 2 diabetes. N Engl J Med. 2020;383(23):2219-29.
21. Pitt B, Filippatos G, Agarwal R, et al.; FIGARO-DKD Investigators. Cardiovascular events with finerenone in kidney disease and type 2 diabetes. N Engl J Med. 2021;385(24):2252-63.

22. Mann JFE, Ørsted DD, Brown-Frandsen K, et al. Liraglutide and renal outcomes in type 2 diabetes. N Engl J Med. 2017;377:839-48.
23. Tsapas A, Karagiannis T, Kakotrichi P, et al. Comparative efficacy of glucose-lowering medications on body weight and blood pressure in patients with type 2 diabetes: a systematic review and network meta-analysis. Diabetes Obes Metab. 2021;23:2116-24.
24. Heidenreich PA, Bozkurt B, Aguilar D, et al. 2022 AHA/ACC/HFSA Guideline for the Management of Heart Failure. Circulation. 2022;145(18): e895-e1032.
25. McDonagh TA, Metra M, Adamo M, et al. 2023 ESC Focused Update on Heart Failure Guidelines: An update of the 2021 ESC Guidelines for the diagnosis and treatment of acute and chronic heart failure. Eur Heart J. 2023;44(36):3423-536.
26. Evén G, Stenfors T, Jacobson SH, et al. Integrated, person-centred care for patients with complex cardiovascular disease, diabetes mellitus and chronic kidney disease: a randomized trial. Clin Kidney J. 2024;17(11):sfae331. Published 2024 Oct 29. doi:10.1093/ckj/sfae331.
27. Narain R, Bijman L, Joshi H, et al. Novel multidisciplinary cardiometabolic clinic in a UK tertiary cardiology centre: early activity, interventions and potential for cardiovascular risk optimization. Eur Heart J. 2021;42(Suppl 1): ehab724.2631.
28. Haleem A, Javaid M, Singh RP, et al. Telemedicine for healthcare: capabilities, features, barriers, and applications. Sens Int. 2021;2:100117.
29. Serrano LP, Maita KC, Avila FR, et al. Benefits and challenges of remote patient monitoring as perceived by health care practitioners: a systematic review. Perm J. 2023;27:100-11.
30. Handelsman Y, Anderson JE, Bakris GL, et al. DCRM 2.0: multispecialty practice recommendations for the management of diabetes, cardiorenal, and metabolic diseases. Metabolism. 2024;159:155931.
31. Katz IJ, Pirabhahar S, Williamson P, et al. iConnect CKD - virtual medical consulting: A web-based chronic kidney disease, hypertension, and diabetes integrated care program. Nephrology (Carlton). 2018;23(7):646-52.
32. Cases A, Broseta JJ, Marqués M, et al. Cardiovascular-kidney-metabolic syndrome definition and its role in the prevention, risk staging, and treatment. An opportunity for the Nephrology. Nefrología (Engl Ed). 2024;44(6): 771-83.
33. Ridker PM, Everett BM, Thuren T, et al.; CANTOS Trial Group. Antiinflammatory therapy with canakinumab for atherosclerotic disease. N Engl J Med. 2017;377(12):1119-31.
34. Thomas EE, Taylor ML, Banbury A, et al. Factors influencing the effectiveness of remote patient monitoring interventions: a realist review. BMJ Open. 2021;11:e051844.

CHAPTER 2

Nanoplastics in Coronary Artery Disease

Rajeev Gupta, Surendra Singh, Madhu Agarwal, Ajeet Bana, Akhilendra Bhushan Gupta

■ INTRODUCTION

Environmental pollution has emerged as an important risk factor for coronary artery disease (CAD). Various forms have been implicated. Plastics, which are common household and industrial items, have microscopic forms [microplastics (MPs) and nanoplastics (NPs)] and have emerged as notable pollutants. Nanoplastics (<0.1 micron) are created from the breakdown of larger plastic debris or are intentionally produced for industry. These particles are found in environmental matrices such as air, water, and food, as well as in human tissues such as blood, lungs, liver, placenta, and breast milk. The cardiovascular system is increasingly recognized as a target for nanoplastic toxicity. Preclinical and clinical studies indicate a link between nanoplastic exposure and cardiovascular diseases (CVDs), including atherosclerosis, myocardial infarction, stroke, and heart failure. Evidence suggests that nanoplastics cause cardiovascular damage through oxidative stress, inflammation, mitochondrial dysfunction, apoptosis, endothelial dysfunction, and thrombogenesis. A study detected nanoplastics in carotid atherosclerotic plaques of patients undergoing carotid endarterectomy. This was associated with higher incidence of major cardiovascular events over the long term. We have initiated a study to detect nanoplastics in coronary atheroma in patients undergoing coronary artery bypass surgery. Standardization of the detection process using Fourier Transform Infrared spectroscopy, Raman spectroscopy, and scanning electron microscopy has been carried out. If nanoplastics are confirmed as a coronary risk factor, their widespread presence in the environment could intensify the global burden of CAD. Public health strategies to mitigate nanoplastic exposure should include reducing plastic pollution through regulatory measures and public awareness campaigns. Future research should focus on large-scale epidemiological studies, standardized detection techniques, environmental exposure models, mechanistic investigations, and intervention trials to guide policy development.

■ CORONARY RISK FACTORS

The South Asian region is home to more than a quarter of the world's population and has high levels of ambient, water and soil pollution.[1] It has recently undergone a rapid epidemiological transition, with an increase in life expectancy and socioeconomic development.[2] This has led to a shift in disease patterns from communicable and maternal-childhood diseases in the last century to the predominance of noncommunicable diseases (NCDs).[3] CVDs, particularly ischemic heart disease (IHD), are the leading NCDs in this region, as reported by multiple national[4] and the Global Burden of Disease (GBD) studies.[5] IHD and stroke epidemiology in India is characterized by significant subnational geographic variation,[5] premature onset of atherosclerosis, and acute IHD events,[6] substantially higher mortality compared

TABLE 1: Cardiovascular risk factors identified in INTERHEART[6] and PURE Studies.[8]

INTERHEART Study (case–control)*	PURE Study (CVD incidence)*	
Acute myocardial infarction	Cardiovascular diseases	Coronary artery disease
Raised ApoB/ApoA$_1$ ratio (47%)	Hypertension (22%)	High non-HDL cholesterol (17%)
Smoking/tobacco (38%)	High non-HDL cholesterol (8%)	Hypertension (13%)
Raised waist–hip ratio (38%)	Household air pollution (7%)	Tobacco use (12%)
Physical inactivity (27%)	Tobacco use (6%)	Abdominal obesity (11%)
Low fruit–vegetable intake (21%)	Poor diet (6%)	Diabetes (8%)
Hypertension (19%)	Low education (6%)	Low education (7%)
Psychosocial factors (16%)	Abdominal obesity (6%)	Low grip strength (7%)
Alcohol intake (16%)	Diabetes (5%)	Household pollution (5%)
Diabetes (12%)	Low grip strength (3%)	Poor diet (4%)
	Low physical activity (2%)	Low physical activity (<1%)
	Depression (<1.0%)	Depression (<1%)
	Excessive alcohol (<1.0%)	Excessive alcohol (<1%)

*Numbers in parentheses are population attributable risk (INTERHEART) and population-attributable fraction (PURE study). Cardiovascular diseases (CVDs) include coronary artery disease (CAD), stroke, and peripheral artery disease.

to higher-income countries,[7] and association with some unique risk factors—diabetes, metabolic syndrome, and indoor air pollution **(Table 1)**.[8]

NANOPLASTICS AS NOVEL RISK FACTORS

The GBD has identified environmental and other forms of pollution as the most important CVD risk factors.[9] Some of these are listed in **Table 2**.[10-12] The pervasive presence of plastic pollution in the environment has emerged as a significant public health concern, with MPs and nanoplastics gaining particular attention due to their potential to infiltrate biological systems.[13] MPs are defined as plastic particles smaller than 5 micron, while nanoplastics are even smaller, typically less than 0.1 micron. Nano- and microplastics (NMPs) are universally pervasive and persistent pollutants in environmental ecosystems and have emerged as a major challenge due to their potential toxicity that threatens biodiversity and ecological stability.

These particles, resulting from the degradation of larger plastic debris or intentionally manufactured for industrial purposes, have been detected in various environmental matrices, including air, water, and food, as well as in human tissues such as blood, lungs, liver, placenta, and breast milk.[13,14] They pose significant ecological risks by transmitting through integrating exposure pathways like bioaccumulation, trophic transfer, and toxicity.

It is important to quantify the distribution of nanoplastics and predict their interactions with biotic and abiotic components to assess their long-term ecological and health consequences. The cardiovascular system is increasingly being recognized as a target for the adverse effects of nanoplastics.[14,15] Emerging evidence from preclinical and clinical studies suggests a potential link between nanoplastic exposure and CVD, including atherosclerosis, myocardial infarction, stroke, and heart failure. This chapter presents the current state of knowledge on the association between nanoplastics and heart disease,

TABLE 2: Pollution-associated risk factors implicated in cardiovascular diseases.

Class	Risk factors
Environmental pollution	• Ambient pollution (PM_{10}, $PM_{2.5}$, NO_2, SO_2, CO, O_3, construction activities, etc.) • Indoor pollution (PM_{10}, $PM_{2.5}$, NO_2, CO, O_3, volatile organic compounds, combustion from cooking (wood, charcoal), heating, second-hand smoke, household chemicals and pesticides, construction materials, etc.)
Food and water pollutants	• *Food pollution:* Organic and inorganic pollutants, heavy metals, endocrine disruptors, fertilizers, etc. • *Water pollution:* Persistent organic pollutants, inorganic pollutants, etc. • *Plastics:* micro- and nanoplastics • Gut microbiome
Climate change leading to increased pollution	• *Air temperature:* Excessive heat or cold • *Climate catastrophes:* Cyclones, storms, earthquakes, forest fires, etc.

exploring exposure pathways, mechanistic insights, clinical evidence, and research gaps.

PATHOBIOLOGY OF NANOPLASTICS IN HUMAN DISEASES

Nanoplastics enter the human body through multiple routes, including ingestion, inhalation, and dermal contact.[13] The major reported exposure routes of nanoplastics into the human body are through inhalation or ingestion. However, the dermal route also cannot be ignored due to the extensive use of personal care products containing nanoplastics. Nanoplastics after entering the human body may translocate from the exposed organ to other parts of the body. Their fate within the human body depends on how nanoplastics can translocate from the primary exposed organs to secondary organs due to naturally occurring defense mechanisms against tissue translocation. Recent studies indicate that a dermal translocation of nanoplastics is rather unlikely, and they generally translocate from the gastrointestinal and respiratory systems to other tissues.[16] Exposure to nanoplastics has been reported to pose several health risks, including mitochondrial impairment and cytomembrane destruction,[17] cytotoxicity, and immunotoxicological effects, especially at higher concentrations and smaller particle sizes.[18] Their small size allows them to penetrate biological barriers, such as the intestinal or pulmonary epithelium, and enter the bloodstream, where they can distribute to various organs, including the heart and blood vessels **(Figs. 1A to E)**.[19,20]

Ingestion: Nanoplastics are prevalent in food and water sources, with studies detecting them in bottled and tap water, seafood, and other consumables. For instance, polyethylene (PE) and polyvinyl chloride (PVC) particles have been identified in drinking water and marine organisms, which are common dietary components.[20] Once ingested, nanoplastics can cross the gastrointestinal barrier, particularly in the small intestine, and enter systemic circulation. Animal studies have demonstrated that polystyrene nanoplastics accumulate in the blood and heart following oral exposure, highlighting the bioavailability of these particles.[15]

Inhalation: Airborne nanoplastics, often associated with particulate matter (PM2.5), are another significant exposure route.[13] These particles are released from sources such as plastic degradation, industrial emissions, and urban pollution. Inhalation allows nanoplastics to translocate from the lungs into the bloodstream,

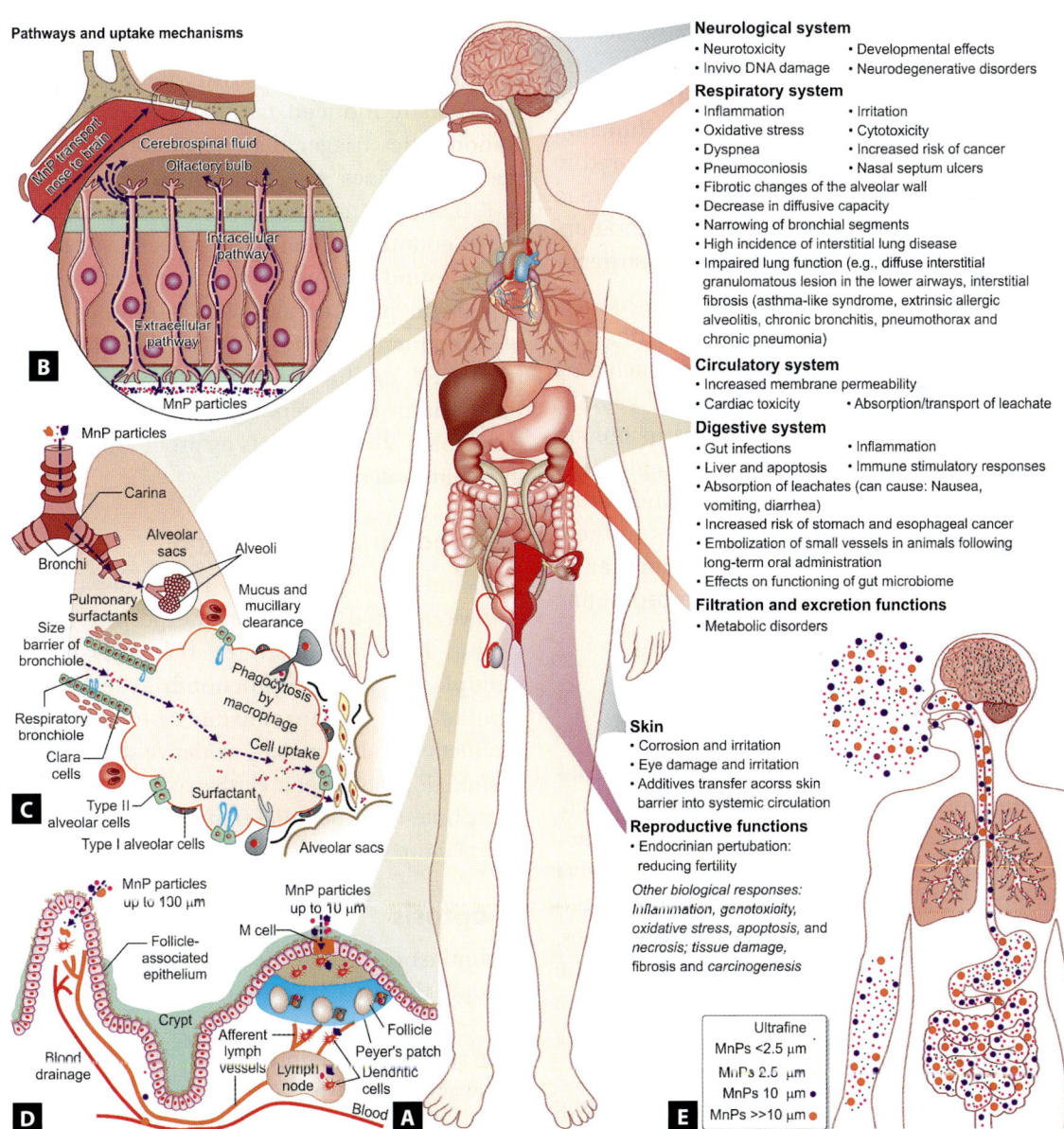

Figs. 1A to E: *Microplastics pathobiology:* Hypothesized uptake mechanisms of nanoparticles in various human organs.
Source: Sun Z, Wen Y, Zhang F, et al. Exposure to nanoplastics induces mitochondrial impairment and cytomembrane destruction in Leydig cells. Ecotoxicol Environ Saf. 2023;255:114796. Published under license: CCBY-NC-ND 4.0.

potentially reaching cardiovascular tissues. Workers exposed to high concentrations of plastics, such as polyethylene terephthalate (PET) and polyamide (PA), have reported respiratory symptoms, suggesting that inhalation is a critical pathway for occupational exposure.

Dermal contact: Although less studied, dermal contact with nanoplastics in cosmetics and personal care products may contribute to systemic exposure. The skin's barrier function is less permeable to nanoplastics compared to ingestion or inhalation, but chronic exposure to nanoscale particles could facilitate penetration, particularly through compromised skin barriers.

Bioaccumulation in cardiovascular tissues: Once in the bloodstream, nanoplastics can accumulate in cardiovascular tissues, including the heart, pericardium, and blood vessels. Studies have detected nanoplastics in human atherosclerotic plaques, pericardial, epicardial adipose tissues, and myocardia, indicating their potential to infiltrate and persist in these critical structures.[14,15,19] This bioaccumulation raises concerns about their role in promoting cardiovascular pathology.

NANOPLASTICS AND CARDIOVASCULAR TOXICITY

The mechanisms by which nanoplastics contribute to CVD are complex and multifaceted, involving oxidative stress, inflammation, mitochondrial dysfunction, apoptosis, and endothelial dysfunction. These pathways, elucidated primarily through in vitro and animal studies, provide a foundation for understanding the potential cardiotoxic effects of nanoplastics.[20]

Oxidative Stress

Nanoplastics induce oxidative stress by generating reactive oxygen species (ROS), which can overwhelm cellular antioxidant defenses. In vitro studies have shown that exposure to polystyrene nanoplastics promotes ROS production in endothelial and vascular smooth muscle cells, leading to oxidative damage. This oxidative stress disrupts cellular homeostasis and contributes to the progression of atherosclerosis by promoting lipid peroxidation and plaque formation.

Inflammation

Inflammation is a central mechanism in nanoplastic-induced cardiovascular toxicity. Nanoplastics trigger the release of proinflammatory cytokines, such as interleukin-1β (IL-1β), IL-6, IL-18, and tumor necrosis factor alpha (TNF-α), in endothelial and immune cells. A human study found that patients with nanoplastics in carotid plaques exhibited elevated levels of inflammatory biomarkers, correlating with increased cardiovascular events.[21] Chronic inflammation driven by nanoplastics may exacerbate atherosclerosis by promoting plaque instability and rupture.[15]

Mitochondrial Dysfunction

Mitochondrial dysfunction is another critical pathway affected by nanoplastic exposure. Animal studies have demonstrated that polystyrene nanoplastics cause mitochondrial lesions in cardiac cells, compromising cellular energy production and increasing oxidative stress.[13] This dysfunction can impair cardiac contractility and contribute to myocardial fibrosis, a precursor to heart failure.

Apoptosis

Nanoplastics induce programmed cell death (apoptosis) in cardiovascular cells, further exacerbating tissue damage. In vitro studies have shown that nanoplastics activate apoptotic pathways, such as the Wnt/β-catenin and NLRP3/caspase-1 signaling cascades, leading to the loss of functional cardiomyocytes and endothelial cells.[15,19] This cell loss can impair cardiac and vascular function, increasing the risk of adverse cardiovascular outcomes.

Endothelial Dysfunction

The endothelial dysfunction, characterized by impaired vasodilation and increased vascular permeability, is a hallmark of nanoplastic toxicity.[14,15] Animal models have shown that nanoplastic exposure reduces vessel flexibility and promotes thrombosis, increasing the risk of vascular occlusion. These effects are mediated by the disruption of nitric oxide signaling and the activation of prothrombotic pathways, contributing to conditions such as hypertension and IHD.

Thrombogenesis and Vascular Damage

Nanoplastics have been linked to increased thrombotic activity, as evidenced by elevated D-dimer levels in exposed individuals. This heightened thrombogenicity can exacerbate existing cardiovascular conditions by promoting blood clot formation, which may lead to myocardial infarction or stroke. Additionally, nanoplastics cause structural abnormalities in cardiac valves and blood vessels, further compromising cardiovascular function.

Preclinical Evidence

Animal models have provided valuable insights into the cardiovascular effects of nanoplastic exposure.[13-15] Studies in zebrafish, mice, and rats have demonstrated that nanoplastics cause a range of adverse effects, including:
- *Altered heart rate:* Exposure to polystyrene nanoplastics in zebrafish embryos resulted in reduced heart rate and impaired cardiac development.
- *Myocardial fibrosis:* Chronic exposure to nanoplastics in rodents led to excessive collagen deposition in the heart, impairing cardiac function and predisposing to heart failure.
- *Cardiac hypertrophy:* In a mouse model of angiotensin II-induced hypertension, ingestion of polystyrene nanoplastics increased cardiac hypertrophy and reduced cardiac output.
- *Vascular inflammation:* Nanoplastics induced vascular inflammation and reduced vessel flexibility in animal models, contributing to atherosclerosis and thrombosis.

These preclinical findings suggest that nanoplastics act as a novel risk factor for CVD, although the translation to human health requires further investigation.

NANOPLASTICS AND ATHEROSCLEROSIS

Recent clinical studies have provided compelling evidence linking nanoplastic exposure to cardiovascular outcomes in humans. A landmark study in the *New England Journal of Medicine* investigated the presence of nanoplastics in carotid artery plaques from 257 patients undergoing carotid endarterectomy.[21] The study found that 58% of patients had detectable nanoplastics, primarily PE and PVC, in their plaques. Over a 34-month follow-up, patients with nanoplastic-contaminated plaques had a 4.5-fold higher risk of experiencing a composite endpoint of myocardial infarction, stroke, or death compared to those without detectable nanoplastics. This increased risk persisted after adjusting for traditional risk factors such as age, sex, body mass index, diabetes, and cholesterol levels. Another prospective observational study involving 142 patients with myocardial infarction found that 95.4% had detectable PVC in coronary blood samples, with higher concentrations associated with increased proinflammatory factors and a higher odds ratio for major adverse cardiac events.[22] Nanoplastics have also been found in blood in patients with acute coronary syndromes.[23] These findings suggest that nanoplastics may exacerbate existing cardiovascular conditions by promoting inflammation and thrombogenesis.

However, these studies have limitations. The observational nature of the research precludes establishing causation, and the patient populations studied (e.g., those undergoing carotid endarterectomy) may not be representative of the general population. Additionally, confounding factors, such as smoking, high cholesterol, and diabetes, which were more prevalent in patients with nanoplastic-containing plaques, complicate the interpretation of results.[10,24]

■ RESEARCH GAPS AND CHALLENGES

Despite the growing body of evidence, several knowledge gaps and methodological challenges persist in the study of nanoplastics and heart disease.

Population-level Data

The generalizability of current findings is limited by the specific populations studied, such as those with preexisting cardiovascular conditions. Future research should include diverse populations to determine whether nanoplastics pose a risk to individuals without known risk factors.

Environmental and Demographic Factors

The role of environmental and demographic factors, such as geographic location, socio-economic status, and occupational exposure, in modulating nanoplastic-related cardiovascular risk remains underexplored. Studies incorporating zip code-level data and environmental exposure profiles could provide valuable insights.

Long-term Effects

Most studies have focused on short-term or intermediate-term outcomes, leaving the long-term cardiovascular effects of chronic nanoplastic exposure poorly understood. Longitudinal studies are needed to assess the cumulative impact of nanoplastics over decades.

Methodological Limitations

The detection and quantification of nanoplastics in biological tissues remain challenging due to their small size and chemical diversity. Techniques such as pyrolysis–gas chromatography–mass spectrometry and electron microscopy are commonly used, but standardized protocols are lacking for the processing of samples and the existence of a well-defined sequence of analytical procedures for extracting information from very small sample sizes and cross-confirming the inferences. Variability in detection methods across studies hinders the comparability of results and the establishment of exposure thresholds.[25]

Ethical Considerations

Ethical constraints limit the ability to conduct controlled human exposure studies, necessitating reliance on observational data and preclinical models. This reliance introduces uncertainty about the direct applicability of findings to humans.

■ PRELIMINARY DATA FROM OUR STUDY

Surge in premature CAD in India has triggered a search for novel coronary risk factors ranging from standard risk factors, social determinants, COVID-19, and pollution **(Table 2)**.[26,27] The term pollution includes ambient pollution, indoor air pollution, water and food pollution with various endocrine disruptors, inorganic pollutants, MPs, and nanoplastics **(Table 2)**.[10,11,24]

To identify the presence of nanoplastics in coronary atheroma harvested during coronary bypass graft surgery (CABG) in CAD patients undergoing coronary atherectomy, we designed a registry-based prospective study. More than 1,200 bypass surgeries are performed annually at our tertiary care center, and endarterectomy samples are abundant. These samples are being assessed for the presence of inflammation using conventional histopathology techniques and nanoparticles, as well as Fourier Transformed Infrared (FTIR) spectroscopy, Raman spectroscopy, and electron microscopy. The FTIR spectrum provides a molecular fingerprint by displaying its absorption and transmission, while Raman spectroscopy uses the vibrational modes of molecules, although rotational and other low-frequency modes of systems may also be observed. These techniques are valuable for identifying molecules, studying their structure, and analyzing the properties of various materials.[27,28]

In a 51-year-old male CAD patient (Patient 1) who underwent coronary atherectomy during coronary bypass surgery, we evaluated the presence of nanoplastics in the atheroma sample using various spectroscopy techniques and scanning electron microscopy **(Figs. 2A and B)**. The spectra obtained reveal minor peaks that may corroborate with MPs or nanoplastics in the sample.

In another patient (Patient 2), a 53-year-old male, the FTIR spectrum revealed a complex mixture of polymeric materials, with prominent peaks aligning with common MPs such as polyethene (PE), polypropylene (PP), PET, and PVC **(Fig. 3A)**. In contrast, the spectrum of the membrane with MPs **(Fig. 3B)** reveals several new or shifted peaks, particularly in the 3,380 cm^{-1} and 1,400–1,000 cm^{-1} regions compared to the fresh membrane. Similar peaks were also observed in the spectra of solid tissue **(Fig. 3C)**. These changes are indicative of the deposition of MPs such as PE, PP, PET, and PVC. The comparison of FTIR spectra of fresh, used, and solid samples **(Fig. 3D)** reveals distinct absorption peaks in the fingerprint region (1,500–500 cm^{-1}), which are characteristic of synthetic polymers. Peaks around 1,450 cm^{-1} and 1,375 cm^{-1} correspond to CH$_2$ and CH$_3$ bending vibrations, confirming the presence of polyethene and polypropylene. Additional peaks near 1,230–1,100 cm^{-1} indicate C–O stretching, consistent with PET or polycarbonate. Low-frequency peaks around 750–600 cm^{-1} suggest C–Cl stretching, indicative of PVC. The used membrane shows distinct signs of MP contamination, evidenced by new peaks and shifts in the C–H and C–O regions. These spectral changes align with known signatures of PE,

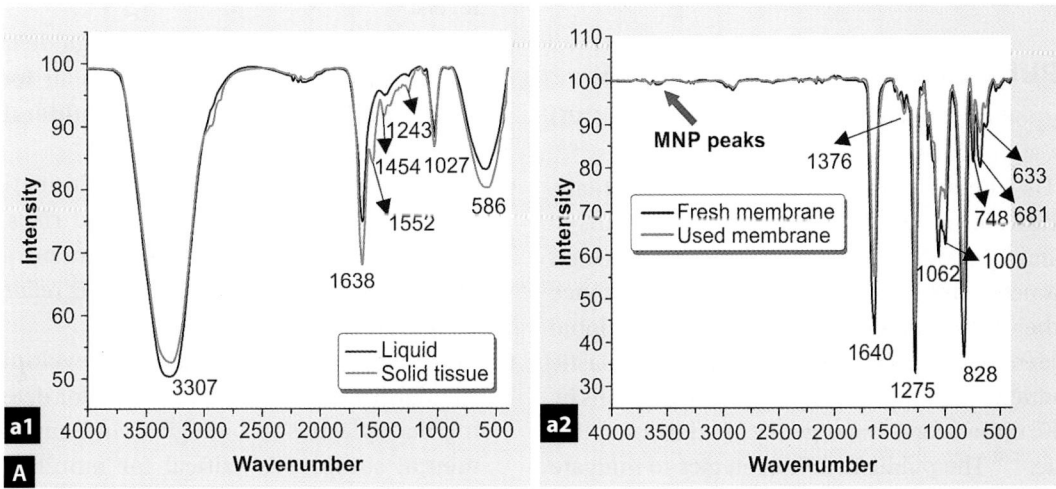

Fig. 2A: Fourier Transformed Infrared (FTIR) findings from an atheroma sample in Patient 1. FTIR analysis using (a1) solid tissue and liquid sample as initially received, and (a2) after filtration with a tissue-digested solution. (MNP: micro-nanoplastics).

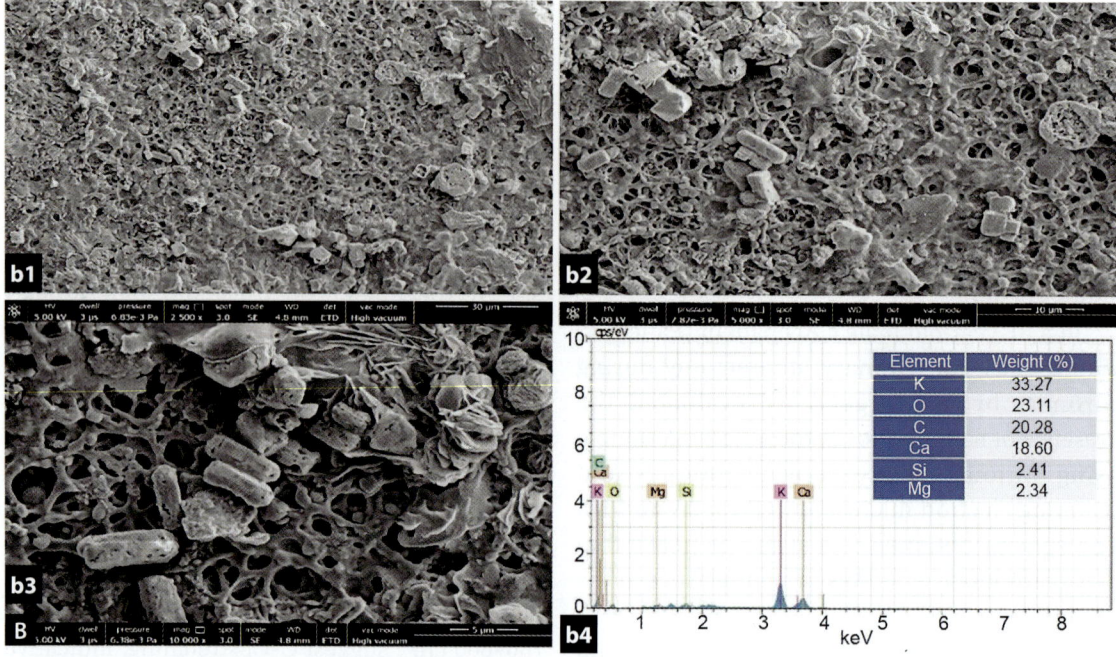

Fig. 2B: Scanning electron microscope images of the membrane after filtration of the tissue-digested solution in Patient 1: (b1) 2,500× magnification with 30 μm, (b2) 5,000× magnification with 10 μm, (b3) 10,000× magnification with 5 μm, and (b4) EDS membrane after filtration of the tissue-digested solution.

polypropylene, and PET, suggesting that MPs have adhered to or penetrated the membrane during use.

PUBLIC HEALTH INTERVENTIONS

The potential link between nanoplastics and CVD has significant public health implications.[12-14] CVDs remain the leading cause of death worldwide, accounting for approximately 30% of global mortality.[5] If nanoplastics are confirmed as a novel risk factor, their ubiquitous presence in the environment could exacerbate the global burden of CVD. The projected increase in plastic production, estimated to reach 13.2 billion tons by 2050, underscores the urgency of addressing this issue.[29,30] The public health strategies to mitigate nanoplastic exposure should include:

- *Policies for reducing plastic pollution:* Implementing policies to reduce single-use plastics and improve waste management could decrease environmental nanoplastic levels.
- *Regulatory measures:* Establishing guidelines for acceptable nanoplastic levels in food, water, and air could protect vulnerable populations.
- *Public awareness campaigns:* Educating the public about the sources and risks of nanoplastic exposure could encourage behavioral changes, such as reducing reliance on plastic-containing products.
- *Improving detection methods:* Developing standardized, sensitive techniques for detecting nanoplastics in biological and environmental samples is critical for monitoring exposure.

To advance our understanding of the relationship between nanoplastics and heart

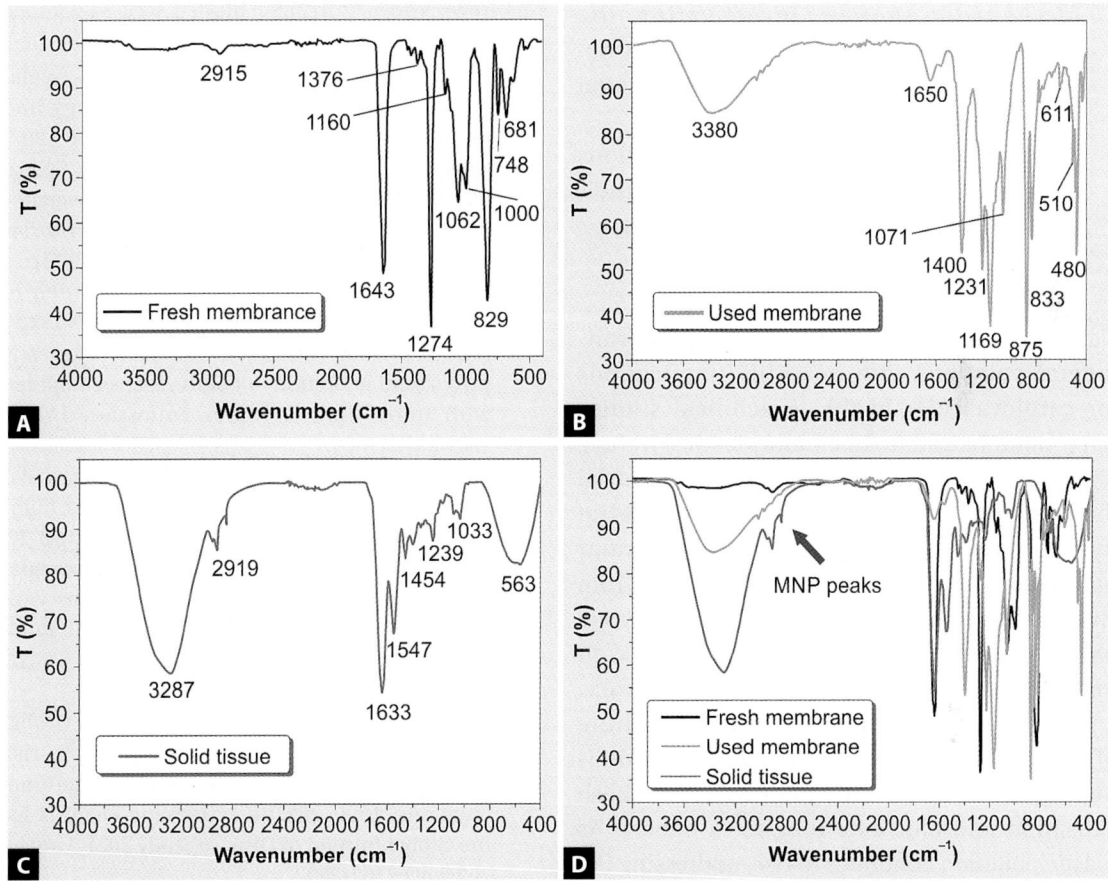

Figs. 3A to D: Fourier Transformed Infrared (FTIR) spectroscopy and Raman spectroscopy findings from the atheroma sample in Patient 2: (A) Fresh membrane; (B) Used membrane after filtration; (C) Solid tissue; and (D) Combined spectra. (MNP: micro-nanoplastics).

disease, future research should focus on the following areas:[31]

- *Large-scale epidemiological studies:* Conducting prospective cohort studies in diverse populations to assess the association between nanoplastic exposure and cardiovascular outcomes.
- *Environmental exposure models:* Integrating environmental and demographic data to model nanoplastic exposure and its cardiovascular impacts at a population level.
- *Standardized detection methods:* Developing consensus protocols for nanoplastic detection to improve the reliability and reproducibility of research findings. In our study, the sample size is very small, a more accurate and sensitive technique for identification is needed. The interference of biological polymers with plastic polymers in detection through FTIR is major hurdle. The most focus and advanced techniques such as LDIR or Py-GC analysis can provide better confirmations. The focus research in developing standard methods for nanoplastics detection with simple technique and instrument is still a challenge to be handled.

- *Mechanistic studies:* Investigating the molecular pathways underlying nanoplastic-induced cardiotoxicity to identify potential therapeutic targets.
- *Intervention studies*: Exploring interventions to reduce nanoplastic exposure and their effects on cardiovascular health outcomes.

CONCLUSION

Nanoplastics represent an emerging environmental pollutant with potential implications for cardiovascular health. Preclinical studies have demonstrated that nanoplastics induce oxidative stress, inflammation, mitochondrial dysfunction, apoptosis, and endothelial dysfunction, contributing to cardiovascular pathology. Clinical evidence, particularly from studies detecting nanoplastics in atherosclerotic plaques, suggests a significant association with increased risks of myocardial infarction, stroke, and death. However, the observational nature of these studies and methodological limitations highlight the need for further research to establish causation and elucidate long-term effects. As plastic pollution continues to rise, addressing the cardiovascular risks of nanoplastics is a critical public health priority.[32] By advancing research and implementing targeted interventions, we can mitigate the impact of this novel risk factor and protect global cardiovascular health.

REFERENCES

1. Tiseo I. (2025). Environmental pollution in India: statistics and facts. [online] Available from https://www.statista.com/topics/6853/environmental-pollution-in-india/#topicOverview [Last accessed November, 2025].
2. Gupta R, Gupta KD. Coronary heart disease in low socioeconomic status subjects in India: An evolving epidemic. Indian Heart J. 2009;61:358-67.
3. India State-Level Disease Burden Collaborators. Nations within a nation: variations in epidemiological transition across the states in India 1990-2016, in the Global Burden of Disease Study. Lancet. 2017;390:2437-60.
4. Prabhakaran D, Jeemon P, Roy A. Cardiovascular diseases in India: current epidemiology and future directions. Circulation. 2016;133:1605-20.
5. GBD 2021 Causes of Deaths Collaborators. Global burden of 288 causes of death and life expectancy decomposition in 204 countries and territories and 811 subnational locations, 1990–2021: a systematic analysis for the Global Burden of Disease Study 2021. Lancet. 2024;403:2100-132.
6. Joshi P, Islam S, Pais P, et al. Risk factors for early myocardial infarction in South Asians compared with individuals in other countries. JAMA. 2007;297:286-94.
7. Yusuf S, Rangarajan S, Teo K, et al. Cardiovascular risk and events in 17 low-, middle- and high-income countries. N Engl J Med. 2014;371:818-27.
8. Joseph P, Kutty VR, Mohan V, et al. Cardiovascular disease, mortality and their associations with modifiable risk factors in a multinational South Asia cohort: a PURE sub-study. Eur Heart J. 2022;43:2831-40.
9. GBD 2021 Risk Factors Collaborators. Global burden and strength of evidence for 88 risk factors in 204 countries and 811 subnational locations, 1990–2021: a systematic analysis for the Global Burden of Disease Study 2021. Lancet. 2024;403:2162-203.
10. Munzel T, Hahad O, Sorenson M, et al. Environmental risk factors and cardiovascular diseases: a comprehensive review. Cardiovasc Res. 2022;118:2880-902.
11. Sagheer U, Al-Kindi S, Abohashem S, et al. Environmental pollution and cardiovascular disease: Part 1. JACC Adv. 2024;3:100805.
12. Daiber A, Rajagopalan S, Kuntic M, et al. Cardiovascular risk posed by the exposome. Atherosclerosis. 2025;405:119222.
13. Thompson RC, Courtene-Jones W, Boucher J, et al. Twenty years of microplastics pollution research—what have we learned? Science. 2025;386:eadl2746.
14. Zhu X, Wang C, Duan X, et al. Micro- and nanoplastics: a new cardiovascular risk factor? Environ Int. 2023;171:107662.
15. Zheng H, Vidili G, Casu G, et al. Microplastics and nanoplastics in cardiovascular disease:

a narrative review with worrying links. Front Toxicol. 2024;6:1479292.
16. Barnes DKA, Galgani F, Thompson RC, et al. Accumulation and fragmentation of plastic debris in global environments. Philos Trans Roy Soc Lond Series B Biol Sci. 2009;364:1985-98.
17. Sun Z, Wen Y, Zhang F, et al. Exposure to nanoplastics induces mitochondrial impairment and cytomembrane destruction in Leydig cells. Ecotoxicol Environ Saf. 2023;255:114796.
18. Beijer NR. Relationship between particle properties and immunotoxicological effects of environmentally-sourced microplastics. Front Water. 2022;4:866732.
19. Goldsworthy A, O'Callaghan LA, Blum C, et al. Micro-nanoplastic induced cardiovascular disease and dysfunction: a scoping review. J Expo Sci Environ Epidemiol. 2025;35(5):746-69.
20. Krause S, Ouellet V, Allen D, et al. The potential of micro- and nanoplastics to exacerbate the health impacts and global burden of noncommunicable diseases. Cell Rep Med. 2024;5:101581.
21. Marfella R, Prattichizzo F, Sardu C, et al. Microplastics and nanoplastics in atheroma and cardiovascular events. N Engl J Med. 2024;390: 900-10.
22. Zhang Y, Gao Q, Gao Q, et al. Microplastics and nanoplastics increase major adverse cardiac events in patients with myocardial infarction. J Hazard Mat. 2025;489:137624.
23. Yang Y, Zhang F, Jiang Z, et al. Microplastics are associated with elevated atherosclerosis risk and increased vascular complexity in acute coronary syndrome patients. Particle Fibre Toxicol. 2024; 21:354.
24. Sagheer U, Al-Kindi S, Abohashem S, et al. Environmental pollution and cardiovascular disease: Part 2. JACC Adv. 2024;3:100815.
25. De Bruin CR, de Rijke E, van Wezel AP, et al. Methodologies to characterise, identify and quantify nano- and sub-micron-sized plastics in relevant media for human exposure. Environ Sci Adv. 2022;1:238-58.
26. Gupta R. Covid-19 and sudden deaths among the young. RUHS J Health Sciences. 2024;9:63-6.
27. Bana A, Sangal A, Mehta N, et al. Off-Pump CABG surgery in left-main coronary artery disease: A single centre prospective registry. Ind J Thor Cardiovasc Surg. 2023;39:446-52.
28. Raman Spectroscopy. Advances in molecular imaging for surgery. [online] Available from https://www.sciencedirect.com/topics/agricultural-and-biological-sciences/raman-spectroscopy#:~:text=Basics%20of%20Raman%20Spectroscopy,be%20used%20for%20their%20identification [Last accessed November, 2025].
29. Ritchie H, Sambroska V, Roser M. Plastic pollution. [online] Available from https://ourworldindata.org/plastic-pollution [Last accessed November, 2025].
30. Winiarska E, Jutel M, Zemelka-Wiacek M, The potential impact of nano- and microplastics on human health: Understanding human health risks. Env Res. 2024;251:118535.
31. Prattichizzo F, Ceriello A, Pellegrini V, et al. Microplastics and cardiovascular diseases: evidence and perspectives. Eur Heart J. 2024;45:4099-110.
32. Landigran PJ, Dunlop S, Treskova M, et al. The Lancet countdown on health and plastics. Lancet. 2025;40(10507):1044-62.

CHAPTER 3

The Lancet Commission: Relooking at Coronary Heart Disease in 2025

Rajeev Gupta

INTRODUCTION

The Lancet Commission (2025) on *Rethinking Coronary Artery Disease: Moving from Ischaemia to Atheroma* has redefined coronary artery disease (CAD) as a process of progressive atherosclerosis across the life course. This report highlights that ischemia, which has so far been the focus of clinical management, addresses the delayed consequences of atherosclerosis. The report recommends restructuring the approach to CAD, shifting the focus to preventing the initiation and progression of atherosclerosis in early childhood and adolescence to improve long-term health outcomes, including the prevention of premature CAD. The Commission also emphasizes the importance of more comprehensive prevention methods related to cardiovascular care, including early detection, prevention, screening, and management of risk factors (primordial and primary prevention), and highlights the most effective strategies to prevent, regress, and cure atherosclerosis. It advocates for a shift from diagnosing CAD after the development of ischemia or a cardiovascular event, toward assessing an individual's lifetime risk at the earliest opportunity. The present review summarizes the Commission report into 10 key messages with a focus on strategies to translate this knowledge to India.

2025 LANCET COMMISSION ON CORONARY ARTERY DISEASE

A significant development in CAD management is the increasing focus on prevention.[1] CAD prevention guidelines emanating from developed countries [American College of Cardiology/American Heart Association (ACC/AHA), European Society of Cardiology (ESC), and others] have advised primary prevention strategies to be initiated at the age of 35–40 years.[2] Indeed, most of their coronary risk stratification tools commence classification of risk at the age of 40 years. The World Health Organization and several national societies, on the other hand, recommend primordial prevention (i.e., prevention of risk factors) from adolescence and early youth.[3,4] Lack of strong evidence and the cost-effectiveness of starting prevention in childhood were considered important barriers to implementation.

The Lancet Commission (2025) has redefined CAD as a process of progressive atherosclerosis and atherothrombosis across the life course.[5] The report calls for redefining the approach to CAD, shifting the focus to preventing disease occurrence and progression in early childhood and adolescence and improving long-term health outcomes, including prevention of premature CAD (so rampant in India) **(Fig. 1)**,[6] to delaying the onset of this condition into the 70s and 80s. The Commission underscores the importance of more comprehensive prevention methods related to cardiovascular care, including early detection and management of risk factors, and highlights the most important strategies to prevent, regress, and cure atherosclerosis.[5] It advocates for a shift from diagnosing CAD after the development of ischemia or a cardiovascular event, toward assessing an individual's lifetime risk at the earliest opportunity. Once ischemia and obstruction develop, prevention is no longer possible, and the

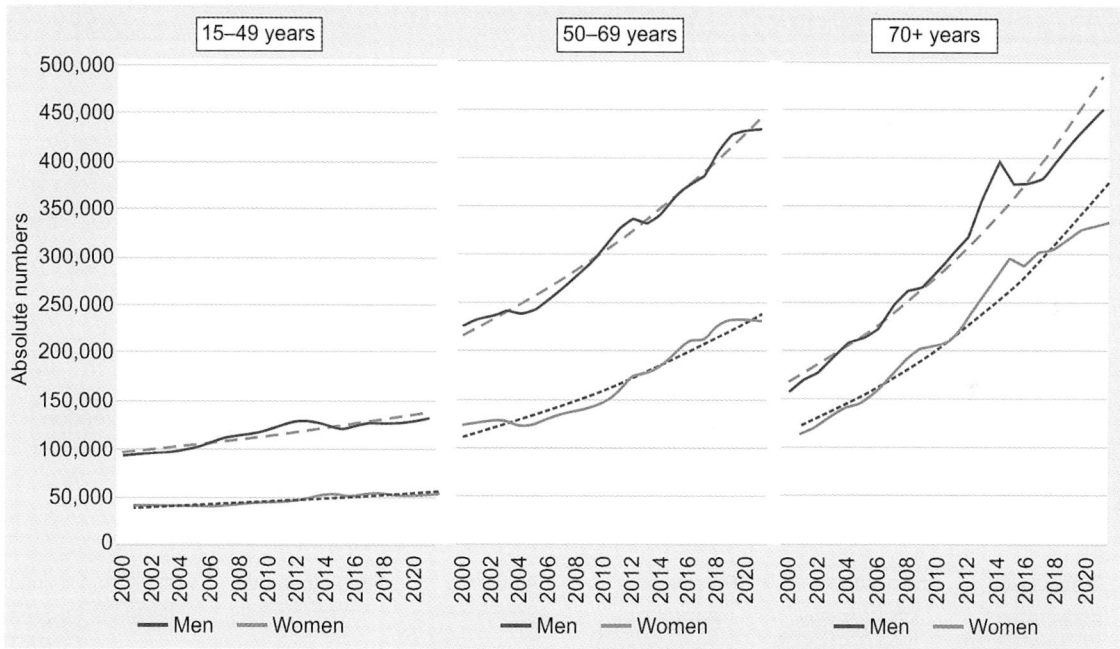

Fig. 1: Secular trends in premature CAD deaths at ages 15–49 and 50–69 years among women and men in India. Global Burden of Disease Study 2021.

effectiveness of interventions in reducing disease and mortality is reduced.[5] The article also suggests focus on healthcare manpower generation and deployment, public health initiatives, and cutting-edge research with proper funding to achieve the target. In the present article, the suggestions of the Lancet Commission are classified into 10 key messages **(Table 1)** and reviewed with a focus on strategies to translate this knowledge to India, the nation with the greatest burden of CAD.[7,8]

PATHOBIOLOGY OF EARLY ATHEROSCLEROSIS

Atherosclerosis is a multifactorial inflammatory disease. The process of atherosclerosis usually begins in childhood and adolescence and continues for decades, leading to both nonfatal and fatal cardiovascular events, including myocardial infarction, stroke, and sudden death **(Fig. 2)**. A surfeit of evidence exists regarding the onset of atherosclerosis in childhood and youth.[9]

There is pathological evidence that fatty streaks, the earliest lesions, can appear in the aorta and coronary arteries as early as infancy, with prevalence increasing through childhood and adolescence.

Autopsy studies, such as the Bogalusa Heart Study, reveal fatty streaks in 50% of children aged 2–15 years, with fibrous plaques in 8% by adolescence.[10] The Pathobiological Determinants of Atherosclerosis in Youth (PDAY) study found that by the age of 15–34 years, advanced lesions are present in 10–20% of individuals, correlating with higher low-density lipoprotein (LDL) cholesterol and lower high-density lipoprotein (HDL) cholesterol levels.[11] Imaging studies, like carotid intima-media thickness (CIMT) measurements, show increased arterial wall thickness in youths with risk factors, indicating early vascular damage.[12]

Lifestyle factors, including poor diet and physical inactivity, exacerbate progression,

TABLE 1: Ten key messages from the 2025 Lancet Commission on CAD.

	Messages
1.	CAD clinical pathways should be focused away from ischemia to atherosclerosis
2.	CAD should be seen as a lifetime continuum from childhood to old age
3.	The onset of CAD can be prevented by early risk factor modification
4.	Effective strategies for early screening and detection of CAD are needed
5.	Implementation of current prevention approaches to be improved
6.	Local and global disparities in prevention, diagnosis, treatment, and outcomes to be addressed
7.	Development of new therapies to eradicate atherosclerosis
8.	Global standard for data collection to be established
9.	The health workforce and research infrastructure must be aligned toward early detection and prevention
10.	Research funding commensurate with the global burden of CAD

(CAD: coronary artery disease)

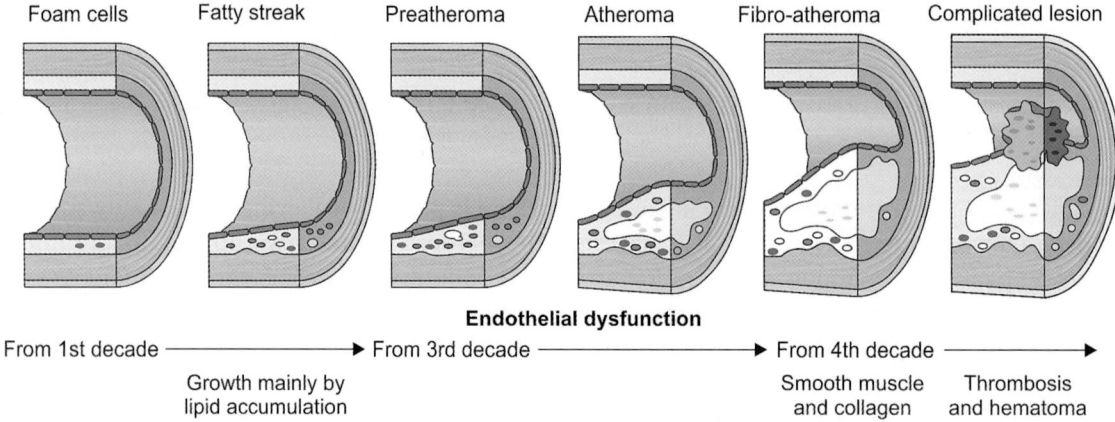

Fig. 2: Early origins of atherosclerosis and its progression.

and risk factors such as obesity, hypertension, dyslipidemia, and diabetes accelerate this process.[1] Early intervention targeting modifiable risk factors can delay the onset of atherosclerosis.

CORONARY ATHEROSCLEROSIS ALONG THE LIFE COURSE

Fatty Streaks

Beginning in childhood, this is the initial stage of the process of atherosclerotic plaque formation. Fatty streaks are characterized by deposition of LDL cholesterol particles in arterial locations prone to atherosclerosis, such as areas of high oscillatory shear, including arterial bifurcation points and inner walls of curvatures.[13] Early fatty streak areas are also characterized by high expression of key inflammatory markers, such as nuclear factor kappa B (NF-κB).[14] Because the endothelium is constantly exposed to the circulation, the initial endothelial dysfunction caused by local inflammation and LDL cholesterol infiltration is augmented by toxins present in the circulation, as occurs during tobacco use, exposure to pollution, diabetes, and dyslipidemia. Hypertension contributes to endothelial dysfunction by increasing the physical force exerted in atherosclerosis-prone areas. Monocytes also begin their migration into the plaque at this stage, turning into macrophages and, after being loaded with chemically modified lipids, becoming foam cells.

Atheroma/Fibroatheroma

This is the progressive stage of plaque formation, characterized by the migration of smooth muscle cells into the intima, attracted by signals from the foam cells. LDL cholesterol particles and macrophages progressively accumulate into a lipid core, while smooth muscle cells produce extracellular matrix proteins that comprise the fibrous cap.[15]

Advancing Atheroma

The final stage of atheroma progression is characterized by a large necrotic core and low smooth muscle cell density, with a thin fibrous cap leading to a vulnerable plaque prone to rupture and thrombosis. Atherosclerotic plaques typically progress to the advancing atheroma stage between the ages of 55 and 65 years.

ATHEROSCLEROSIS RISK FACTORS AND EARLY LIFE PREVENTION

India has undergone a rapid epidemiological transition due to an increase in life expectancy and socioeconomic development.[8] Cardiovascular diseases (CVDs), particularly CAD, are the leading noncommunicable diseases (NCDs) in this region, as reported by multiple national and the Global Burden of Disease (GBD) studies.[7] CAD epidemiology in India is characterized by premature onset of atherosclerosis and acute coronary events, substantially higher mortality compared to higher-income countries, and association with some unique risk factors—diabetes, metabolic syndrome, and indoor air pollution, along with others.[6] All these factors have been discussed in the global context in the 2025 Lancet Commission report.[5]

The study of causal risk factors for CAD in India has had a circuitous path.[16] In the early and mid-20th century, there were multiple theories and hypotheses to explain the premature CAD occurrence in Indians. The risk factors proposed were genetics, obesity, stress, and other social factors.[16] Early case-control studies in India reported that unhealthy lifestyles (smoking, poor diet, stress, smokeless tobacco, etc.) and obesity-related factors (hypertension, diabetes, insulin resistance, and dyslipidemias) are important.[17] Studies that evaluated urban-rural differences in CAD risk factors reported the importance of standard modifiable risk factors (smoking, hypertension, diabetes, and dyslipidemias).[18] Two large studies, the case-control INTERHEART[19] and the prospective PURE (Prospective Urban Rural Epidemiology),[20,21] provide critical insights **(Table 2)**.

INTERHEART Study

This large international case-control study was conducted in 52 countries on all continents and was developed and initiated in India.[19] More than 15,000 men and women ($n = 15,152$) hospitalized with their first myocardial infarction and matching controls ($n = 14,820$) were recruited in the international study. Case-control comparison showed that nine common modifiable risk factors were responsible for more than 90% of acute myocardial infarctions. Five South Asian countries (India, Pakistan, Bangladesh, Nepal, and Sri Lanka) participated in the study with 1,732 cases and 2204 controls.[19] Risk factors important in South Asian patients were dyslipidemias (increased apolipoprotein B/A$_1$ ratio), smoking, hypertension, diabetes, abdominal adiposity,

TABLE 2: Atherosclerotic CVD risk factors identified in INTERHEART and PURE studies.

INTERHEART study (case–control)*	PURE study (CVD incidence)*	
Acute myocardial infarction	*Cardiovascular diseases*	*Coronary artery disease*
Raised ApoB/ApoA$_1$ ratio (47%)	Hypertension (22%)	High non-HDL cholesterol (17%)
Smoking/tobacco (38%)	High non-HDL cholesterol (8%)	Hypertension (13%)
Raised waist–hip ratio (38%)	Household air pollution (7%)	Tobacco use (12%)
Physical inactivity (27%)	Tobacco use (6%)	Abdominal obesity (11%)
Low fruit–vegetable intake (21%)	Poor diet (6%)	Diabetes (8%)
Hypertension (19%)	Low education (6%)	Low education (7%)
Psychosocial factors (16%)	Abdominal obesity (6%)	Low grip strength (7%)
Alcohol intake (16%)	Diabetes (5%)	Household pollution (5%)
Diabetes (12%)	Low grip strength (3%)	Poor diet (4%)
	Low physical activity (2%)	Low physical activity (<1%)
	Depression (<1.0%)	Depression (<1%)
	Excessive alcohol (<1.0%)	Excessive alcohol (<1%)

*Numbers in parentheses are population attributable risk (INTERHEART) and population-attributable fraction (PURE study). Cardiovascular diseases (CVD) include coronary artery disease (CAD), stroke, and peripheral artery disease.

psychosocial factors, physical inactivity, and low fruit and vegetable consumption. An important finding in the INTERHEART study was a 10-year gap in the age of first myocardial infarction in South Asians compared to other countries.[19] The mean age of presentation among participants in South Asian countries was 51 years compared to 61 years in the more developed countries. This study also reported that the CAD risk factors occurred earlier in South Asian participants compared to developed countries, commensurate with the earlier onset of acute coronary events, the focus of the 2025 Lancet Commission. Thus, this study confirmed the importance of all the classical CHD risk factors for the occurrence of an acute coronary event in India, with the main difference being the earlier (premature) occurrence of risk factors.

PURE Study

The PURE study is the first large-scale population-based prospective study to identify cardiovascular risk factors in many lower-income countries, including India.[20,21] The study began in Bangalore urban and rural locations with about 10,000 participants and is presently being conducted in 26 countries across the globe with more than 200,000 participants. The PURE study has identified that 12 common risk factors are responsible for 65–70% of incident CVD and CAD events in the South Asian cohort **(Fig. 3)**.[21] The 10 important risk factors identified in the PURE study for CVD are hypertension, non-HDL cholesterol, diabetes, low educational status, abdominal obesity, indoor air pollution, smoking/tobacco use, sedentary lifestyle, frailty, and depression. For the incident acute coronary event, raised non-HDL cholesterol (>120 mg/dL) is the most important risk factor, followed by indoor air pollution, hypertension, and diabetes **(Table 2)**.[20] All these risk factors are similar to the INTERHEART study. An important difference is that, while the INTERHEART study attributed 90% of the population attributable risk to nine common risk factors, in the PURE

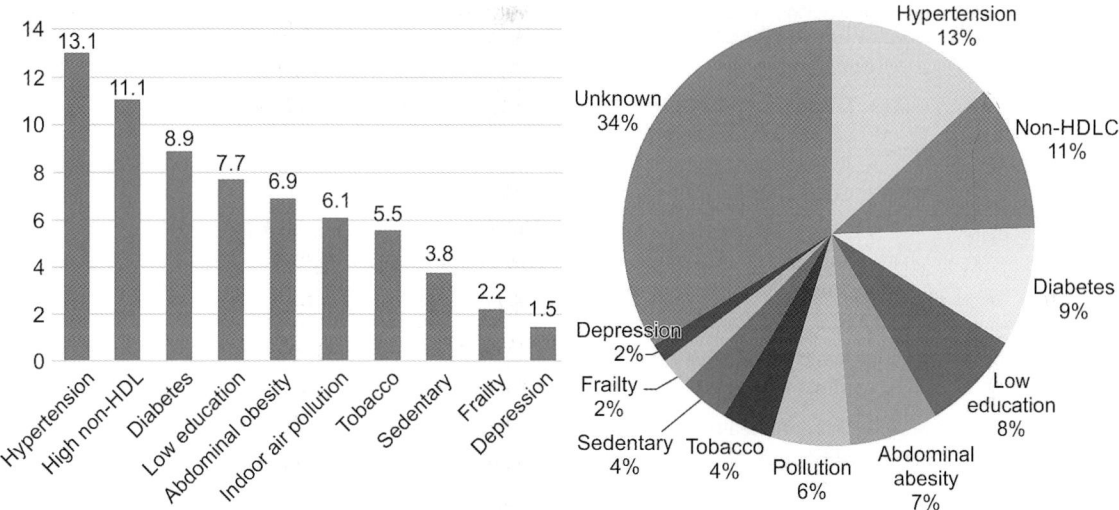

Fig. 3: Population proportionate attributable fractions (PAF, %) for various cardiovascular risk factors and incidence of cardiovascular diseases in the PURE-South Asia cohort (n = 33,583; median follow-up 11.5 years).

study, only 60–65% of the population attributable fraction was attributable to them.

Risk Factor Control in the Young

The process of atherosclerosis begins in childhood; therefore, it is important to resort to primordial and primary prevention strategies as highlighted in the *Lancet Commission*.[5] Although clinical trial evidence has shown convincingly that pharmacological treatment of risk factors can prevent events.[1] The data are less definitive but also highly suggestive that appropriate public policy and lifestyle interventions aimed at eliminating tobacco use, limiting salt consumption, encouraging physical exercise, and improving diet during childhood can prevent events.[1] There has been concern about whether efforts aimed at primordial and primary prevention provide value or are cost-effective.[4] Although questions about the value of therapeutics for acute disease may be addressed by cost-effectiveness analysis, the long-time frames involved in evaluating preventive interventions make cost-effectiveness analysis difficult and flawed. I believe that widespread implementation of healthy policies using a health-in-all-policies approach, population-wide community efforts, and pharmacological interventions is likely to be cost-effective and often cost-saving.[1]

Primordial Prevention

Primordial prevention of atherosclerosis focuses on preventing the development of its risk factors in childhood to reduce the incidence of CVD later in life.[3] Unlike primary or secondary prevention, which address existing risk factors or disease, primordial prevention targets healthy populations to maintain low-risk profiles. Childhood is a critical period for establishing lifelong health behaviors, as early lifestyle patterns significantly influence future cardiovascular health **(Table 3)**. Key risk factors for CAD, such as obesity, hypertension, dyslipidemia, and insulin resistance, often begin in childhood. Some of these risk factors begin *in utero* and, therefore, also require a focus on maternal health.[1]

Primordial prevention emphasizes healthy lifestyle habits to mitigate these risks before they

TABLE 3: Primordial prevention strategies in the 2025 Lancet Commission Report.

Strategy	Intervention
Healthy diet	• Emphasis on fruits, vegetables, whole grains, dairy products, fish, complex carbohydrates, and millets • Avoid sugars, refined carbohydrates, ultraprocessed foods, trans fats, and saturated fats • Creation of healthy food environment
Physical activity	• Encourage moderate intensity physical activity, 60 minutes daily • Weight training exercises to prevent sarcopenia • Conducive environment for physical activity
Tobacco avoidance	• Prevent smoking initiation • Avoid second-hand smoke and vaping • Implementation of tobacco control policies
Family-based interventions	• Promote healthy lifestyles within families • Mitigation of indoor environmental pollution • Creation of role models
Community programs	• Implementation of school-based nutrition and physical activity initiatives
Screening	• Monitor body mass index, blood pressure, and lipids in at-risk children • Consider cascade screening for lipids and blood pressure in high-risk families • Genetic screening using polygenic risk scores in high-risk families
Social determinants	• Focus on UN Sustainable Development Goals for the elimination of poverty, hunger, illiteracy, gender inequality, pollution (ambient, indoor, water, soil, etc.), social inequality, etc. • Promotion of sustainable cities and communities, decent work and economic growth, affordable and clean energy, and climate action • Health-in-all-policies approach

emerge. A balanced diet rich in fruits, vegetables, whole grains, and lean proteins, while limiting processed foods high in sugar, sodium, and trans fats, is foundational. The AHA recommends children consume less than 25 g of added sugars daily and avoid trans fats to support heart health.[4] Encouraging regular physical activity of at least 60 minutes of moderate-to-vigorous intensity exercise daily helps maintain healthy body weight, blood pressure (BP), and lipid profiles.[4] Tobacco exposure, including second-hand smoke, is a significant risk factor for CAD.[4] Preventing smoking initiation in childhood through education and smoke-free environments is critical. Schools and families play a pivotal role in delivering antitobacco messaging and modeling healthy behaviors.[1] Additionally, managing stress and promoting mental health through supportive family dynamics and social connections can reduce the likelihood of adopting harmful coping mechanisms, such as overeating or substance use, later in life.[1]

Family-based interventions are highly effective for primordial prevention.[4,22] Parents influence children's dietary and activity habits, making family-wide adoption of healthy lifestyles essential. Community programs, such as school-based nutrition education and physical activity initiatives, reinforce these efforts. For example, programs like the Coordinated Approach to Child Health (CATCH) have shown success in improving children's dietary habits and physical fitness. Policy-level interventions, such as regulating food marketing to children and ensuring access to healthy school meals, further support primordial prevention.[23]

Primary Prevention

Primary prevention of CAD aims to reduce the incidence of disease by addressing modifiable risk factors across the lifespan.[1] Unlike primordial prevention, which prevents risk factor development, primary prevention targets individuals with existing risk factors but no established CAD.[4] Effective strategies evolve with age, emphasizing lifestyle modifications, risk factor management, and, when necessary, medical interventions to mitigate risks like hypertension, dyslipidemia, diabetes, obesity, and smoking. In childhood and adolescence, primary prevention focuses on establishing healthy habits to address early risk factors such as obesity or elevated BP. Encouraging a diet low in saturated fats and high in fruits, vegetables, and whole grains, alongside at least 60 minutes of daily physical activity, helps maintain a healthy weight and lipid profiles. The AHA recommends limiting sodium and added sugars to prevent hypertension and insulin resistance **(Table 4)**. Anti-smoking education is critical, as adolescence is a common period for smoking initiation.[24,25]

In young adulthood (20–39 years), primary prevention emphasizes maintaining healthy behaviors and screening for risk factors.[26] Regular monitoring of BP, cholesterol, and glucose levels allows early intervention. For example, statins may be considered for individuals with persistently high LDL cholesterol levels (>100 mg/dL). Stress management and mental health support are vital, as chronic stress can exacerbate risk factors like hypertension. Middle age (40–59 years) is a critical period, as CAD risk increases with age-related physiological changes. Lifestyle interventions remain central, but medical management intensifies. BP control (target <130/80 mm Hg) and diabetes management (HbA1c <7%) are prioritized. Smoking cessation programs,

TABLE 4: Primary prevention across the life course.

Life stage	Primary prevention strategies
Childhood and adolescence	• Healthy diet and regular physical activity • Antismoking education and avoidance of pollution • Monitoring of body mass index
Young adulthood	• Screening for hypertension, dyslipidemia, and diabetes • Promote stress management and sleep
Middle age	• Control blood pressure to targets • Control LDL cholesterol, triglycerides, and diabetes • Smoking cessation • Weight loss using lifestyle intervention ± drugs • Exercise
Older adulthood	• Exercise • Dietary adjustments • Selective medication use • Manage comorbidities

including counseling and pharmacotherapy, are highly effective, reducing CAD risk by up to 50% within a year of quitting. Weight management is crucial, as obesity amplifies other risk factors. In older adulthood (60+ years), primary prevention balances risk reduction with quality of life. Low-dose aspirin is not recommended by guidelines,[24,25] but may be considered for select individuals with high cardiovascular risk but low bleeding risk.[1] Regular exercise, such as walking or resistance training, supports cardiovascular health, while dietary adjustments address age-related metabolic changes. Polypharmacy using polypills focuses on careful management of medications like antihypertensives or statins.[27]

EARLY SCREENING AND DETECTION OF ATHEROSCLEROSIS

Screening for early risk factors, such as elevated body mass index (BMI) or BP, allows for timely interventions **(Table 3)**. The American Academy of Pediatrics (AAP) recommends lipid screening for children with a family history of CAD or other risk factors between the age of 9 and 11 years.[28] Early identification enables targeted lifestyle modifications to prevent progression to clinical disease. Below are the key strategies for early screening, focusing on identifying risk factors such as hypercholesterolemia, hypertension, and other modifiable and nonmodifiable factors, supported by evidence from relevant studies.

Targeted Screening

Targeted screening focuses on children and adolescents with known risk factors for atherosclerosis, such as a family history of premature CVD (before the age of 55 years in men or 65 years in women), familial hypercholesterolemia (FH), obesity, diabetes, or hypertension. The AAP recommends lipid screening for children with these risk factors starting after the age of 2 years but no later than age of 10 years.[29] Screening involves measuring lipid profiles (total cholesterol, LDL cholesterol, HDL cholesterol, and triglycerides) with a follow-up confirmation test if abnormalities are detected. This strategy is cost-effective and focuses on high-risk groups. For example, children with a family history of FH or premature CVD are prioritized for lipid screening and genetic testing if indicated. For example, the Simon Broome or Dutch Lipid Clinic Network Score integrates LDL cholesterol levels, family history, and physical findings (e.g., xanthomas) to identify FH in children.

Cascade Screening

This strategy involves screening family members of individuals diagnosed with FH, leveraging genetic or lipid testing to identify affected relatives. This can be implemented when a child or parent is diagnosed with FH, cascade screening uses DNA testing or lipid profiles to screen first-degree relatives. This is particularly effective in settings with genetic testing availability, as 50% of first-degree relatives inherit FH mutations. It is highly cost-effective, as it targets families with a high likelihood of FH. The European Atherosclerosis Society (EAS) Consensus recommends cascade screening in countries with FH registries and to develop such registries where none exist.[30] However, it requires access to genetic testing and family cooperation, which may not be universally available.

Universal Screening

Universal screening involves testing all children for lipid abnormalities, typically between the age of 9 and 11 years, when lipid levels are stable before puberty. The National Heart, Lung, and Blood Institute (NHLBI) endorses universal lipid screening in this age group to detect FH and other dyslipidemias early.[31] A nonfasting lipid panel can be used initially, followed by fasting tests for confirmation. It captures cases missed by targeted screening, especially in populations with high FH prevalence (e.g., India). Early detection can lead to lifestyle interventions or pharmacotherapy, such as statins, which are safe and effective in children. The cost-effectiveness of this strategy is debated, and there is limited evidence on the long-term outcomes of universal screening.

Reverse Screening

This approach starts with screening children and, if abnormalities are found, extends to parents and siblings to identify familial risk factors. It can be used in settings where pediatric screening is routine, such as during well-child visits. If a child has elevated LDL cholesterol (>150 mg/dL), parents are screened for FH or other risk factors. It identifies undiagnosed FH in families and promotes family-wide interventions but relies on pediatrician's awareness and willingness to initiate screening, which may be low due to limited knowledge about pediatric atherosclerosis.

Noninvasive Imaging for Risk Assessment

Noninvasive methods, such as CIMT measurement via ultrasound or coronary artery calcium (CAC) scoring, assess early structural changes in arteries.[32] CIMT is currently used in research settings to detect subclinical atherosclerosis in high-risk children, such as those with FH, diabetes, or chronic kidney disease (CKD). It is not routine in clinical practice due to limited pediatric data, but shows promise for identifying at-risk individuals. It provides direct evidence of arterial changes, correlating with risk factors like LDL cholesterol, obesity, and hypertension. CAC scoring requires specialized equipment and expertise, and is not relevant in childhood and adolescence. Its use is primarily reserved for research or high-risk cases such as those with homozygous FH.

Integration with Lifestyle and Risk Factor Assessment

Screening is combined with evaluating lifestyle factors (e.g., diet, physical activity, and smoking) and other risk conditions (e.g., obesity, diabetes, and CKD) to provide a comprehensive risk profile. The pediatrician assesses BMI, BP, and glucose levels alongside lipid profiles during routine check-ups. The Bogalusa Heart Study and other cohort studies show that multiple risk factors (e.g., obesity and hypertension) increase atherosclerosis severity in youth. Such a holistic approach supports primordial prevention through lifestyle interventions, such as promoting a Mediterranean diet, but requires coordinated care and patient/family adherence to lifestyle changes.

There are a number of challenges for screening, including limited awareness among pediatricians and general practitioners and the public about the importance of early atherosclerosis screening that hinders implementation. Universal screening's cost-effectiveness is under scrutiny, with targeted and cascade screening often preferred in resource-limited settings. There are ethical concerns regarding screening children, with concerns about stigmatization and the psychological impact of diagnosing a chronic condition early in life. Screening strategies vary by country, with some adopting universal screening due to high FH prevalence, while others rely on targeted approaches. In India, no such public health strategy exists, although it has been recommended by the lipid management guidelines.[33]

ADDRESSING LOCAL AND GLOBAL DISPARITIES IN PREVENTION

Socioeconomic factors also influence primordial prevention, and a focus on social determinants is essential **(Table 5)**.[1] Children in low-income communities may face barriers to access healthy foods or safe spaces for physical activity. Addressing these disparities through public health initiatives, such as subsidized healthy food programs or community recreation facilities, is crucial for equitable prevention. Focusing on the United Nations Sustainable Development Goals is important for primordial prevention.[1] By fostering healthy habits in childhood, primordial prevention lays the foundation for lifelong cardiovascular health, reducing the burden of CAD in adulthood.[31]

Social determinants, such as access to healthcare and socioeconomic status, influence the success of the primary prevention.[1] Community programs, workplace wellness initiatives, and policy measures—like tobacco taxes or healthy food subsidies—enhance adherence to preventive strategies.[34] Digital health tools, such as wearable devices, support self-monitoring of physical activity and heart rate.[35] By addressing risk factors proactively across the life course, primary

TABLE 5: Social determinants of health and CAD prevention: Lessons from the Lancet Commission.

UN SDG number	CAD-relevant UN SDG – SDG domain	Public health response and interventions for CAD prevention and control
1.	No poverty	• Prioritizing health needs of the poor
2.	Zero hunger	• Addressing causes and consequences of all forms of malnutrition • Focus on under- and overnutrition, frailty, etc.
3.	Good health and well-being	• Ensure healthy lives • Promote well-being across the life course • Primordial prevention • Primary prevention • Secondary prevention • Ensure availability, affordability, and adherence to medicines
4.	Quality education	• General literacy • Population level health literacy • Focuses on physicians' and health professionals' education for NCD prevention and control
5.	Gender equality	• Women-specific policies for CAD prevention
8.	Decent work and economic growth	• Gainful employment • Inclusive economic growth • Reduction of social and economic disparities
10.	Reducing inequalities	• Equitable access to health promotion • Access to healthcare and medicines • Strong primary care services
11.	Sustainable cities and communities	• Focus on urban planning for creating healthy cities • Cleaner air, water, and green spaces • Safe and walkable areas
12.	Responsible consumption and production	• Responsible consumption of foods • Evidence-based consumption of medicines • Avoid overmedicalization and unnecessary placebos
13.	Climate action	• Protecting health from climate risks • Promoting health through low-carbon development

(CAD: coronary artery disease; NCD: noncommunicable diseases; SDG: sustainable development goals)

prevention significantly reduces CAD incidence, promoting long-term cardiovascular health: A key message of 2025 Lancet Commission.[5]

DEVELOPMENT OF NEW THERAPIES TO ERADICATE ATHEROSCLEROSIS

There are a number of strategies to prevent the development of initial atherosclerosis and eradicate it.[15] These range from preimplantation tools, gene-modifying approaches using CRISPR-CAS technology to nanotechnology.[36] The new therapies to eradicate atherosclerosis focus on reversing plaque build-up, inflammation, and lipid retention in arteries, moving beyond symptom management **(Table 6)**. Eight genes have been identified as key to myocardial infarction resistance: *PCSK9, NPC1L1, LPA, APOC3, ANGPTL3, ANGPTL4, ASGRI1,* and

TABLE 6: New therapies to eradicate atherosclerosis.

Therapy type	Mechanism	Development stage	Potential benefits
PCSK9 inhibitors (evolocumab, alirocumab, inclisiran, etc.)	Enhance LDL receptor activity, promotes plaque regression	Approved	Reduce atherosclerosis, reduces MACE in clinical trials, stabilizes plaques, and widely available
Anti-inflammatory drugs (IL-2 inhibitors, colchicine, IL-6 inhibitors, etc.)	Reduce vascular inflammation and cytokine-driven plaque progression. Inhibit NLRP3 inflammasome, reducing inflammation and plaque instability	Colchicine available. Others in trials	
Nanozyme therapy	Mimic antioxidant enzymes to scavenge ROS, reducing oxidative stress and plaque size	Preclinical	0–65% plaque reduction, nontoxic, dual anti-inflammatory/antioxidative effects
Immunotherapy	Blocks ApoB-lipoprotein retention in arterial walls to halt plaque formation	Preclinical	Prevents progression, potential for early-stage intervention
Nucleic acid-based therapies	Target genetic pathways (e.g., lncRNAs, miRNAs) to regulate lipid metabolism and inflammation	Early-stage research	Personalized treatment, high specificity, potential for long-term plaque regression
Gene-based therapies. Focus on *PCSK9*, *ANGPTL3*, *APOC3*, and *LDLR* genes	CRISPR-CAS-based therapies lead to a reduction in target molecules in cholesterol and triglyceride pathways	Preclinical and early-stage research	60–90% reduction in target molecules. Atherosclerosis reduction in mouse models

APOB. CRISPR therapies target lipid metabolism genes (*PCSK9, ANGPTL3, APOC3,* and *LDLR*) to reduce LDL cholesterol and triglycerides, showing promise in preclinical models.[37,38] Challenges include delivery efficacy, off-target effects, and ethical concerns. Clinical translation requires further safety and efficacy trials.[39,40]

Current lipid-lowering drugs such as statins and PCSK9 inhibitors reduce LDL cholesterol and promote plaque regression, as seen in lipid trials.[41] However, residual risk persists, prompting innovative approaches. Anti-inflammatory therapies that target cytokines: Canakinumab, an interleukin (IL)-1β inhibitor, reduced major adverse cardiovascular events (MACE) by 15% in the CANTOS trial, though there was a risk of increased incidence of infections.[42] Colchicine, now guideline-recommended, lowered MACE by 31% in LoDoCo2.[43] IL-6 inhibitors like ziltivekimab are in phase 3 trials (ZEUS) for high-risk patients.[43] Nanotechnology offers precision: Nanozymes, such as cerium oxide NPs, mimic enzymes to scavenge ROS, reducing plaque by 60–65% in mouse models via antioxidative and anti-inflammatory effects. MSU's nanoparticle infusion activates immune cells to eat plaque cores, decreasing inflammation in pig arteries without side effects. Novel immunotherapies include chP3R99 mAb, which blocks ApoB-lipoprotein retention, halting progression in preclinical studies.[36] Nucleic acid-based treatments and precision medicine, leveraging genomics, promise personalized eradication.[36-39] Ongoing trials emphasize safety, with potential to transform cardiovascular care by 2030.

These therapies aim to eradicate atherosclerosis by targeting its root causes—lipid accumulation, inflammation, and oxidative stress. PCSK9 inhibitors and colchicine are clinically available, while others, like nanozymes and immunotherapies, show promise in preclinical studies. Challenges include safety, scalability, and long-term efficacy. Funding is required for new drug development. The field of molecular sciences in India has just started, and we may likely identify important atherosclerosis-modifying agents from our country.

GLOBAL STANDARD OF DATA COLLECTION

Global standardized data collection for atherosclerosis prevention and management is critical for reducing the global burden of atherosclerotic CVD. The PURE study (mentioned earlier) in 27 countries with more than 200,000 participants has provided a template for global data collection using uniform pragmatic methodology.[20] Uniform data protocols enable consistent risk assessment, treatment evaluation, and cross-country comparisons, addressing disparities in low- and middle-income countries (LMICs) where 80% of CVD cases occur.[44] The key components include:

- *Risk factor monitoring*: Standardized metrics for LDL cholesterol, non-HDL cholesterol, BP, BMI, smoking, and diabetes are essential. The WHO's Global HEARTS Initiative promotes uniform risk assessment tools, such as the WHO risk charts, to identify high-risk individuals.[45]
- *Clinical data harmonization*: Protocols like those in the Atherosclerosis Risk in Communities (ARIC) study collect standardized lipid profiles, CIMT, and CAC scores to track subclinical atherosclerosis.[46]
- *Electronic health records (EHRs)*: Integrating EHRs with standardized coding (e.g., ICD-10) ensures data comparability. The Multi-Ethnic Study of Atherosclerosis (MESA)[47] validates EHRs against cohort data for accuracy.
- *Global registries*: PURE study[48] and other cardiovascular registries standardize genetic and clinical data and aid screening.
- *Surveillance systems*: WHO's Global Burden of Disease Study data tools track CVD prevalence, incidence, and mortality, using age-standardized rates.[49,50]

There are a number of challenges that include variations in healthcare infrastructure, data privacy regulations, and computerization levels complicate global standardization. Paper-based tools are used in low-resource settings to bridge gaps. However, standardized data enhances guideline development, improves resource allocation, and supports precision medicine. For example, consistent LDL cholesterol data inform statin therapy thresholds. Collaborative efforts drive evidence-based prevention and management strategies globally.[50]

HEALTH AND RESEARCH WORKFORCE ALIGNED TO PREVENTION

For long, the prevention strategies have been physician-driven, with limited success.[35,51] A robust health and research workforce is essential for preventing CVD. Aligning this workforce to prioritize prevention involves strategic training, task shifting, and research integration to address risk factors such as hypertension, dyslipidemia, and lifestyle behaviours.[51]

Health Workforce Strategies

- *Training primary care providers:* General practitioners and nurses should be trained in evidence-based prevention protocols, such as the WHO's Global HEARTS Initiative,[45] which emphasizes BP control and lipid management. Programs like Canada's hypertension management model, achieving world-leading detection rates, highlight the impact of skilled primary care.[47]

- *Task shifting:* Nonphysician health workers (NPHWs), including community health workers, can screen for risk factors and promote lifestyle interventions. Studies show task shifting in LMICs improves hypertension control by 5–20%.[51]
- *Multidisciplinary teams:* Integrating dietitians, pharmacists, and social workers enhances holistic prevention. The AHA's barbershop intervention, leveraging pharmacists for BP counselling, reduced CVD risk in high-risk communities.[52]

Research Workforce Strategies

- *Translational research:* Researchers should focus on primordial and primary prevention, studying social determinants and novel interventions like CRISPR therapies targeting PCSK9.
- *Global collaboration:* Initiatives like the Lancet Commission on Hypertension foster research in LMICs, enhancing evidence for scalable interventions.[53]
- *Data standardization:* Researchers must adopt standardized data collection, as in the Global Burden of Disease Study, to inform policy and track prevention outcomes.[50]

Health workforce shortages and limited training in LMICs, such as India, hinder progress.[54,55] Cultural mistrust and inadequate funding also impede implementation. Aligning the workforce requires upskilling primary care, empowering NPHWs, and fostering multidisciplinary and research-driven approaches. These strategies, rooted in global initiatives, can significantly reduce the CVD burden.

■ RESEARCH FUNDING

Improving research funding for atherosclerosis prevention in LMICs is critical to address the disproportionate burden of CVDs, which cause 80% of global CVD deaths in these regions. Strategic approaches can enhance funding and research capacity and include:

- *Innovative financing models:* Implement taxes on tobacco, alcohol, and sugary beverages to generate revenue for CVD research, as demonstrated in countries like Mexico, where soda taxes fund public health initiatives. Public-private partnerships, such as those with pharmaceutical companies, can cofund trials for low-cost interventions like generic statins.[51,55]
- *International collaborations:* Foster partnerships between LMICs and high-income countries (HICs) to share resources, expertise, and infrastructure. The Prospective Urban Rural Epidemiology (PURE) study exemplifies multicountry collaboration, providing data on CVD risk factors across 27 LMICs.[48] Global health organizations, and the WHO, can facilitate these networks.[45]
- *LMIC-led research:* Prioritize funding for local researchers through grants from various international agencies that support capacity-building in LMICs. Empowering local institutions ensures culturally relevant research and sustainable outcomes.[56]
- *Reducing barriers:* Address financial and logistical barriers by offering reduced publication fees, hybrid conference formats, and language support to enhance LMIC researchers' global participation. Open-access platforms can further democratize knowledge sharing. Advocacy and policy change for increased national health budgets allocated to NCD research, leverage frameworks like the WHO's Global Action Plan for NCDs[57] and the United Nations Global Summit on NCDs.[58]

The challenges for conducting high-quality research in India and other LMICs are multiple and include limited infrastructure, competing health priorities (e.g., infectious diseases), and brain-drain.[55,57] Coordinated global efforts and sustained investment are essential to bridge these gaps and accelerate atherosclerosis prevention.

■ CONCLUSION

The Lancet Commission (2025) on *Rethinking Coronary Artery Disease: Moving from Ischaemia to Atheroma* has redefined CAD as a process of progressive atherosclerosis across the life course.[5] The report calls for restructuring the approach to CAD via shifting the focus to prevent CAD in early childhood and adolescence for improving long-term health outcomes, including the prevention of premature CAD, which is rampant in our country.[16] In this article, we have summarized 10 key messages from the report and contextualized them for our country. Recognition that atherosclerosis is a life-course disease with roots in childhood and adolescence is important. Prevention strategies, including primordial and primary prevention, as well as screening, should be initiated early and maintained throughout a person's lifetime **(Table 1)**. Implementation of these strategies is crucial and should address local and global disparities in prevention, diagnosis, and treatment to improve outcomes. The healthcare workforce should be augmented accordingly. Focus on the development of new therapies to eradicate atherosclerosis, supported by proper research, high-quality research infrastructure and funding, is essential. Overall, this is a herculean task, but the *Lancet Commission* has provided a clear direction not only for developed countries, but also for developing countries such as India.

■ REFERENCES

1. Gupta R, Wood DA. Primary prevention of ischemic heart disease: populations, individuals, and healthcare professionals. Lancet. 2019;394: 685-96.
2. Khanji MY, Bicalho VVS, van Waardhuizen CN, et al. Cardiovascular risk assessment: a systematic review of guidelines. Ann Intern Med. 2016;165: 713-22.
3. WHO. Primordial prevention of coronary heart disease. Technical Report Series. 1994.
4. Weintraub WS, Daniels SR, Burke LE, et al. Value of primordial and primary prevention for cardiovascular disease: A policy statement from the American Heart Association. Circulation. 2011;124:967-90.
5. Zaman S, Wasfy JH, Kapil V, et al. The Lancet Commission on rethinking coronary artery disease: moving from ischaemia to atheroma. Lancet. 2025;405:1264-312.
6. Gupta R, Gaur K. Epidemiology of coronary heart disease in India and risk factors: recent evidence. In: Tyagi S (Ed). CSI Cardiology Update 2024. New Delhi. Jaypee Brothers Medical Publishers & Cardiological Society of India; 2024. pp. 8-18.
7. Gupta R, Gaur K. Epidemiology of ischemic heart disease and diabetes in India: An overview of the twin epidemic. Curr Diabetes Rev. 2020; e100620186664.
8. Kalra A, Jose AP, Prabhakaran P, et al. The burgeoning cardiovascular disease epidemic in Indians: perspectives on contextual factors and potential solutions. Lancet Reg Health SE Asia. 2023;12:100156.
9. Ridker PM, Libby P, Buring JE. Risk markers and the primary prevention of cardiovascular disease. In: Zipes D, Libby P, Bonow RO (Eds). Braunwald's Heart Disease: A Textbook of Cardiovascular Medicine, 11th edition. New York: Elsevier; 2019. pp. 876-909.
10. Berenson GS, Srinivasan SR, Bao W, et al. Association between multiple cardiovascular risk factors and atherosclerosis in children and young adults. N Eng J Med. 1998;338:1650-6.
11. McGill HC, McMahan A, Zieske AWS, et al. Associations of coronary heart disease risk factors with the intermediate lesion of atherosclerosis in youth. Arterioscler Thromb Vasc Biol. 2000;20:1998-2007.
12. Strong JP, Malcom GT, McMahan A, et al. Prevalence and extent of atherosclerosis in adolescents and young adults. JAMA. 1999;281:727-35.

13. Ross R. Atherosclerosis - an inflammatory disease. N Engl J Med. 1999;340:115-26.
14. Libby P. The changing landscape of atherosclerosis. Nature. 2021;592:524-33.
15. Libby P. The changing nature of atherosclerosis: what we thought we knew, what we think we know, and what we have to learn. Eur Heart J. 2021;47:4781-82.
16. Gupta R. Genetics-based risk scores for prediction of premature coronary artery disease. Indian Heart J. 2023;75:327-34.
17. Gupta R, Mohan I, Narula J. Trends in coronary heart epidemiology in India. Ann Glob Health. 2016;82:307-15.
18. Gupta R, Gupta VP. Lessons for prevention from a coronary heart disease epidemiology study in western India. Curr Sci. 1998;74:1074-7.
19. Joshi P, Islam S, Pais P, et al. Risk factors for early myocardial infarction in South Asians compared with individuals in other countries. JAMA. 2007; 297:286-94.
20. Yusuf S, Joseph P, Rangarajan S, et al. Modifiable risk factors, cardiovascular disease, and mortality in 155,722 individuals from 21 high-income, middle-income, and low-income countries (PURE): a prospective cohort study. Lancet. 2020; 395:795-808.
21. Joseph P, Kutty VR, Mohan V, et al. Cardiovascular diseases, mortality and their associations with modifiable risk factors in a multinational South Asia cohort: A PURE Substudy. Eur Heart J. 2022; 43:2831-40.
22. Lloyd-Jones DM, Albert MA, Elkind M. The American Heart Association's focus on primordial prevention. Circulation. 2021;144:e233-235.
23. Perry CL, Sellers DE, Cook K, et al. The child and adolescent trial for cardiovascular health (CATCH): intervention, implementation, and feasibility for elementary schools in the United States. Health Edu Behav. 1997;24:716-35.
24. Arnett DK, Blumenthal RS, Albert MA, et al. 2019 ACC/AHA guideline on the primary prevention of cardiovascular disease: Executive summary. J Am Coll Cardiol. 2019;74:1376-414.
25. Visseren GLJ, Mach F, Smulders YM, et al. 2021 ESC Guidelines on cardiovascular disease prevention in clinical practice: developed by the Task Force for cardiovascular disease prevention in clinical practice with representatives of the European Society of Cardiology and 12 medical societies with the special contribution of the European Association of Preventive Cardiology (EAPC). Eur Heart J. 2021;42:3227-337.
26. WHO. Prevention in childhood and youth of adult cardiovascular diseases: time for action. Report of a WHO Expert Committee. WHO Tech Rep Series. 1990;792:1-105.
27. Chow CK, Meng Q. Polypills for primary prevention of cardiovascular disease. Nature Rev Cardiol. 2019;16:602-11.
28. Brady TM, Altemose K, Urbina EM. Impact of the 2017 American Academy of Pediatrics' clinical practice guideline on the identification and risk stratification of youth at increased cardiovascular risk. Hypertension. 2021;77:1815-24.
29. Schipper HS, de Ferranti S. Atherosclerotic cardiovascular risk as an emerging priority in pediatrics. Pediatrics. 2022;150:e2022057956.
30. Stock J. New EAS consensus statement on FH: improving the care of FH patients. Atherosclerosis. 2103;231:69-71.
31. De Feranti SD, Daniels SR, Gillman M, et al. NHLBI integrated guidelines on cardiovascular disease risk reduction: can we clarify the controversy about cholesterol screening and treatment in childhood? Clin Chem. 2012;58:1626-30.
32. Urbina EM, Williams RV, Alpert BS, et al. Noninvasive assessment of subclinical atherosclerosis in children and adolescents: recommendations for standard assessment for clinical research: a scientific statement from the American Heart Association. Hypertension. 2009;54:919-50.
33. Sawhney JPS, Madan K. Familial hypercholesterolemia. Indian Heart J. 2024;76(Suppl 1): S108-112.
34. Marmot M. Social determinants of health inequalities. Lancet. 2005;1099-104.
35. Gupta R. Primary prevention of coronary heart disease: Public health perspective. In: Heart Disease Prevention: Essays on Preventive Cardiology in India. Jaipur, Jaipur Heart Watch Foundation; 2025. pp. 1-40.
36. Zheng WC, Chan W, Dart A, et al. Novel therapeutic targets and emerging treatments for atherosclerotic cardiovascular disease. Eur Heart J Cardiovasc Pharmacother. 2024; 10:53067.

37. Beznosov E, Chernyi N, Saruhanyan M, et al. Gene therapy approaches for atherosclerosis focusing on targeting lipid metabolism and inflammation. Int J Mol Sci. 2025;26:6950.
38. Bonowicz K, Jerka D, Peirska K, et al. CRISPR-Cas9 in cardiovascular medicine: unlocking new potential for treatment. Cells. 2025;14:e131.
39. Mitsis A, Khattab E, Kyriakou M, et al. Genomic and precision medicine approaches in atherosclerotic cardiovascular disease: from risk prediction to therapy—a review. Biomedicines. 2025;13:1723.
40. Gu B, Li M, Li D, et al. CRISOR-Cas9 targeting PCSK9: a promising therapeutic approach for atherosclerosis. J Cardiovasc Transl Res. 2025;18:424-41.
41. Karatasakis A, Danek BA, Karacsonyi J, et al. Effect of PCSK9 inhibitors on clinical outcomes in patients with hypercholesterolemia: a meta-analysis of 35 randomised controlled trials. J Am Heart Assoc. 2017;6:e006910.
42. Ridker PM, Everett BM, Thuren T, et al. Anti-inflammatory therapy with canakinumab for atherosclerotic disease. N Engl J Med. 2017;377:1119-31.
43. Tucker B, Goonetilleke N, Patel S, et al. Colchicine in atherosclerotic cardiovascular disease: a review. Heart. 2024;110:618-25.
44. World Health Organization. The Global Health Observatory. [online] Available from https://www.who.int/data/gho [Last accessed November, 2025].
45. World Health Organization. (2020). HEARTS: Technical package for cardiovascular disease management in primary health care: Risk-based CVD management. [online] Available from https://www.who.int/publications/i/item/9789240001367 [Last accessed November, 2025].
46. ARIC Investigators. The Atherosclerosis Risk in Community (ARIC) study: design and objectives. Am J Epidemiol. 1989;129:687-702.
47. Olson JL, Bild DE, Kronmal RA, et al. Legacy of MESA. Global Heart. 2016;11:269-74.
48. Teo KK, Chow CK, Vaz M, et al. The Prospective Urban Rural Epidemiology (PURE) study: Examining the impact of societal influences on chronic non-communicable diseases in low, middle and high-income countries. Am Heart J. 2009;158:1-7.
49. GBD 2023 Cardiovascular Disease Collaborators. Global, regional and national burden of cardiovascular diseases and risk factors in 204 countries and territories, 1990-2023. J Am Coll Cardiol. 2025;S0735-1097(25)07428-5.
50. Global Burden of Disease Study 2019 Viewpoint Collaborators. Five insights from the Global Burden of Disease Study 2019. Lancet. 2020;396: 1135-59.
51. Gupta R, Yusuf S. Challenges in management and prevention of ischemic heart disease in low socioeconomic status people in LLMICs. BMC Med. 2019;17:e209.
52. Victor RG, Lynch K, Li N, et al. A cluster randomised trial of blood pressure reduction in black barbershops. N Engl J Med. 2018;378:1291-301.
53. Olsen MH, Angell SY, Asma S, et al. A call to action and a life-course strategy to address the global burden of raised blood pressure on current and future generations: the Lancet Commission on hypertension. Lancet. 2016;388:2665-712.
54. Tsolekile LP, Abrahams-Gessel S, Puoane T. Healthcare professional shortage and task shifting to prevent cardiovascular disease: implications for low- and middle-income countries. Curr Cardiol Rep. 2015;17:e115.
55. Dandona L, Katoch VM, Dandona R. Research to achieve health care for all in India. Lancet. 2011;377:1055-7.
56. Engelgou MM, Sampson UK, Rabadan-Diehl C, et al. Tackling NCD in LMIC: achievements and lessons learned from the NHLBI-United Health global health centers of excellence program. Global Heart. 2016;11:5-15.
57. Banatvala N, Akselrod S, Bovet P, et al. (2023). The WHO Global action plan for the prevention and control of NCDs 2013-2030. [online] Available from https://www.taylorfrancis.com/chapters/oa-edit/10.4324/9781003306689-36/global-action-plan-prevention-control-ncds-2013%E2%80%932030-nick-banatvala-svetlana-akselrod-pascal-bovet-shanthi-mendis.[Last accessed November, 2025].
58. Alleyne G, CollpSeck AM, Frieden TR, et al. Fourth time a charm? How to make the UN high-level meeting on noncommunicable diseases effective. JAMA. 2025;333:1485-31.

CHAPTER 4

Are SGLT2 Inhibitors New Wonder Drugs? Effects Beyond Their Task

Mohd Akram, Suman Bhandari

INTRODUCTION

Sodium–glucose cotransporter 2 inhibitors (SGLT2i) offer health benefits that extend beyond lowering blood glucose levels. A variety of proposed cellular and physiological mechanisms may explain these additional effects. Clinical trials involving individuals with diabetes mellitus have demonstrated a decrease in cardiovascular (CV) mortality.[1] Further ongoing research is investigating whether these CV advantages also apply to individuals without diabetes but who possess heightened CV risk.[2]

Sodium–glucose cotransporter 2 inhibitors have become integral to the treatment of both heart failure (HF)[3] and kidney disease,[4] irrespective of a patient's diabetic status. Current and future clinical trials are likely to broaden the range of patients who may gain from SGLT2i therapy and to provide insights into their optimal use, including among those suffering from kidney failure.

MECHANISMS OF ACTION OF SODIUM–GLUCOSE COTRANSPORTER 2 INHIBITORS

They act by targeting the SGLT2 protein, primarily expressed on the luminal surface of epithelial cells within the proximal convoluted tubules of the kidney. This protein is also present, to a lesser extent, in organs such as the brain, liver, thyroid gland, and skeletal muscle.[5] Under normal physiological conditions, SGLT2 is responsible for reabsorbing approximately 90–97% of the glucose filtered by the glomerulus. This reabsorption occurs through a sodium-dependent mechanism, where each glucose molecule is cotransported with a Na ion. The process is driven by the Na^+ gradient sustained by the energy-consuming Na^+/K^+ ATPase pump located on the basolateral membrane of epithelial cells.[6] Additional glucose uptake is mediated by the high-affinity transporter SGLT1, which is situated further along the proximal tubule. SGLT1 is also present in several other organs, including the small intestine and the heart.[7]

GLYCOSURIC EFFECTS

Sodium–glucose cotransporter 2 inhibition in the kidneys promotes urinary glucose and sodium loss, lowering blood glucose levels.[8] In people with diabetes, this leads to a reduction in HbA1c by 0.6–0.9% (7–10 mmol/mol), though the effect diminishes with declining kidney function and is minimal at estimated glomerular filtration rate (eGFR) <30 mL/min/1.73 m^2.[9] These modest glycemic effects alone do not fully explain the broad clinical benefits observed, prompting deeper investigation into underlying mechanisms. SGLT2i can boost urinary glucose excretion by up to 50%,[10] lowering glucose independently of insulin. Increased SGLT1 expression may also reduce hypoglycemia risk.[7] In diabetic rat models, SGLT2 inhibition reduces advanced glycation end-products (AGEs),[11] thereby limiting oxidative stress and kidney damage **(Flowchart 1)**.

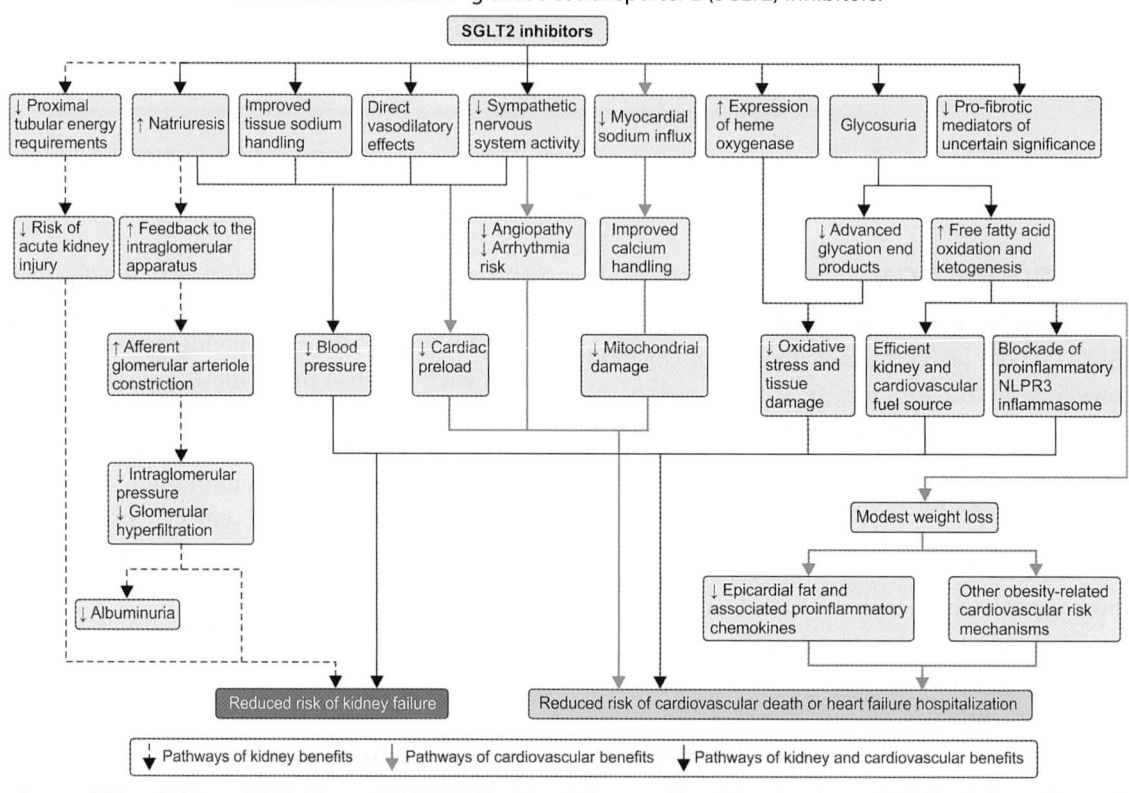

Flowchart 1: Sodium–glucose cotransporter 2 (SGLT2) inhibitors.

Source: O'Hara DV, Lam CS, McMurray JJV, Yi TW, Hocking S, Dawson J, et al. Applications of SGLT2 inhibitors beyond glycaemic control. Nat Rev Nephrol. 2024;20(8):513-29.

EFFECTS ON NATRIURESIS AND SODIUM HANDLING

Sodium–glucose cotransporter 2 inhibitors induce natriuresis by blocking SGLT2 and inhibiting Na^+/H^+ exchanger 3 (NHE3), reducing proximal sodium reabsorption.[7] This increases Na delivery to the macula densa, enhancing afferent arteriolar tone and lowering intraglomerular pressure—a reversible effect that reduces proteinuria.[7] Reduced protein uptake by tubular cells also limits tubulointerstitial injury.[12] These effects are amplified in diabetes, where SGLT2 overactivity impairs tubuloglomerular feedback.[5] In Na^+ retentive states like diabetes or HF, SGLT2i lower tissue Na, as shown by 23Na MRI[13] scan. Compared to loop diuretics, they preferentially reduce interstitial fluid with less impact on blood volume,[14] contributing to plasma volume reduction noted early in treatment.[8] Additionally, they may inhibit myocardial NHE1, lowering intracellular Na and improving calcium balance, mitochondrial health, and contractility.[15]

ANTIOXIDANT AND ANTI-INFLAMMATORY EFFECTS

Sodium–glucose cotransporter 2 inhibitors may reduce oxidative stress by upregulating hem oxygenase via ROS-NRF2 signaling, protecting against inflammation and mitochondrial damage.[16] They also lower proinflammatory cytokines through TLR4/NF-κB inhibition,[17] reduce ICAM1 and MCP1,[18] and promote ketone production, notably β-hydroxybutyrate, which suppresses the NLRP3 inflammasome.[19] Ketogenesis may also inhibit mTORC1 activity, reducing tubular and podocyte injury.[20]

ANTIFIBROTIC EFFECTS

Markers of fibrosis remained stable or improved with SGLT2i versus glimepiride in a trial,[21] possibly through anti-inflammatory or vascular endothelial growth factor (VEGFA)-mediated pathways.

ENERGY AND METABOLIC EFFICIENCY

By reducing SGLT2 and NHE3 activity, these agents lower proximal tubule energy demands and oxygen use.[18] They also shift metabolism toward ketones and fatty acids, which are more oxygen-efficient.[22]

SYMPATHETIC NERVOUS SYSTEM AND RENIN-ANGIOTENSIN-ALDOSTERONE SYSTEM MODULATION

Sodium–glucose cotransporter 2 inhibitors may blunt sympathetic activity, commonly elevated in diabetes and chronic kidney disease (CKD), by reducing oxidative stress and renal afferent signaling.[23] Their effects appear independent of renin-angiotensin-aldosterone system (RAAS) modulation.[24]

EPICARDIAL FAT AND VASCULAR EFFECTS

They reduce epicardial fat and its inflammatory secretions in T2DM and promote vasodilation by enhancing nitric oxide availability and reducing vascular resistance, contributing to improved cardiac remodeling and reduced left ventricular mass.[25]

BENEFITS OF SODIUM–GLUCOSE COTRANSPORTER 2 INHIBITORS

Originally developed in the 1990s for glucose-lowering, SGLT2i have shown unexpected benefits beyond glycemic control, especially in CV and renal outcomes.[26] The EMPA-REG OUTCOME trial showed that empagliflozin (EMPA), an SGLT2 inhibitor, significantly reduced CV deaths, all-cause mortality, HF hospitalizations, and slowed kidney disease progression in people with type 2 diabetes. These results, confirmed by further trials in diabetic and nondiabetic patients, led to expanded use of SGLT2i in managing both types of HF.[27-29]

KIDNEY PROTECTION

Sodium–glucose cotransporter 2 inhibitors slow CKD progression and reduce risks of acute kidney injury (AKI) and hyperkalemia.[30] Their role in diabetic kidney disease (DKD) was established early through reductions in albuminuria and eGFR decline. Cardiovascular outcome trials (CVOTs) such as CANVAS and DECLARE-TIMI 58 showed consistent kidney benefits, though VERTIS CV and SCORED had more limited findings due to trial design and shorter follow-up.[31] Dedicated trials like CREDENCE confirmed that canagliflozin significantly reduced risks of kidney failure and CV death in high-risk DKD patients.[29] These studies demonstrate that kidney protection is a key therapeutic benefit of SGLT2i.

CHRONIC KIDNEY DISEASE

The DAPA-CKD and EMPA-KIDNEY trials expanded evidence for the renal benefits of SGLT2i by including individuals without diabetes. Both trials included participants with lower eGFRs down to 25 mL/min/1.73 m² in DAPA-CKD and 20 mL/min/1.73 m² in EMPA-KIDNEY and expanded albuminuria criteria. EMPA-KIDNEY also included participants with eGFR 20–45 mL/min/1.73 m² without albuminuria.[32] Dapagliflozin reduced the composite kidney outcome by 44% in DAPA-CKD [hazard ratio (HR): 0.56, 95% confidence interval (CI): 0.45–0.68],[32] while empagliflozin reduced a broader outcome by 28% in EMPA-KIDNEY (HR: 0.72, 95% CI: 0.64–0.82).[33] Kidney failure incidence was also significantly reduced in both trials. The benefits for prevention of the kidney composite outcome were similar across glycemic strata. A meta-analysis including 90,409 participants (15,605 without diabetes) found a 37% reduction in kidney disease progression (HR: 0.63, 95% CI: 0.58–0.69), with no difference by diabetes status ($p = 0.31$).[34] Benefits were consistent across eGFR levels[33] and primary kidney disease.[34] However, individuals with ADPKD, kidney transplants, or on high-dose immunosuppression were excluded. Renal benefits appeared regardless of baseline albuminuria. Greater eGFR preservation was noted in those with higher albuminuria in CANVAS, CREDENCE, DAPA-CKD, and EMPA-KIDNEY. In EMPA-KIDNEY, among those with eGFR 20–45 mL/min/1.73 m² and no proteinuria (20% of cohort), empagliflozin had no significant effect on the composite outcome (HR: 1.01, 95% CI: 0.66–1.55), likely due to limited power (84 events), though eGFR slope was improved (difference 0.78 mL/min/1.73 m²).[33]

ESTIMATED GLOMERULAR FILTRATION RATE PRESERVATION

Sodium–glucose cotransporter 2 inhibitors slow eGFR decline despite an initial drop of 3–5 mL/min/1.73 m² on initiation.[35] Both DAPA-CKD and EMPA-KIDNEY showed improved eGFR slopes with treatment.[33] In DAPA-CKD, even >10% acute eGFR reductions were not linked to adverse outcomes.[36] Greater benefit in eGFR slope was seen in patients with diabetes than those without (2.26 vs. 1.29 mL/min/1.73 m²); EMPA-KIDNEY showed similar trends.[33] Also they were associated with a 23% reduced risk of AKI in major clinical trials.[34]

PREVENTION OF HYPERKALEMIA

A meta-analysis of six large trials in people with diabetes found a 16% lower risk of serious hyperkalemia with SGLT2 inhibitor use.[37] Although the average reduction in serum potassium was minimal (−0.04 mmol/L), the benefit likely stems from increased Na delivery to the distal nephron, enhancing potassium excretion via increased tubular electronegativity.[37] No significant rise in hypokalemia has been observed.

REMAINING KNOWLEDGE GAPS IN SGLT2 INHIBITOR USE FOR KIDNEY DISEASE

In the EMPA-KIDNEY trial, empagliflozin was shown to be safe down to an eGFR of 20 mL/min/1.73 m²,[33] but individuals with lower eGFR values, including those on dialysis, were excluded from this and other major trials.[34] Preclinical studies in polycystic kidney disease (PKD) have yielded mixed outcomes. For instance, the dual SGLT1/SGLT2 inhibitor phlorizin improved kidney function without affecting cyst development in a rat model, whereas dapagliflozin worsened albuminuria and cyst growth in a recessive PKD model, and canagliflozin showed no benefit in a mouse model of ADPKD.[38]

Although 2.2% of participants in EMPA-KIDNEY had T1DM, specific efficacy and safety data for this subgroup were not reported. Larger kidney outcome studies are lacking, and concerns persist regarding the potential for ketoacidosis.[39]

CARDIOPROTECTION AND ROLE IN HEART FAILURE

The EMPA-REG OUTCOME trial showed a reduced CV death by 38% (HR: 0.62), major adverse cardiovascular event (MACE) by 14% (HR: 0.86), and hospitalization for heart failure (HFH) by 35% (HR: 0.65), despite only a modest HbA1c reduction (−0.24 percentage points). These benefits were consistent across HbA1c levels and independent of baseline CV risk factor control. Other SGLT2i canagliflozin, dapagliflozin, and ertugliflozin—have also demonstrated CV benefit.[27] The DAPA-HF and EMPEROR-Reduced trials showed that SGLT2i, when added to standard therapy, effectively reduced HF hospitalizations, CV death, and improved patient symptoms in HFrEF.[40]

A combined meta-analysis of these studies, involving 2,637 events, demonstrated a 25% reduction in the composite of CV death or HFH (HR: 0.75, 95% CI: 0.68–0.84). First HF hospitalizations were reduced by nearly 31% (HR: 0.69, 95% CI: 0.62–0.78), and CV death declined by 14% (HR: 0.86, 95% CI: 0.76–0.98). These benefits were consistent across subgroups including age, sex, diabetes status, HF severity, renal function, and concurrent medications.[41] In terms of symptom improvement, SGLT2i led to greater odds of meaningful NYHA class improvement.[3]

A meta-analysis of EMPEROR-Preserved and DELIVER trials revealed a 26% reduction in hospitalization for worsening HF (HR: 0.74, 95% CI: 0.67–0.83) and a borderline reduction in CV mortality (HR: 0.88, 95% CI: 0.77–1.00) in HFpEF patients. The DELIVER trial also demonstrated benefit in patients with heart failure with improved ejection fraction (HFimpEF)—those whose left ventricular ejection fraction (LVEF) had improved to >40% prior to randomization (HR: 0.74, 95% CI: 0.56–0.97).[42] Guidelines now recommend hospitalization as a key opportunity to start SGLT2i in eligible HF patients.[3]

SODIUM–GLUCOSE COTRANSPORTER 2 INHIBITORS IN ACUTE MYOCARDIAL INFARCTION

Nikolaou et al. investigated the effects of empagliflozin (EMPA) following acute myocardial infarction (AMI) and found that oral administration of the drug modulates endothelial gene expression and protects the coronary microvasculature. EMPA treatment, initiated after reperfusion, reduced inflammation by limiting immune cell infiltration and suppressing intercellular adhesion molecule 1 (ICAM-1), matrix metalloproteinase-2 (MMP-2), and phosphorylated STAT-3 within 48 hours of reperfusion. In animal models, EMPA lessened infarct size and improved overall cardiac function. In patients with diabetes who had STEMI, post-AMI oral EMPA also enhanced endothelial glycocalyx integrity and improved flow-mediated vasodilation. These findings suggest that initiating EMPA after reperfusion may help to prevent microvascular damage and highlight the potential for further research into SGLT2i as part of AMI management strategies (Fig. 1).[13]

SODIUM–GLUCOSE COTRANSPORTER 2 INHIBITORS—ANTIARRHYTHMIC EFFECT

Clinical studies and meta-analyses indicate that SGLT2i lower the rates of atrial fibrillation (AF), atrial flutter, ventricular tachycardia (VT), and sudden cardiac death (SCD) in a wide range of patients, regardless of diabetes or HF status. While no large prospective trials have focused solely on their antiarrhythmic effects, observed benefits are attributed to mechanisms beyond glucose lowering, including the reduction of intracellular

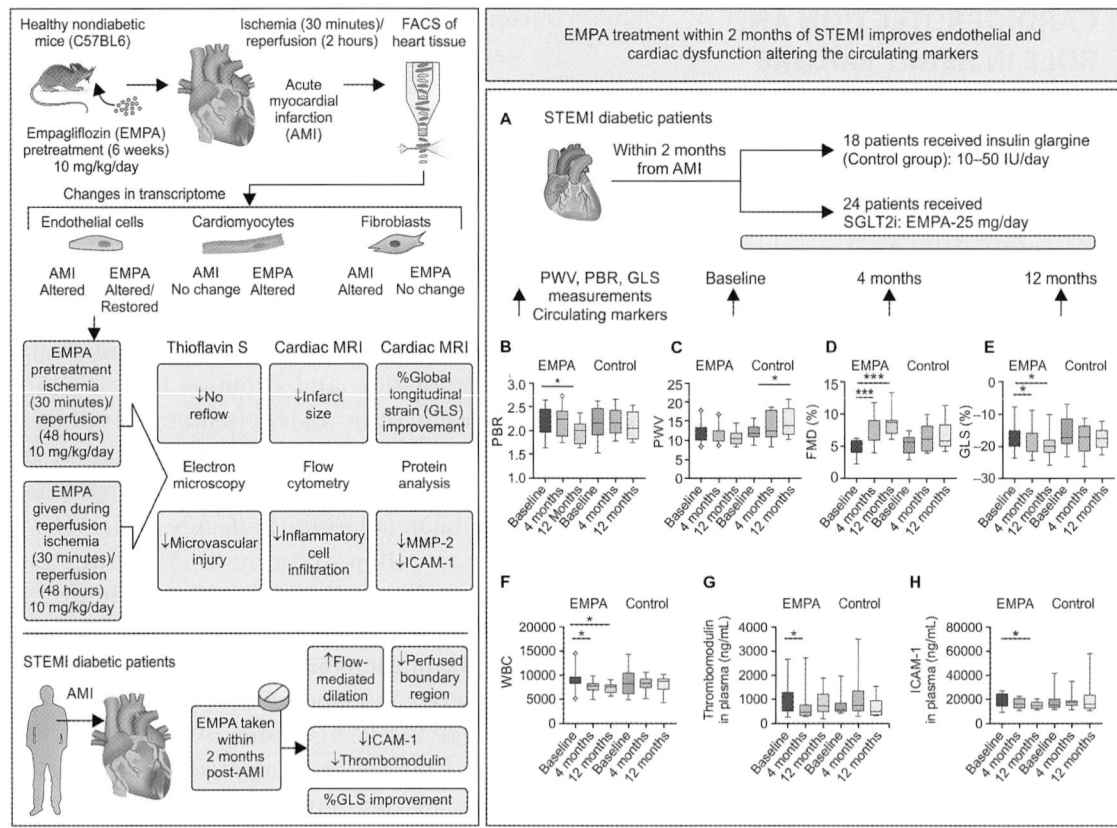

Fig. 1: SGLT2 inhibitors in AMI. (GLS: global longitudinal strain; MMP: matrix metalo protienases; PBR: perfused boundary region; PWV: pulse wave velocity; SGLT2: sodium–glucose cotransporter 2; STEMI: ST-elevation myocardial infarction; WBC: white blood cells)
Source: Nikolaou PE, Konijnenberg LSF, Kostopoulos IV, Miliotis M, Mylonas N, Georgoulis A, et al. Empagliflozin in Acute Myocardial Infarction Reduces No-Reflow and Preserves Cardiac Function by Preventing Endothelial Damage. JACC Basic Transl Sci. 2024;10(1):43-61.

Na and calcium overload (via inhibition of late Na currents and Na-hydrogen exchanger 1 in cardiomyocytes) and the induction of favorable metabolic and autophagic changes that decrease inflammation and fibrosis—key drivers of arrhythmia **(Fig. 2)**.

These combined acute and chronic cellular effects make SGLT2i compelling candidates for arrhythmia prevention and management, though further dedicated research is needed to fully validate and elucidate these actions.[44]

SODIUM–GLUCOSE COTRANSPORTER 2 INHIBITOR IN AMYLOIDOSIS[45]

Sodium–glucose cotransporter 2 inhibitor treatment in transthyretin amyloid cardiomyopathy (ATTR-CM) patients was well tolerated and associated with favorable effects on HF symptoms, renal function, and diuretic agent requirement over time. SGLT2i treatment was associated with reduced risk of HF hospitalization and CV and all-cause mortality, regardless of the ejection fraction, despite the effect size being likely overestimated.

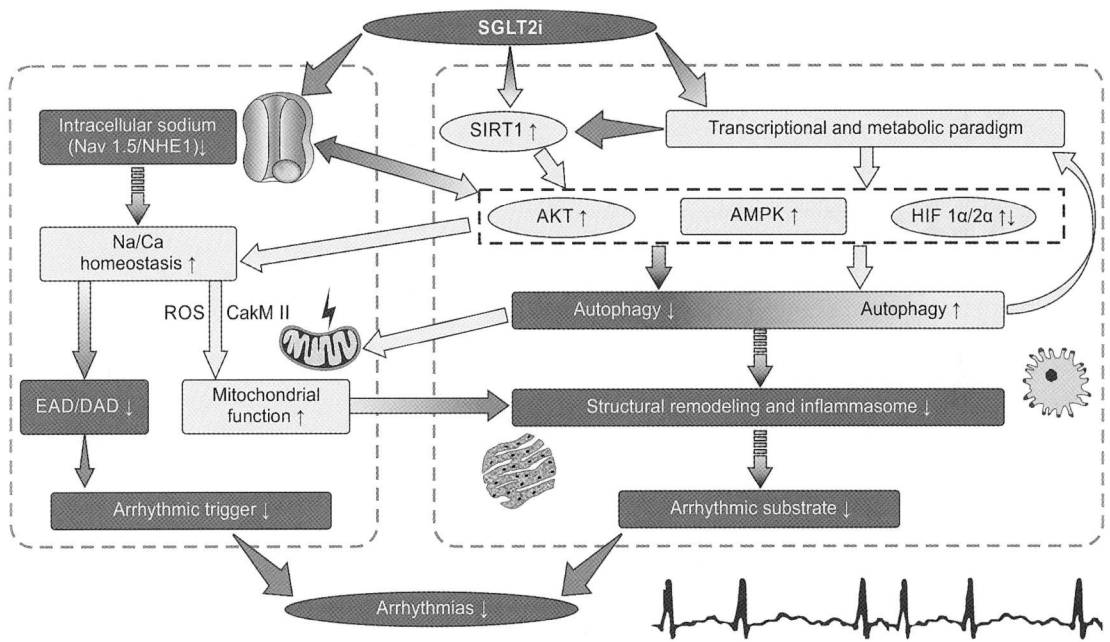

Fig. 2: Possible mechanism of sodium–glucose cotransporter 2 inhibitor (SGLT2i) therapy for arrhythmia.[44] (AKT: protien kinase B; AMPK: AMP-activated protien kinase; HIF: hypoxia inducible factor; DAD: delayed after depolarisation; EAD: early after depolarisation; NHE: sodium hydeogen exchanger; SIRT1: sirtuin 1)

In the absence of randomized trials, these data may inform clinicians regarding the use of SGLT2i in patients with ATTR-CM **(Fig. 3)**.

SODIUM–GLUCOSE COTRANSPORTER 2 INHIBITION MECHANISMS IN AORTIC STENOSIS AND FOLLOWING TRANSCATHETER AORTIC VALVE REPLACEMENT[46]

Sodium–glucose cotransporter 2 inhibitors, commonly used for diabetes, may slow aortic stenosis progression by reducing endothelial dysfunction, inflammation, fibrosis, and calcification in the valve. These drugs also lower oxidative stress and act directly on disease-affected cells in the valve. Early clinical evidence shows improved heart function and slower disease progression in patients taking SGLT2 inhibitors, but more research and clinical trials are needed to confirm their optimal use, especially in early disease stages or after valve replacement procedures. Overall, SGLT2 inhibitors are promising for aortic stenosis but further study is necessary.

ADVERSE EFFECTS OF SODIUM–GLUCOSE COTRANSPORTER 2 INHIBITORS

Sodium-glucose cotransporter 2 inhibitors are generally well tolerated, with large trials like CREDENCE, DECLARE-TIMI 58, and DAPA-CKD showing fewer serious adverse events than placebo. Importantly, they do not increase the risk of major hypoglycemia, even in nondiabetic patients.

Ketoacidosis, while rare, can occur in people with diabetes—most notably with sotagliflozin.[31] Though extremely rare, a few cases have occurred in nondiabetics.[33]

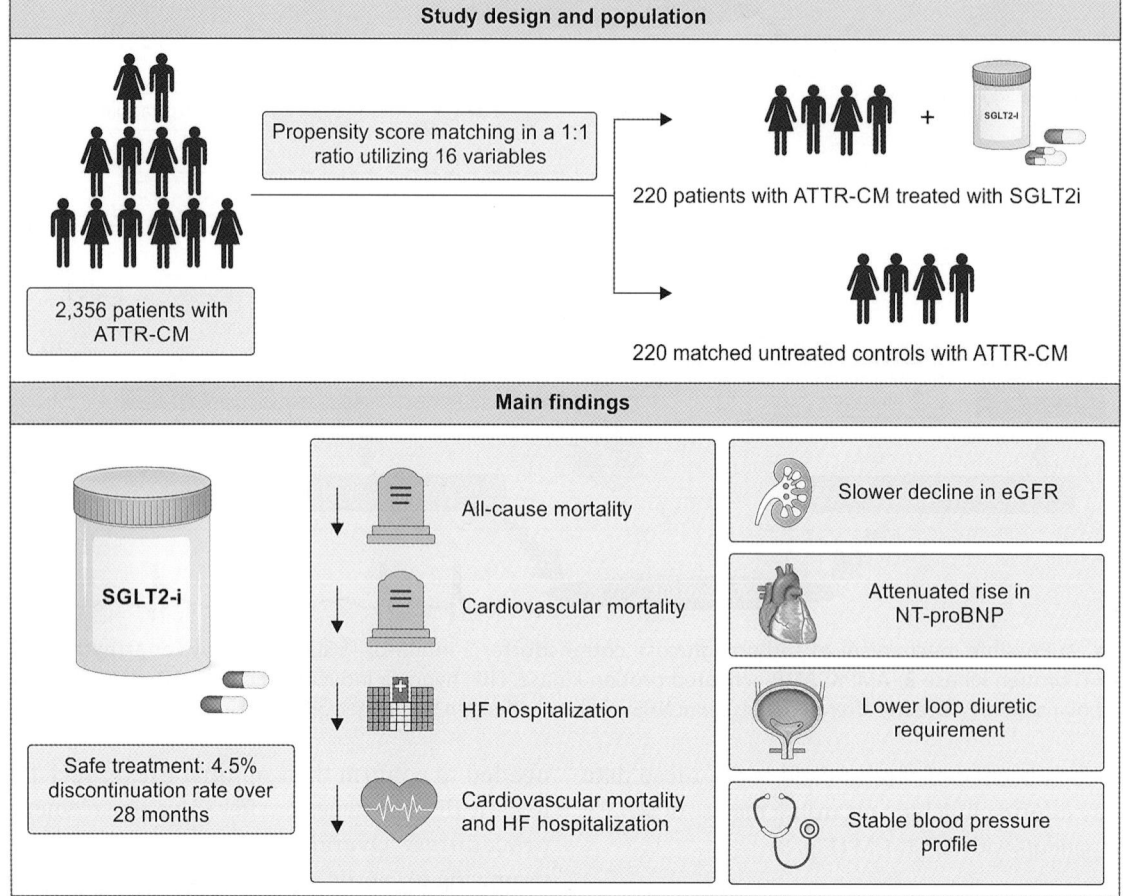

Fig. 3: Sodium–glucose cotransporter 2 inhibitors in amyloidosis. (ATTR-CM: transthyretin amyloid cardiomyopathy; HF: heart failure; SGLT2i: sodium glucose like transporter 2 inhibitors)
Source: Porcari A, Cappelli F, Nitsche C, Tomasoni D, Sinigiani G, Longhi S, et al. SGLT2 Inhibitor Therapy in Patients With Transthyretin Amyloid Cardiomyopathy. J Am Coll Cardiol. 2024;83(24):2411-22.

Hypotension and volume depletion were not significantly increased in meta-analyses or trials involving HF and CKD.[33]

Genital infections occur more frequently in diabetics (2.3–6.4%), especially in women and those with higher BMI.[28] The risk is lower and inconsistently reported in nondiabetics.[33]

Amputation and fracture risks remain debated (CANVAS reported higher amputation and fracture rates with canagliflozin).

CONCLUSION

Initially developed to lower blood glucose in type 2 diabetes, SGLT2i have rapidly evolved into multifunctional agents with significant CV, renal, and metabolic benefits. Their mechanisms of action extend well beyond glycemic control, involving improvements in natriuresis, inflammation, oxidative stress, and vascular health. SGLT2i are no longer just antidiabetic drugs—they are becoming essential tools in modern therapeutic strategy, earning their place among the most promising pharmacologic advances in recent decades.

REFERENCES

1. McGuire DK, Shih WJ, Cosentino F, et al. Association of SGLT2 Inhibitors With Cardiovascular and Kidney Outcomes in Patients With Type 2 Diabetes: A Meta-analysis. JAMA Cardiol. 2021;6(2):148-58.
2. ClinicalTrials.gov. (2023). EMPA-KIDNEY: The Study of Heart and Kidney Protection With Empagliflozin. [online] Available from https://clinicaltrials.gov/study/NCT03594110 [Last accessed November, 2025].
3. McDonagh TA, Metra M, Adamo M, et al. 2021 ESC Guidelines for the diagnosis and treatment of acute and chronic heart failure. Eur Heart J. 2021;42(36):3599-726. Erratum in: Eur Heart J. 2021;42(48):4901.
4. UK Kidney Association. (2026). UK Kidney Association clinical practice guideline: sodium-glucose co-transporter-2 (SGLT-2) inhibition in adults with kidney disease [online] Available from https://www.ukkidney.org/sites/renal.org/files/UKKA%20guideline_SGLT2i%20in%20adults%20with%20kidney%20disease%20v1%2020.10.21.pdf [Last accessed November, 2025].
5. Cowie MR, Fisher M. SGLT2 inhibitors: mechanisms of cardiovascular benefit beyond glycaemic control. Nat Rev Cardiol. 2020;17(12):761-72.
6. Youssef ME, Yahya G, Popoviciu MS, et al. Unlocking the Full Potential of SGLT2 Inhibitors: Expanding Applications beyond Glycemic Control. Int J Mol Sci. 2023;24(7):6039.
7. Hou YC, Zheng CM, Yen TH, et al. Molecular Mechanisms of SGLT2 Inhibitor on Cardiorenal Protection. Int J Mol Sci. 2020;21(21):7833.
8. Heerspink HJ, Perkins BA, Fitchett DH, et al. Sodium Glucose Cotransporter 2 Inhibitors in the Treatment of Diabetes Mellitus: Cardiovascular and Kidney Effects, Potential Mechanisms, and Clinical Applications. Circulation. 2016;134(10):752-72.
9. Cherney DZ, Kanbay M, Lovshin JA. Renal physiology of glucose handling and therapeutic implications. Nephrol Dial Transplant. 2020;35(Suppl 1):i3-i12.
10. DeFronzo RA, Hompesch M, Kasichayanula S, et al. Characterization of renal glucose reabsorption in response to dapagliflozin in healthy subjects and subjects with type 2 diabetes. Diabetes Care. 2013;36(10):3169-76.
11. Ojima A, Matsui T, Nishino Y, et al. Empagliflozin, an Inhibitor of Sodium-Glucose Cotransporter 2 Exerts Anti-Inflammatory and Antifibrotic Effects on Experimental Diabetic Nephropathy Partly by Suppressing AGEs-Receptor Axis. Horm Metab Res. 2015;47(9):686-92.
12. Cravedi P, Remuzzi G. Pathophysiology of proteinuria and its value as an outcome measure in chronic kidney disease. Br J Clin Pharmacol. 2013;76(4):516-23.
13. Karg MV, Bosch A, Kannenkeril D, et al. SGLT-2-inhibition with dapagliflozin reduces tissue sodium content: a randomised controlled trial. Cardiovasc Diabetol. 2018;17(1):5.
14. Hallow KM, Helmlinger G, Greasley PJ, et al. Why do SGLT2 inhibitors reduce heart failure hospitalization? A differential volume regulation hypothesis. Diabetes Obes Metab. 2018;20(3):479-87.
15. Uthman L, Baartscheer A, Bleijlevens B, et al. Class effects of SGLT2 inhibitors in mouse cardiomyocytes and hearts: inhibition of Na+/H+ exchanger, lowering of cytosolic Na+ and vasodilation. Diabetologia. 2018;61(3):722-6.
16. Peyton KJ, Behnammanesh G, Durante GL, et al. Canagliflozin Inhibits Human Endothelial Cell Inflammation through the Induction of Heme Oxygenase-1. Int J Mol Sci. 2022;23(15):8777.
17. Oraby MA, El-Yamany MF, Safar MM, et al. Dapagliflozin attenuates early markers of diabetic nephropathy in fructose-streptozotocin-induced diabetes in rats. Biomed Pharmacother. 2019;109:910-20.
18. Androutsakos T, Nasiri-Ansari N, Bakasis AD, et al. SGLT-2 Inhibitors in NAFLD: Expanding Their Role beyond Diabetes and Cardioprotection. Int J Mol Sci. 2022;23(6):3107.
19. Lupsa BC, Kibbey RG, Inzucchi SE. Ketones: the double-edged sword of SGLT2 inhibitors? Diabetologia. 2023;66:23-32.

20. Heerspink HJL, Perco P, Mulder S, et al. Canagliflozin reduces inflammation and fibrosis biomarkers: a potential mechanism of action for beneficial effects of SGLT2 inhibitors in diabetic kidney disease. Diabetologia. 2019;62(7):1154-66.
21. Zhang Y, Nakano D, Guan Y, et al. A sodium-glucose cotransporter 2 inhibitor attenuates renal capillary injury and fibrosis by a vascular endothelial growth factor-dependent pathway after renal injury in mice. Kidney Int. 2018;94(3):524-35.
22. Sano M. A new class of drugs for heart failure: SGLT2 inhibitors reduce sympathetic overactivity. J Cardiol. 2018;71:471-6.
23. Sano M. Sodium glucose cotransporter (SGLT)-2 inhibitors alleviate the renal stress responsible for sympathetic activation. Ther Adv Cardiovasc Dis. 2020;14:1753944720939383.
24. Seidu S, Kunutsor SK, Topsever P, et al. Benefits and harms of sodium-glucose co-transporter-2 inhibitors (SGLT2-I) and renin-angiotensin-aldosterone system inhibitors (RAAS-I) versus SGLT2-Is alone in patients with type 2 diabetes: A systematic review and meta-analysis of randomized controlled trials. Endocrinol Diabetes Metab. 2022;5(1):e00303.
25. Herrington WG, Savarese G, Haynes R, et al. Cardiac, renal, and metabolic effects of sodium-glucose co-transporter 2 inhibitors: a position paper from the European Society of Cardiology ad-hoc task force on sodium-glucose co-transporter 2 inhibitors. Eur J Heart Fail. 2021;23(8):1260-75.
26. Cefalu WT, Kaul S, Gerstein HC, et al. Cardiovascular Outcomes Trials in Type 2 Diabetes: Where Do We Go From Here? Reflections From a Diabetes Care Editors' Expert Forum. Diabetes Care. 2018;41(1):14-31.
27. Wanner C, Inzucchi SE, Lachin JM, et al. Empagliflozin and Progression of Kidney Disease in Type 2 Diabetes. N Engl J Med. 2016;375(4):323-34.
28. Nuffield Department of Population Health Renal Studies Group; SGLT2 inhibitor Meta-Analysis Cardio-Renal Trialists' Consortium. Impact of diabetes on the effects of sodium glucose co-transporter-2 inhibitors on kidney outcomes: collaborative meta-analysis of large placebo-controlled trials. Lancet. 2022;400(10365): 1788-1801.
29. Heerspink HJL, Stefánsson BV, Correa-Rotter R, et al. Dapagliflozin in Patients with Chronic Kidney Disease. N Engl J Med. 2020;383(15):1436-46.
30. Heerspink HJL, Greene T, Tighiouart H, et al. Change in albuminuria as a surrogate endpoint for progression of kidney disease: a meta-analysis of treatment effects in randomised clinical trials. Lancet Diabetes Endocrinol. 2019;7(2):128-39.
31. Mosenzon O, Wiviott SD, Cahn A, et al. Effects of dapagliflozin on development and progression of kidney disease in patients with type 2 diabetes: an analysis from the DECLARE-TIMI 58 randomised trial. Lancet Diabetes Endocrinol. 2019;7(8):606-17. Erratum in: Lancet Diabetes Endocrinol. 2019; 7(8):e20.
32. The EMPA-KIDNEY Collaborative Group; Herrington WG, Staplin N, et al. Empagliflozin in Patients with Chronic Kidney Disease. N Engl J Med. 2023;388(2):117-27.
33. Packer M, Anker SD, Butler J, et al. Cardiovascular and Renal Outcomes with Empagliflozin in Heart Failure. N Engl J Med. 2020;383(15):1413-24.
34. Perkovic V, Jardine MJ, Neal B, et al. Canagliflozin and Renal Outcomes in Type 2 Diabetes and Nephropathy. N Engl J Med. 2019;380(24): 2295-306.
35. Kraus BJ, Weir MR, Bakris GL, et al. Characterization and implications of the initial estimated glomerular filtration rate 'dip' upon sodium-glucose cotransporter-2 inhibition with empagliflozin in the EMPA-REG OUTCOME trial. Kidney Int. 2021;99(3):750-62.
36. Jongs N, Chertow GM, Greene T, et al. Correlates and Consequences of an Acute Change in eGFR in Response to the SGLT2 Inhibitor Dapagliflozin in Patients with CKD. J Am Soc Nephrol. 2022; 33(11):2094-107.
37. Neuen BL, Oshima M, Agarwal R, et al. Sodium-Glucose Cotransporter 2 Inhibitors and Risk of Hyperkalemia in People With Type 2 Diabetes: A Meta-Analysis of Individual Participant Data From Randomized, Controlled Trials. Circulation. 2022;145(19):1460-70.
38. Afsar B, Kanbay M, Ortiz A. Sodium–glucose cotransporter inhibition in polycystic kidney disease: fact or fiction. Clin Kidney J. 2022;15(7): 1275-83.

39. Maffei P, Bettini S, Busetto L, et al. SGLT2 Inhibitors in the Management of Type 1 Diabetes (T1D): An Update on Current Evidence and Recommendations. Diabetes Metab Syndr Obes. 2023;16:3579-98.
40. Anker SD, Butler J, Filippatos G, et al. Empagliflozin in heart failure with a preserved ejection fraction. N Engl J Med. 2021;385:1451-61.
41. Zannad F, Ferreira JP, Pocock SJ, et al. SGLT2 inhibitors in patients with heart failure with reduced ejection fraction: a meta-analysis of the EMPEROR-Reduced and DAPA-HF trials. Lancet. 2020;396(10254):819-29.
42. Vaduganathan M, Docherty KF, Claggett BL, et al. SGLT-2 inhibitors in patients with heart failure: a comprehensive meta-analysis of five randomised controlled trials. Lancet. 2022;400(10354):757-67. Erratum in: Lancet. 2023;401(10371):104.
43. Nikolaou PE, Konijnenberg LSF, Kostopoulos IV, et al. Empagliflozin in acute myocardial infarction reduces no-reflow and preserves cardiac function by preventing endothelial damage. Basic to Translational Science. 2025;10(1):43-61.
44. Duan HY, Barajas-Martinez H, Antzelevitch C, et al. The potential anti-arrhythmic effect of SGLT2 inhibitors. Cardiovasc Diabetol. 2024;23:252.
45. Porcari A, Cappelli F, Nitsche C, et al. SGLT2 inhibitor therapy in patients with transthyretin amyloid cardiomyopathy. J Am Coll Cardiol. 2024;83(24):2411-22.
46. Trimaille A, Hmadeh S, Marchandot B, et al. SGLT2 Inhibition Mechanisms in Aortic Stenosis and Following Transcatheter Aortic Valve Replacement. JACC Cardiovasc Interv. 2025; 18(14):1831.

Atherosclerosis: Newer Concepts

Akhilesh Kumar, Suman Bhandari

INTRODUCTION

Cardiovascular diseases (CVDs) account for approximately one-third of all deaths globally.[1,2] Despite significant advances in preventive cardiology, interventional therapies, and surgical techniques, the burden of atherosclerotic disease, aortic pathology, and peripheral artery disease (PAD) remains high. Current standard therapies—statins, antiplatelets, β-blockers, antihypertensives, and surgical interventions—have dramatically improved outcomes but fail to address residual risk.[3,4]

Several factors underlie this residual burden. First, atherosclerosis is increasingly recognized as a chronic inflammatory disease, not merely a lipid storage disorder.[5] Second, inherited and acquired abnormalities of the aortic wall are only partially mitigated by blood pressure control, with a need for targeted therapies that modulate vascular remodeling.[6] Third, PAD continues to be underdiagnosed and undertreated, with event rates comparable to or higher than coronary disease.[7]

In this context, the search for *new therapeutic targets* has become central to contemporary cardiovascular medicine. These targets include:
- *Inflammation* [targeting interleukin-1β (IL-1β), interleukin-6 (IL-6), and NLRP3 inflammasome]
- *Residual lipoprotein risk* [lipoprotein(a) and remnant cholesterol]
- *Thrombosis beyond platelets* (dual-pathway inhibition with factor Xa blockade)
- *Vascular extracellular matrix remodeling* [matrix metalloproteinases (MMPs) and TGF-β signaling].

This review summarizes key advances across three interrelated entities—atherosclerosis, aortic dissection, and PAD—with emphasis on clinical trial data, mechanistic rationale, and practical implications for the clinician.

ATHEROSCLEROSIS: PATHOBIOLOGY RECAP

Atherosclerosis arises from a complex interplay between lipid accumulation, endothelial dysfunction, immune cell infiltration, and maladaptive remodeling.[8] Modified lipoproteins, low-density lipoprotein (LDL) and Lp(a), trigger chronic inflammation, leading to plaque formation and eventual clinical sequelae including myocardial infarction and stroke.[9]

Steps in Plaque Formation

Consequent to the initial lesion to the endothelium, both innate and adaptive immune responses are triggered (**Fig. 1**, Initial lesion). Circulating monocytes infiltrate subendothelial regions upon binding to adhesion molecules upregulated on the endothelial cells, leading to the accumulation of intimal macrophages.[10] Furthermore, disturbed endothelial homeostasis facilitates the transportation and entrapment of LDL into the subendothelial space, where it undergoes oxidation and is subsequently taken up by macrophages, leading to the development of foam cells (**Fig. 1**, Initial lesion). Additionally,

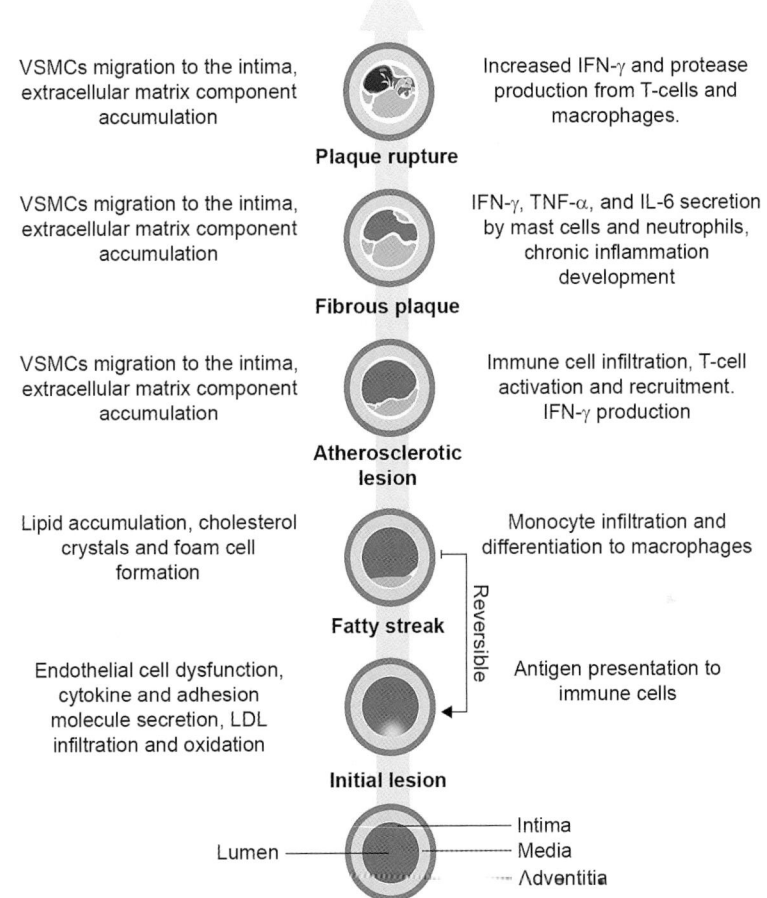

Fig. 1: Atherosclerosis is a metabolic and chronic inflammatory disease. Damage to endothelial cells results in the release of adhesion molecules and the accumulation of intimal macrophages. The oxidation of LDL and the subsequent formation of foam cells intensify inflammation and the development of plaques. Plaque advancement occurs through lipid accumulation and production of extracellular matrix components, resulting in arterial wall thickening and the formation of fibrous caps. Concurrently, chronic inflammation ensues, as immune cells are recruited to the plaque site, secreting elevated levels of inflammatory mediators. Finally, plaque rupture leads to clinical complications. (IFN-γ: interferon-γ; IL-6: interleukin-6; LDL: low-density lipoprotein; TNF-α: tumor necrosis factor-α; VSMCs: vascular smooth muscle cells)

foam cells derived from vascular smooth muscle cells (VSMCs) exacerbate the vascular inflammatory response.[11]

The accumulation of necrotic foam cells, cholesterol crystals, and cellular debris forms the lipid core of the atherosclerotic plaque. The consequent upregulation of multiple chemokines and cytokines stimulates VSMCs to undergo proliferation and migration toward the intima, resulting in the synthesis of extracellular matrix components such as collagen and elastin.[12] This process contributes to the formation of the fibrous cap and thickening of the arterial wall.

Subsequently, the plaques expand as fibrous tissues proliferate, thereby restricting blood flow. In some cases, the fibrous cap thins because there is a decrease in the synthesis of extracellular matrix macromolecules, while in other cases, plaques may progress to accumulate a higher proportion of matrix and a lower proportion of lipid over time.[13] Both types of plaques eventually culminate in thrombosis, either through plaque rupture or superficial erosion, consequently leading to ST-elevated myocardial infarction (STEMI) or non-ST-elevated myocardial infarction (NSTEMI).[14]

Plaque formation and vulnerability are not solely propelled by lipids but also by inflammation. Changes in the composition of numerous immune cells, including macrophages, dendritic cells, T cells, B cells, mast cells, and neutrophils, as well as the modified release of cytokines, chemokines, and other bioactive molecules, disrupt the balance between inflammation and anti-inflammation at plaque formation sites.[15] For instance, vulnerable plaques have fewer regulatory T cells and more effector T cells compared with stable plaques.[16]

Current Standard Therapies

- *Lipid lowering:* Statins remain first-line, achieving ≈25–35% reduction in events.[17] Ezetimibe and PCSK9 inhibitors add incremental benefits.[3,4]
- *Antithrombotic therapy:* Aspirin and P2Y12 inhibitors reduce recurrent ischemic events, though bleeding risk persists.[18]
- *Lifestyle and risk factor control:* Smoking cessation, diabetes management, and hypertension control remain essential.[19]

Despite aggressive therapy, patients continue to experience residual cardiovascular events, fueling research into new mechanisms.

ATHEROSCLEROSIS NEWER CONCEPTS

The past decade has seen an integration of immunology, hematology, microbiology, and systems biology into cardiovascular science.

Today, atherosclerosis is described as a *chronic maladaptive inflammatory and immune-metabolic disease of the arterial wall* rather than a static lipid storage disorder.[12] It is a dynamic ecosystem of immune cells, vascular cells, lipoproteins, extracellular matrix, and microbiota-derived signals. Newer concepts in atherosclerosis and their mechanisms are summarized in **Table 1**.

Immunity and Inflammation: The Core Driver

The Inflammatory Hypothesis

Pathological and experimental studies consistently demonstrate that inflammation, not just lipid retention, drives lesion initiation and progression.[20] LDL particles undergo oxidative modification, acting as neoantigens that stimulate both innate and adaptive immune responses. Activated endothelial cells upregulate adhesion molecules VCAM-1 and ICAM-1, facilitating leukocyte recruitment.[21] Monocytes differentiate into macrophages that ingest modified lipids, generating foam cells. The inflammatory milieu perpetuates further leukocyte recruitment, extracellular matrix degradation, and necrotic core expansion.[10]

Clinical Validation

The *CANTOS trial* (2017) provided definitive proof-of-principle: *canakinumab*, an IL-1β inhibitor, reduced recurrent cardiovascular events by 15% independent of lipid lowering.[22] Similarly, *colchicine* in COLCOT and LoDoCo2 trials, reduced events by broadly dampening inflammatory responses, with hazard ratios of 0.69 (95% CI: 0.57–0.83) in LoDoCo2 trail and 0.77 (95% CI: 0.61–0.96) in COLCOT trial.[23,24] However, anti-inflammatory therapy is not universally effective—increased infection risk, cost, and lack of broad applicability highlight the need for precision immunomodulation.[25]

TABLE 1: Newer concepts in atherosclerosis and their mechanisms.

Concept	Key mechanism	Translational relevance
Trained immunity	Epigenetic/metabolic reprogramming of innate cells	Explains residual inflammatory risk
Clonal hematopoiesis (CHIP)	Somatic mutations in HSCs → proinflammatory myeloid clones	Genetic risk marker; potential target for inflammasome blockade
Immunometabolism	Glycolysis vs. OXPHOS balance in immune cells	Druggable pathways; links diabetes/obesity to CVD
VSMC plasticity	Dedifferentiation into foam-like, osteogenic, and fibroblast-like cells	Drivers of calcification and instability
EndoMT	Endothelial cells → mesenchymal-like cells under TGF β, shear stress	Contributes to fibrosis and restenosis
Gut microbiome	TMAO, bile acids, and SCFAs	Dietary and microbiota-targeted therapies
Lipoprotein(a)	Prothrombotic, proinflammatory, and carries oxidized phospholipids	RNA therapies in late-phase trials
Plaque ecosystem	Interacting multicellular system	Imaging-based risk stratification

(CHIP: clonal hematopoiesis of indeterminate potential; CVD: cardiovascular disease; EndoMT: endothelial-to-mesenchymal transition; HSCs: hematopoietic stem cells; OXPHOS: oxidative phosphorylation; SCFAs: short-chain fatty acids; TMAO: trimethylamine N-oxide; VSMC: vascular smooth muscle cell)

Trained Immunity—Memory in Innate Cells

Traditionally, immunologic memory was attributed only to adaptive cells T and B lymphocytes). However, it is now clear that innate immune cells—monocytes, macrophages, NK cells—can undergo epigenetic reprogramming after exposure to stimuli such as oxidized LDL, β-glucan, or microbial products.[26]

- *Mechanism:* Epigenetic marks (e.g., histone methylation/acetylation) and metabolic rewiring (shift to glycolysis and mevalonate pathway activation) prime progenitor cells in bone marrow to generate hyperresponsive monocytes/macrophages.[27]
- *Impact in atherosclerosis:* Even after clearance of the initial insult, trained cells maintain heightened inflammatory capacity, perpetuating vascular inflammation.[28]
- *Clinical relevance:* This explains residual inflammatory risk in patients who achieve LDL-C goals but continue to suffer events. It also provides rationale for therapies targeting metabolic checkpoints (e.g., mevalonate pathway and glycolysis inhibitors).[29]

Clonal Hematopoiesis of Indeterminate Potential

- *Concept:* CHIP refers to the age-related expansion of hematopoietic stem cell clones carrying mutations in genes such as *TET2, DNMT3A, ASXL1,* and *JAK2*.[30] While initially described as a precursor state to hematologic malignancy, CHIP is now firmly linked to CVD.[31]
- *Mechanism:* Mutant clones produce monocytes/macrophages with heightened inflammatory responses, increased IL-1β, IL-6, and NLRP3 inflammasome activation.[32] Animal

models of TET2 deficiency show accelerated atherosclerosis.[32]
- Clinical implications:
  - *Risk magnitude:* CHIP carriers have two-fold higher risk of coronary heart disease and all-cause mortality.
  - *Independence from traditional risk factors:* The association persists after adjusting for LDL-C, hypertension, smoking, etc.[33]
  - *Future directions:* Screening for CHIP may refine risk stratification, and therapies aimed at mutant clone suppression (e.g., hypomethylating agents and inflammasome inhibitors) are under exploration.[34]

Immunometabolism—Metabolic Control of Immunity

Immune cells dynamically adjust their metabolism to suit function.[35]
- *Proinflammatory macrophages (M1):* Shift to glycolysis, succinate accumulation, and ROS generation.
- *Anti-inflammatory macrophages (M2):* Rely on oxidative phosphorylation and fatty acid oxidation.

This metabolic plasticity intersects with trained immunity, diabetes, and obesity—linking systemic metabolic disorders to vascular inflammation.[36] Drugs modulating metabolism (e.g., metformin, glutamine antagonists, and statins beyond lipid lowering) may exert antiatherosclerotic effects partly via immunometabolic pathways.[37,38]

Vascular Smooth Muscle Cells Phenotypic Switching

Vascular smooth muscle cells, traditionally viewed as contractile structural cells, can adopt diverse phenotypes under stress.[39,40]
- *Foam cell-like phenotype:* Express macrophage markers and ingest lipids.[41,42]
- *Osteogenic phenotype:* Promote vascular calcification.[39,43]
- *Fibroblast-like phenotype:* Contribute to fibrous cap and matrix deposition.

This plasticity underlies plaque calcification and instability. Importantly, *lineage tracing studies* demonstrate that a substantial proportion of plaque "macrophage-like cells" originate from VSMCs, not monocytes.[44]

Endothelial-to-Mesenchymal Transition

Endothelial cells exposed to inflammatory cytokines, disturbed shear stress, or TGF-β signaling can lose endothelial markers (VE-cadherin and CD31) and gain mesenchymal markers (α-SMA and vimentin).[45,46] Endothelial-to-mesenchymal transition (EndoMT) contributes to intimal thickening, fibrosis, and neointimal hyperplasia.[47] Therapeutically, inhibiting EndoMT or stabilizing endothelial identity may limit early lesion development and restenosis after interventions.[48]

Gut Microbiome and Atherosclerosis

Trimethylamine N-oxide Pathway

Gut bacteria metabolize dietary choline, carnitine, and phosphatidylcholine into trimethylamine (TMA), converted by hepatic flavin-containing monooxygenase 3 (FMO3) into trimethylamine N-oxide (TMAO).[49,50]

Elevated TMAO promotes:[51,52]
- Enhanced platelet reactivity
- Impaired cholesterol transport and bile acid metabolism
- Endothelial dysfunction and vascular inflammation.

Other Microbial Metabolites

- *Short-chain fatty acids (SCFAs):* Generally protective, improve gut barrier integrity, and anti-inflammatory tone.[53,54]
- *Secondary bile acids:* Can signal through FXR/TGR5, influencing lipid metabolism and vascular inflammation.[54,55]

Therapeutic Approaches

Microbiome-targeted interventions (dietary modulation, pre-/probiotics, antibiotics, and enzyme inhibitors of TMA lyase) are being explored, though translation into human benefit remains preliminary.[49,50,52]

Lipoprotein(a) and Oxidized Phospholipids

Lipoprotein(a) [Lp(a)] is a genetically determined LDL-like particle with apolipoprotein(a).[56] Its atherogenicity stems from:[57,58]
- Carriage of oxidized phospholipids
- Structural homology to plasminogen, impairing fibrinolysis and promoting thrombosis
- Induction of inflammatory responses in vascular cells

Residual risk: Elevated Lp(a) explains why some patients with optimal LDL-C still develop premature coronary disease.

"Plaque Ecosystem" Model

Plaques are not homogeneous—they are *ecosystems* where immune cells, VSMCs, endothelial cells, lipids, extracellular matrix, and microcalcifications interact dynamically.[59]

The fate of a plaque (stable versus vulnerable) depends less on size/stenosis and more on ecosystem balance:
- Necrotic core versus fibrous cap integrity
- Inflammatory versus reparative macrophages
- Microcalcification versus macrocalcification
- Intraplaque angiogenesis and hemorrhage

Advanced intravascular imaging (OCT and NIRS-IVUS) and molecular PET tracers (targeting inflammation, protease activity, and microcalcification) allow in vivo characterization of these features, paving the way for biology-driven risk stratification.[60,61]

NOVEL THERAPEUTIC TARGETS

The contemporary management of atherosclerotic CVD has entered an unprecedented era of molecular precision, marked by the emergence of innovative therapeutic agents that transcend traditional lipid-lowering paradigms. While statins remain foundational therapy, achieving substantial reductions in cardiovascular events, the persistent residual risk observed in optimally treated patients has catalyzed the development of next-generation therapeutics targeting distinct pathophysiological mechanisms underlying atherosclerosis. These novel interventions represent a paradigm shift from conventional "one-size-fits-all" approaches to precision medicine strategies that address the complex interplay between lipid metabolism, chronic inflammation, immune dysregulation, and emerging pathways such as clonal hematopoiesis and microbiome modulation. The clinical pipeline features groundbreaking agents such as olpasiran and lepodisiran for lipoprotein(a) reduction, ziltivekimab for IL-6 inhibition, and evinacumab for ANGPTL3 blockade, each representing first-in-class mechanisms with the potential to address previously "untreatable" cardiovascular risk factors.

Lipoprotein Metabolism

- *PCSK9 inhibitors (monoclonal antibodies):*
  - Evolocumab and alirocumab → inhibit PCSK9, ↑LDL receptor recycling → ↓LDL-C.[62]
  - *Clinical evidence:* FOURIER[63] (HR: 0.85, 95% CI: 0.79–0.92), ODYSSEY OUTCOMES[64] (HR: 0.85, 95% CI: 0.78–0.93).
- *PCSK9 siRNA:* Inclisiran → blocks PCSK9 synthesis RNA interference → LDL-C lowering with twice-yearly dosing.[65]
- *Lp(a)-targeted agents:*
  - *Pelacarsen (antisense oligonucleotide):* Lowers Lp(a) ~80%.[66]

- *siRNA therapies (olpasiran, lepodisiran, and zerlasiran):* Durable reductions >90%.[67]
- *Outcome trials:* Ongoing [Lp(a)HORIZON and OCEAN(a)-DOSE trial] to prove cardiovascular benefit.
- ANGPTL3 inhibitors:
  - *Evinacumab* (mAb) → inhibits ANGPTL3, ↓ LDL, TG, and HDL.
  - Approved for homozygous familial hypercholesterolemia.[68]

Inflammation and Immunomodulation

- *IL-1β inhibition: Canakinumab* → neutralizes IL-1β; landmark CANTOS trial[22] showed MACE reduction independent of lipid levels.
- *IL-6 pathway blockade:*
  - *Ziltivekimab* → anti-IL-6 ligand mAb; RESCUE-2 trial[69] (hs-CRP lowering); (ZEUS trial for CV outcomes ongoing).
  - *Tocilizumab* (anti-IL-6R, approved for rheumatology) under investigation in ACS.[70]
- *NLRP3 inflammasome inhibitors: Dapansutrile (oral), MCC950 (experimental)* → directly block inflammasome activation.[71]
- *Colchicine (repurposed):* Low dose (0.5 mg daily) → broad anti-inflammatory effects; LoDoCo2 and COLCOT showed CV benefit.[23,24]

Endothelial Dysfunction and Oxidative Stress

- *eNOS enhancers/NO donors* (experimental)
- *NADPH oxidase inhibitors* (preclinical)
- *Antioxidant mimetics* (limited translation to CV endpoints so far).

Clonal Hematopoiesis of Indeterminate Potential

- *Targeting proinflammatory cytokines* (IL-1β and IL-6 blockade particularly relevant in TET2/ASXL1 mutations).
- *Future: Clone-directed therapies* under investigation (precision immunotherapy).

Metabolic and Microbiome Modulation

- *FXR agonists and bile acid sequestrants* → improve lipid/inflammatory signaling.
- *Gut microbiome-targeted therapies* (e.g., inhibitors of TMAO generation, and probiotics) are experimental but promising.

CONCLUSION

- *Established and late-stage:* PCSK9 inhibition, Lp(a)-lowering (ASO/siRNA), IL-1β, and IL-6 blockade.
- *Emerging:* NLRP3 inhibitors, NETosis modulators, CHIP-directed immunotherapies, and microbiome interventions.
- The field is *moving beyond lipid lowering* to *multi-target molecular therapy*, integrating lipid, inflammatory, immune, and thrombotic pathway. Novel therapeutic targets have been summarized in **Table 2**.

Aortic Dissection: Targeting the Vascular Wall

Pathophysiology

Acute aortic dissection results from medial degeneration, elastin fragmentation, and abnormal matrix turnover. Genetic syndromes [Marfan, Loeys–Dietz, and vascular Ehlers–Danlos syndrome (vEDS)] and hypertension are key contributors.

Current Management

- *Medical therapy:* Blood pressure and shear stress reduction with β-blockers and ARBs.
- *Surgical/endovascular repair:* Indicated for type A and complicated type B dissections.

Atherosclerosis: Newer Concepts

TABLE 2: Novel therapeutic targets.

Molecular target	Mechanism	Key drugs	Trial status
PCSK9	Prevents LDLR degradation → ↓LDL-C	Evolocumab, alirocumab, and inclisiran	Approved, large RCTs (FOURIER, ODYSSEY, and ORION)
Lipoprotein(a)	Silencing apo(a) → ↓Lp(a)	Pelacarsen, olpasiran, and lepodisiran	Phase 2–3 [OCEAN(a)-DOSE, HORIZON, ALPACA]
ANGPTL3	Inhibition of ANGPTL3 → ↓LDL and TG	Evinacumab and ANGPTL3 siRNA	Approved for HoFH; early siRNA in phase 2
IL-1β	Neutralizes IL-1β → ↓vascular inflammation	Canakinumab	Phase 3 (CANTOS, positive outcomes)
IL-6 pathway	Blocks IL-6/IL-6R signaling	Ziltivekimab and tocilizumab	Phase 2–3 (RESCUE, ZEUS ongoing)
NLRP3 inflammasome	Blocks inflammasome activation	Dapansutrile and MCC950	Phase 2 (early development)
Inflammation (broad)	Broad anti-inflammatory action	Colchicine	Approved (LoDoCo2, COLCOT)
Endothelial dysfunction/oxidative stress	Restores NO and reduces ROS	NADPH oxidase inhibitors and eNOS enhancers	Preclinical/early clinical
Clonal hematopoiesis (CHIP)	Reduces cytokine-driven inflammation from mutant clones	IL-1/IL-6 blockers (precision use)	Conceptual/early translational
Platelet activation	Inhibits platelet PAR-1 and dual pathway	Vorapaxar, novel antiplatelets	Phase 3 (vorapaxar), new agents in phase 2
Metabolism and microbiome	Targets TMAO, bile acid, and metabolic signaling	FXR agonists, TMAO inhibitors, and probiotics	Preclinical/early translational

(IL-6: interleukin-6; LDL: low-density lipoprotein; TMAO: trimethylamine N-oxide)

Novel Therapeutic Targets (Table 3)

TGF-β Pathway Modulation

- The ARB-TGF-β interaction demonstrates tissue-specific therapeutic effects:
  - *Cardiac tissue:* Reduced myocardial fibrosis and improved cardiac function.
  - *Vascular tissue:* Prevention of adverse vascular remodeling and aortic dilatation.
- *ARBs (losartan and irbesartan):* The AIMS trial[72] showed irbesartan reduced aortic root dilatation versus placebo in Marfan syndrome (difference of 0.22 mm/year, $p = 0.013$). Meta-analyses confirm ARBs reduce aortic growth rate by 50% compared to placebo. Ongoing evidence supports ARBs as standard in heritable aortopathies.

β-blockade with Vasodilating Properties

Celiprolol: The BBEST trial[73] demonstrated reduced rupture/dissection in vEDS patients. Celiprolol is recommended where available, though not globally approved.

Matrix Metalloproteinase Inhibition

Doxycycline: Early promise as an MMP inhibitor was not confirmed in randomized AAA trials. Not recommended in practice.[74]

TABLE 3: Medical strategies in aortic syndromes.

Target pathway	Agent	Evidence/trials	Clinical role
Hemodynamic load	β-blockers	Reduced mortality in dissection	First-line
TGF-β modulation	Losartan and irbesartan	Slowed aortic root growth in Marfan/LDS	Preferred in heritable aortopathy
Vascular wall strength	Celiprolol	BBEST: ↓ rupture in vEDS	For vEDS patients (where available)
MMP inhibition	Doxycycline	Failed AAA trials	Not recommended

TABLE 4: Landmark PAD trials with novel therapies.

Trial	Intervention	Population	Outcome
COMPASS (PAD subset)	Rivaroxaban 2.5 mg + ASA	Stable PAD	↓ MACE, ↓ limb events
VOYAGER-PAD	Rivaroxaban 2.5 mg + ASA	Post lower-extremity revascularization PAD	↓ acute limb ischemia, ↓ MACE
FOURIER PAD sub-study	PCSK9i (evolocumab)	PAD patients	↓ MACE, ↓ limb events
ODYSSEY OUTCOMES PAD sub-study	PCSK9i (alirocumab)	PAD + ACS	↓ MACE, limb events

(PAD: peripheral artery disease)

Peripheral Artery Disease: Expanding Horizons

Burden and Clinical Challenge

Peripheral artery disease affects >200 million people worldwide. Morbidity includes claudication, chronic limb-threatening ischemia, and high rates of cardiovascular events. Event rates often rival those of CAD.

Current Therapies

- Antiplatelet therapy (aspirin or clopidogrel)
- Statin plus ezetimibe
- Exercise therapy and smoking cessation
- Antihypertensive [angiotensin-converting enzyme (ACE) inhibitors/angiotensin receptor blockers (ARB) preferred].[75]

Novel Therapeutic Targets (Table 4)

Dual-pathway Inhibition

- *VOYAGER-PAD trial:* Rivaroxaban 2.5 mg bid + aspirin reduced acute limb ischemia and MACE after lower extremity revascularization.[76]

- *COMPASS PAD subset:* Similar benefit in stable PAD.[77]

PCSK9 Inhibitors

Peripheral artery disease subanalyses of FOURIER[78] and ODYSSEY[64] showed reduced limb events and MACE.

Inflammation and Lp(a)

Mechanistic rationale for colchicine and Lp(a) lowering in PAD; definitive trials awaited.

Regenerative Approaches

Stem-cell and angiogenic therapies under exploration but not yet established in clinical practice.

REFERENCES

1. Roth GA, Mensah GA, Johnson CO, et al. Global Burden of Cardiovascular Diseases and Risk Factors, 1990-2019: Update from the GBD 2019 Study. J Am Coll Cardiol. 2020;76(25):2982-3021.

2. Virani SS, Alonso A, Aparicio HJ, et al. Heart Disease and Stroke Statistics-2021 Update: A Report From the American Heart Association. Circulation. 2021;143(8): e254-e743.
3. Cannon CP, Blazing NA, Giugliano RP, et al. Ezetimibe Added to Statin Therapy after Acute Coronary Syndromes. N Engl J Med. 2015;372(25): 2387-97.
4. Sabatine MS, Giugliano RP, Keech AC, et al. Evolocumab and Clinical Outcomes in Patients with Cardiovascular Disease. N Engi J Med. 2017; 376(18):1713-22.
5. Libby P, Ridker PM, Hansson GK. Progress and challenges in translating the biology of atherosclerosis. Nature. 2011;473(7347):317-25.
6. Milewicz DM, Prakash SK, Ramirez F. Therapeutics Targeting Drivers of Thoracic Aortic Aneurysms and Acute Aortic Dissections: Insights from Predisposing Genes and Mouse Models. Circ Res. 2017;121(9):1055-9.
7. Fowkes FG, Rudan D, Rudan I, et al. Comparison of global estimates of prevalence and risk factors for peripheral artery disease in 2000 and 2010: a systematic review and analysis. Lancet. 2013;382(9901):1329-40.
8. Hansson GK, Hermansson A. The immune system in atherosclerosis. Nat Immunol. 2011;12(3): 204-12.
9. Nordestgaard BG, Chapman MJ, Ray K, et al. Lipoprotein(a) as a cardiovascular risk factor: current status. Eur Heart J. 2010;31(23):2844-53.
10. Moore KJ, Sheedy FJ, Fisher EA. Macrophages in atherosclerosis: a dynamic balance. Nat Rev Immunol. 2013;13(10):709-21.
11. Allahverdian S, Chehroudi AC, McManus BM, et al. Contribution of intimal smooth muscle cells to cholesterol homeostasis and inflammatory responses in atherosclerosis. Circ Res. 2014; 114(9):1400-9.
12. Libby P, Buring JE, Badimon L, et al. Atherosclerosis. Nat Rev Dis Primers. 2019;5(1):56.
13. Bentzon JF, Otsuka F, Virmani R, et al. Mechanisms of plaque formation and rupture. Circ Res. 2014; 114(12):1852-66.
14. Davies MJ. Stability and instability: two faces of coronary atherosclerosis. The Paul Dudley White Lecture 1995. Circulation. 1996;94(8):2013-20.
15. Hansson GK, Libby P. The immune response in atherosclerosis: a double-edged sword. Nat Rev Immunol. 2006;6(7):508-19.
16. Ait-Oufella H, Salomon BL, Potteaux S, et al. Natural regulatory T cells control the development of atherosclerosis in mice. Nat Med. 2006; 12(2):178-80.
17. Cholesterol Treatment Trialists' (CTT) Collaboration. Efficacy and safety of more intensive lowering of LDL cholesterol: a meta-analysis of data from 170,000 participants in 26 randomised trials. Lancet. 2010;376(9753):1670-81.
18. Antithrombotic Trialists' (ATT) Collaboration. Aspirin in the primary and secondary prevention of vascular disease: collaborative meta-analysis of individual participant data from randomised trials. Lancet. 2009;373(9678):1849-60.
19. Piepoli MF, Hoes AW, Agewall S, et al. 2016 European Guidelines on cardiovascular disease prevention in clinical practice: The Sixth Joint Task Force of the European Society of Cardiology and Other Societies on Cardiovascular Disease Prevention in Clinical Practice. Eur Heart J. 2016; 37(29):2315-81.
20. Libby P, Ridker PM, Maseri A. Inflammation and atherosclerosis. Circulation. 2002;105(9):1135-43.
21. Davies MJ, Gordon JL, Gearing AJ, et al. The expression of the adhesion molecules ICAM-1, VCAM-1, PECAM, and E-selectin in human atherosclerosis. J Pathol. 1993;171(3):223-9.
22. Ridker PM, Everett BM, Thuren T, et al. Antiinflammatory Therapy with Canakinumab for Atherosclerotic Disease. N Engl J Med. 2017; 377(12):1119-31.
23. Nidorf SM, Fiolet ATL, Mosterd A, et al. Colchicine in Patients with Chronic Coronary Disease. N Engl J Med. 2020;383(19):1838-47.
24. Tardif JC, Kouz S, Waters DD, et al. Efficacy and Safety of Low-Dose Colchicine after Myocardial Infarction. N Engl J Med. 2019;381(26):2497-505.
25. Ridker PM, MacFadyen JG, Thuren T, et al. Effect of interleukin-1β inhibition with canakinumab on incident lung cancer in patients with atherosclerosis: exploratory results from a randomised, double-blind, placebo-controlled trial. Lancet. 2017;390(10105):1833-42.
26. Netea MG, Dominguez-Andrés J, Barrero LB, et al. Defining trained immunity and its role in health and disease. Nat Rev Immunol. 2020;20(6):375-88.
27. Bekkering S, Quintin J, Joosten LA, et al. Oxidized low-density lipoprotein induces long-term

proinflammatory cytokine production and foam cell formation via epigenetic reprogramming of monocytes. Arterioscler Thromb Vasc Biol. 2014;34(8):1731-8.
28. Christ A, Günther P, Lauterbach MAR, et al. Western Diet Triggers NLRP3-Dependent Innate Immune Reprogramming. Cell. 2018;172(1-2):162-175.e14.
29. Bekkering S, Arts RJW, Novakovic B, et al. Metabolic induction of trained immunity through the mevalonate pathway. Cell. 2018;172(1-2):135-146.e9.
30. Jaiswal S, Fontanillas P, Flannick J, et al. Age-related clonal haematopoiesis associated with adverse outcomes. N Engl J Med. 2014;371(26):2488-98.
31. Jaiswal S, Natarajan P, Silver AJ, et al. Clonal Haematopoiesis and Risk of Atherosclerotic Cardiovascular Disease. N Engl J Med. 2017; 377(2): 111-21.
32. Fuster JJ, MacLauchlan S, Zuriaga MA, et al. Clonal haematopoiesis associated with TET2 deficiency accelerates atherosclerosis development in mice. Science. 2017;355(6327):842-7.
33. Dorsheimer L, Assmus B, Rasper T, et al. Association of Mutations Contributing to Clonal Hematopolesis of Indeterminate Potential With Prognosis in Chronic Ischemic Heart Failure. JAMA Cardiol. 2019;4(1):25-33.
34. Wang Y, Sano S, Yura Y, et al. CHIP promoting cardiac dysfunction and arrhythmias. Basic Res Cardiol. 2020;115(1):8.
35. O'Neill LA, Kishton RJ, Rathmell J. A guide to immunometabolism for immunologists. Nat Rev Immunol. 2016;16(9):553-65.
36. Viola A, Munari F, Sánchez-Rodriguez R, et al. The Metabolic Signature of Macrophage Responses. Front Immunol. 2019;10:1462.
37. Shirakawa K, Endo J, Kataoka M, et al. IL (Interleukin)-10-STAT3-Galectin-3 Axis Is Essential for Osteopontin-Producing Reparative Macrophage Polarization After Myocardial Infarction. Circulation. 2018;138(18):2021-35.
38. Salnikova D, Orekhova V, Grechko A, et al. Mitochondrial Dysfunction in Vascular Wall Cells and Its Role in Atherosclerosis. Int J Mol Sci. 2021;22(16):8990.
39. Zhang F, Guo X, Xia Y, et al. An update on the phenotypic switching of vascular smooth muscle cells in the pathogenesis of atherosclerosis. Cell Mol Life Sci. 2021;79(1):6.
40. Sorokin V, Vickneson K, Kofidis T, et al. Role of Vascular Smooth Muscle Cell Plasticity and Interactions in Vessel Wall Inflammation. Front Immunol. 2020;11:599415.
41. Li Y, Zhu H, Zhang Q, et al. Smooth muscle-derived macrophage-like cells contribute to multiple cell lineages in the atherosclerotic plaque. Cell Discov. 2021;7(1):111.
42. Zhao L, Zhao L, Liu D, et al. Vascular Smooth Muscle Cells: A Therapeutic Target in Atherosclerosis. Rev Cardiovasc Med. 2025;26(6):28240.
43. Grootaert MOJ, Bennett MR. Vascular smooth muscle cells in atherosclerosis: time for a re-assessment. Cardiovasc Res. 2021;117(11): 2326-39.
44. Bentzon JF, Majesky MW. Lineage tracking of origin and fate of smooth muscle cells in atherosclerosis. Cardiovasc Res. 2018;114(4):492-500.
45. Souilhol C, Harmsen MC, Evans PC, et al. Endothelial-mesenchymal transition in atherosclerosis. Cardiovasc Res. 2018;114(4): 565-77.
46. Evrard SM, Lecce L, Michelis KC, et al. Endothelial to mesenchymal transition is common in atherosclerotic lesions and is associated with plaque instability. Nat Commun. 2016;7:11853. Erratum in: Nat Commun. 2017;8:14710.
47. Huang Q, Gan Y, Yu Z, et al. Endothelial to Mesenchymal Transition: An Insight in Atherosclerosis. Front Cardiovasc Med. 2021;8: 734550.
48. Chen PY, Schwartz MA, Simons M. Endothelial-to-Mesenchymal Transition, Vascular Inflammation, and Atherosclerosis. Front Cardiovasc Med. 2020;7:53.
49. Zhu Y, Li Q, Jiang H. Gut microbiota in atherosclerosis: focus on trimethylamine N-oxide. APMIS. 2020;128(5):353-66.
50. Oktaviono YH, Dyah Lamara A, Saputra PBT, et al. The roles of trimethylamine-N-oxide in atherosclerosis and its potential therapeutic aspect: A literature review. Biomol Biomed. 2023; 23(6):936-48.
51. Nam HS. Gut Microbiota and Ischemic Stroke: The Role of Trimethylamine N-Oxide. J Stroke. 2019;21(2):151-9.

52. Wang B, Qiu J, Lian J, et al. Gut Metabolite Trimethylamine-N-Oxide in Atherosclerosis: From Mechanism to Therapy. Front Cardiovasc Med. 2021;8:723886.
53. Callender C, Attaye I, Nieuwdorp M. The Interaction between the Gut Microbiome and Bile Acids in Cardiometabolic Diseases. Metabolites. 2022;12(1):65.
54. Zhang Z, Lv T, Wang X, et al. Role of the microbiota-gut-heart axis between bile acids and cardiovascular disease. Biomed Pharmacother. 2024;174:116567.
55. Fogelson KA, Dorrestein PC, Zarrinpar A, et al. The Gut Microbial Bile Acid Modulation and Its Relevance to Digestive Health and Diseases. Gastroenterology. 2023;164(7):1069-85. Erratum in: Gastroenterology. 2024;166(1):228.
56. Rehberger Likozar A, Zavrtanik M, Šebeštjen M. Lipoprotein(a) in atherosclerosis: from pathophysiology to clinical relevance and treatment options. Ann Med. 2020;52(5):162-77.
57. Gilliland TC, Liu Y, Mohebi R, et al. Lipoprotein(a), Oxidized Phospholipids, and Coronary Artery Disease Severity and Outcomes. J Am Coll Cardiol. 2023;81(18):1780-92.
58. Mohammadnia N, van Broekhoven A, Bax WA, et al. Interleukin-6 modifies Lipoprotein(a) and oxidized phospholipids associated cardiovascular disease risk in a secondary prevention cohort. Atherosclerosis. 2025;405:119211.
59. Eligini S, Gianazza E, Mallia A, et al. Macrophage Phenotyping in Atherosclerosis by Proteomics. Int J Mol Sci. 2023;24(3):2613.
60. Hammad B, Evans NR, Rudd JHF, et al. Molecular imaging of atherosclerosis with integrated PET imaging. J Nucl Cardiol. 2017;24(3):938-43.
61. Grandjean CE, Pedersen SF, Christensen C, et al. Imaging of atherosclerosis with [64Cu]Cu-DOTA-TATE in a translational head-to-head comparison study with [18F]FDG, and Na[18F]F in rabbits. Sci Rep. 2023;13(1):9249.
62. Ma H, Ma W, Liu Y, et al. Effects of Alirocumab and Evolocumab on Cardiovascular Mortality and LDL-C: Stratified According to the Baseline LDL-C Levels. Rev Cardiovasc Med. 2025;26(4):26980.
63. Kang YM, Giugliano RP, Ran X, et al. Cardiovascular Outcomes and Efficacy of the PCSK9 Inhibitor Evolocumab in Individuals With Type 1 Diabetes: Insights From the FOURIER Trial. Diabetes Care. 2025;48(9):1512-6.
64. Schwartz GG, Gabriel Steg P, Bhatt DL, et al. Clinical Efficacy and Safety of Alirocumab After Acute Coronary Syndrome According to Achieved Level of Low-Density Lipoprotein Cholesterol: A Propensity Score-Matched Analysis of the ODYSSEY OUTCOMES Trial. Circulation. 2021;143(11):1109-22.
65. Di Giacomo-Barbagallo F, Andreychuk N, Scicali R, et al. Inclisiran, Reasons for a Novel Agent in a Crowded Therapeutic Field. Curr Atheroscler Rep. 2025;27(1):25.
66. Bhatia HS, Bajaj A, Goonewardena SN, et al. Pelacarsen: Mechanism of action and Lp(a)-lowering effect. J Clin Lipidol. 2025:S1933-2874(25)00322-8.
67. Kanbay M, Ozbek L, Guldan M, et al. siRNA-based therapeutics for lipoprotein (a) lowering: A path toward precision cardiovascular medicine. Eur J Clin Invest. 2025;55(9):e70079.
68. Sosnowska B, Adach W, Surma S, et al. Evinacumab, an ANGPTL3 Inhibitor, in the Treatment of Dyslipidemia. J Clin Med. 2022;12(1):168.
69. Wada Y, Jensen C, Meyer ASP, et al. Efficacy and safety of interleukin-6 inhibition with ziltivekimab in patients at high risk of atherosclerotic events in Japan (RESCUE-2): A randomized, double-blind, placebo-controlled, phase 2 trial. J Cardiol. 2023;82(4):279-85.
70. d'Aiello A, Filomia S, Brecciaroli M, et al. Targeting Inflammatory Pathways in Atherosclerosis: Exploring New Opportunities for Treatment. Curr Atheroscler Rep. 2024;26(12):707-19.
71. Chhunchha B, Kubo E, Lchri D, et al. NLRP3 Inflammasome and Inflammatory Response in Aging Disorders: The Entanglement of Redox Modulation in Different Outcomes. Cells. 2025;14(13):994.
72. Mullen M, Jin XY, Child A, et al. Irbesartan in Marfan syndrome (AIMS): a double-blind, placebo-controlled randomised trial. Lancet. 2019;394(10216):2263-70.
73. Baderkhan H, Wanhainen A, Stenborg A, et al. Celiprolol Treatment in Patients with Vascular Ehlers-Danlos Syndrome. Eur J Vasc Endovasc Surg. 2021;61(2):326-31.

74. Gouveia E Melo R, Rodrigues M, Caldeira D, et al. Doxycycline is not Effective in Reducing Abdominal Aortic Aneurysm Growth: A Mini Systematic Review and Meta-Analysis of Randomised Controlled Trials. Eur J Vasc Endovasc Surg. 2021;61(5):863-4.
75. Abraham AT, Mojaddedi S, Loseke IH, et al. Hypertension in Patients With Peripheral Artery Disease: An Updated Literature Review. Cureus. 2024;16(6):e62246.
76. Bauersachs RM, Szarek M, Brodmann M, et al. Total Ischemic Event Reduction With Rivaroxaban After Peripheral Arterial Revascularization in the VOYAGER PAD Trial. J Am Coll Cardiol. 2021; 78(4):317-26.
77. Steffel J, Eikelboom JW, Anand SS, et al. The COMPASS Trial: Net Clinical Benefit of Low-Dose Rivaroxaban Plus Aspirin as Compared With Aspirin in Patients With Chronic Vascular Disease. Circulation. 2020; 142(1):40-8. Erratum in: Circulation. 2020; 142(1):e23.
78. Bonaca MP, Nault P, Giugliano RP, et al. Low-Density Lipoprotein Cholesterol Lowering With Evolocumab and Outcomes in Patients With Peripheral Artery Disease: Insights From the FOURIER Trial (Further Cardiovascular Outcomes Research With PCSK9 Inhibition in Subjects With Elevated Risk). Circulation. 2018;137(4): 338-50.

CHAPTER 6

Late Myocardial Infarction Presentation: Current Strategy for Best Practices 2025

Atul Kaushik, Suman Bhandari

INTRODUCTION

Current practice supports the primary percutaneous coronary intervention (PCI) in cases with STEMI within 90 minutes of first medical contact as it has a significant absolute mortality reduction of ~12.5% **(Fig. 1)**.[2] If PCI is not available, then thrombolysis can be done unless interhospital transport and PCI is not possible within 120 minutes of first medical contact **(Table 1)**.[3] However, late presentation MI has differing timeline, up to 24 hours in American guidelines[3] and up to 48 hours in European guidelines.[4] A prior history of AMI has shown to reduce probability of late arrival by 35%, probably caused by the patients' awareness of AMI symptoms; while diabetes mellitus, age, prior history of heart failure, and atypical chest pain are also independent predictors of late arrival in STEMI.[5]

TABLE 1: Recent guidelines for PCI in late presenters.

2025 ACC/AHA/ACEP/NAEMSP/SCAI guidelines for ACS[3]	COR	LOE
STEMI: With *cardiogenic shock or hemodynamic instability*, emergency revascularization by PCI or CABG is indicated to improve survival, *irrespective of time from symptom onset*[2]	1	B
STEMI: Up to *12–24 hours after symptom onset*, routine *PPCI is reasonable* to improve clinical outcomes	2a	B
STEMI: *>24 hours after symptom onset* with the presence of *ongoing ischemia* or life-threatening *arrhythmia, PPCI is reasonable* to improve clinical outcomes	2a	C
Routine PCI of an occluded IRA is not recommended in STEMI presenting *>24 hours after without persistent symptoms*	3	B
2023 ESC guidelines for the management of ACS[4]	COR	LOE
In patients with a working diagnosis of *STEMI* and a time from symptom onset *>12 hours*, a PPCI strategy is recommended in the presence of ongoing symptoms suggestive of *ischemia, hemodynamic instability, or life-threatening arrhythmias*	1	C
A routine PPCI strategy should be considered in *STEMI* patients presenting *late (12–48 hours)* after symptom onset	2a	B
Routine PCI of an occluded IRA is *not recommended in STEMI* patients presenting *>48 hours* after symptom onset and without persistent symptoms	3	A

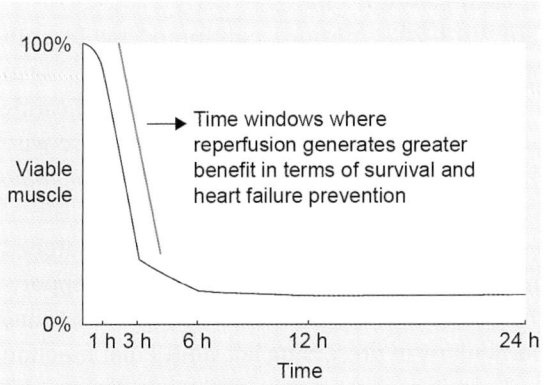

Fig. 1: Relationship between time, extent of myocardial salvage, and mortality reduction.
Source: Reproduced from Farah et al.[1]

Current evidence, however, points to significant viability in patients with no symptoms up to 72 hours.[6] This chapter attempts to focus on the evidence of PCI in late presenters up to 72 hours.

Current evidence for early revascularization is based on BRAVE-2[7] trial which included 365 patients with acute STEMI between 12 and 48 hours after symptom onset and demonstrated that the final left ventricular infarct size was significantly smaller in the invasive compared to the conservative group ($p < 0.001$), and DECOPI[8] trial with late recanalization (2–15 days post-MI) which found improved left ventricular ejection fraction (5% higher LVEF) at 6 months in the intervention group. However, both the trials did not demonstrate any long-term clinical outcomes, but they do demonstrate the benefit of early invasive therapy in late presenters.

The OAT[9] trial which was not a well-planned trial had left an unclear message with respect to the early invasive versus medical therapy in patients presenting with late MI. But it has long been the basis of current practices including the ACC guidelines. It demonstrated no clinical benefit in terms of death, reinfarction, or heart failure from routine PCI compared to optimal medical therapy in patients with persistent occlusion of the infarct-related artery (IRA) 3–28 days post-myocardial infarction (MI) in 2,166 stable patients. This could be since median time to randomization was 8 days in both PCI with medical therapy and medical therapy only group. Therefore, most patients underwent PCI considerably late which could be a reason for similar outcome in both groups. Moreover, this was done earlier in the century and the progress in interventional techniques, devices (drug-eluting stents, etc.), and medications may have affected the outcomes in current scenario. OAT trial was not comparable with the results from BRAVE-2 trial because the median time of angioplasty was <24 hours in BRAVE-2 as compared to 8 days in OAT trial.

However, based on investigations by Nepper-Christensen et al.,[6] who involved 865 STEMI patients with signs of ongoing ischemia presenting between 12 and 72 hours ($n = 58$) after symptom onset, outcomes were compared with those presenting within 12 hours ($n = 807$), the use of MRI after primary PCI and again at 3 months revealed a substantial myocardial salvage index (≥ 0.50) in STEMI patients with signs of ongoing ischemia presenting between 12 and 72 hours after symptom.

In a study by Busk et al.,[10] late presenters (12–72 hours) were compared with early presenters (<12 hours) of STEMI by myocardial perfusion imaging to assess area at risk before angioplasty and was repeated after 30 days to assess final infarct size, salvage index, and LVEF. They found that in patients with TIMI flow 0, late presenters had lower salvage index than early presenters (44% vs. 57%, $p = 0.03$), but there was substantial salvage (>50% of AAR) in 41% of later presenters despite of total infarct-related occlusion.

Furthermore, an analysis of late-presenting STEMI patients (12–48 hours and >48 hours after symptom onset) from the biennial Acute Coronary Syndrome Israeli Surveys (ACSIS) and time-dependent changes (early 2000–2010 vs. late 2013–2021 period) conducted by Tarabih et al.[11] demonstrated that patients presenting at 12–48 hours who underwent PCI had significantly better adjusted 1-year survival than those who presented beyond 48 hours (HR: 0.49, 95% CI: 0.29–0.82; $p = 0.01$).

The retrospective propensity score-matched analysis by Xue and colleagues[12] further supports the notion that late PCI retains prognostic value, particularly in preserving left ventricular function and reducing long-term adverse cardiovascular events. Their analysis indicated that delayed PCI (performed 3–14 days post-symptom onset) in patients presenting with STEMI was associated

TABLE 2: Summary of trials/study on late presenter of MI.

Trial/study	Year	Design	Population	Intervention	Main findings
DECOPI[8]	2004	RCT, multicenter	212 patients (2–15 days post-MI)	PCI of occluded artery versus conservative	↑ LVEF at 6 months; no difference in clinical outcomes
BRAVE-2[7]	2005	RCT, multicenter, open-label	365 STEMI patients (12–48 hours post-onset)	Invasive strategy versus conservative	↓ Infarct size in PCI group; no difference in mortality, recurrent MI, or stroke
OAT[9]	2011	RCT, multicenter	2,166 stable patients (3–28 days post-MI)	Routine PCI versus medical therapy	No benefit in death, reinfarction, or heart failure
Bouisset et al.[4]	2021	Observational cohort	1,169 late STEMI patients (12–48 hours)	PCI versus no PCI	↓ 30-day and long-term mortality in revascularized group
Xue et al.[12]	2021	Retrospective, propensity-matched	STEMI patients (3–14 days post-onset)	Delayed PCI versus medical therapy	↓ MACCE and preserved LV function with PCI
Ki et al.[13]	2021	Retrospective analysis	STEMI patients (≥12 hours post-onset)	Immediate versus delayed PCI	No significant outcome difference between immediate and delayed PCI
Cho et al.[14]	2021	Observational cohort	STEMI patients (late versus early presenters)	Comparison by timing	Late presenters had higher 180-day and 3-year mortality
ACSIS (Tarabih et al.)[11]	2024	Registry analysis	STEMI patients (12–48 hours and >48 hours)	PCI versus no PCI	PCI at 12–48 hours → better adjusted 1-year survival than >48 hours

with a significantly lower incidence of major adverse cardiovascular and cerebrovascular events (MACCE) compared to medical therapy alone. Specifically, the incidence of MACCE was 32.2% in the medical therapy group versus 43.5% in the delayed PCI group ($p < 0.001$) **(Table 2)**.

CONCLUSION

Based on all above evidence, we suggest that PCI could be done up to 48 hours of symptom onset in STEMI and for those presenting after 48–72 hours, a myocardial viability test may guide better regarding the possibility of benefit from PCI, if substantial myocardium is salvageable on the scan. This is in contrary to the OAT trials which has long been viewed as the basis of our practice till now.

REFERENCES

1. Farah A, Barbagelata A. Unmet goals in the treatment of Acute Myocardial Infarction: Review. F1000Res. 2017;6:F1000 Faculty Rev-1243.
2. Cequier Á, Ariza-Solé A, Elola FJ, et al. Impact on Mortality of Different Network Systems in the Treatment of ST-segment Elevation Acute Myocardial Infarction. The Spanish Experience. Rev Esp Cardiol (Engl Ed). 2017;70(3):155-61.
3. Rao SV, O'Donoghue ML, Ruel M, et al. 2025 ACC/AHA/ACEP/NAEMSP/SCAI Guideline for the Management of Patients With Acute Coronary Syndromes: A Report of the American College

of Cardiology/American Heart Association Joint Committee on Clinical Practice Guidelines. Circulation. 2025;151(13):e771-862.
4. Byrne RA, Rossello X, Coughlan JJ, et al.; ESC Scientific Document Group. 2023 ESC Guidelines for the management of acute coronary syndromes. Eur Heart J. 2023;44(38):3720-826.
5. Bouisset F, Gerbaud E, Bataille V, et al. Percutaneous myocardial revascularization in late-presenting patients with STEMI. J Am Coll Cardiol. 2021;78(13):1291-305.
6. Nepper-Christensen L, Lønborg J, Høfsten DE, et al. Benefit From Reperfusion With Primary Percutaneous Coronary Intervention Beyond 12 Hours of Symptom Duration in Patients With ST-Segment-Elevation Myocardial Infarction. Circ Cardiovasc Interv. 2018;11(9):e006842.
7. Schömig A, Mehilli J, Antoniucci D, et al. Mechanical reperfusion in patients with acute myocardial infarction presenting more than 12 hours from symptom onset: a randomized controlled trial. JAMA. 2005;293(23):2865-72.
8. Steg PG, Thuaire C, Himbert D, et al. DECOPI (DEsobstruction COronaire en Post-Infarctus): a randomized multi-centre trial of occluded artery angioplasty after acute myocardial infarction. Eur Heart J. 2004;25(24):2187-94.
9. Hochman JS, Reynolds HR, Dzavík V, et al. Long-term effects of percutaneous coronary intervention of the totally occluded infarct-related artery in the subacute phase after myocardial infarction. Circulation. 2011;124(21):2320-8.
10. Busk M, Kaltoft A, Nielsen SS, et al. Infarct size and myocardial salvage after primary angioplasty in patients presenting with symptoms for <12 h vs. 12-72 h. Eur Heart J. 2009;30(11):1322-30.
11. Tarabih M, Ovdat T, Karkabi B, et al. Characteristics, management and outcome of patients with late-arrival STEMI in the Acute Coronary Syndrome Israeli Surveys (ACSIS). Int J Cardiol Heart Vasc. 2024;53:101476.
12. Xue YL, Ma YT, Gao YP, et al. Long-term outcomes of delayed percutaneous coronary intervention for patients with ST-segment elevation myocardial infarction: A propensity score-matched retrospective study. Medicine (Baltimore). 2021;100(46):e27474.
13. Ki YJ, Kang J, Yang HM, et al.; investigators for Korea Acute Myocardial Infarction Registry-National Institute of Health (KAMIR-NIH). Immediate Compared With Delayed Percutaneous Coronary Intervention for Patients With ST-Segment-Elevation Myocardial Infarction Presenting ≥12 Hours After Symptom Onset Is Not Associated With Improved Clinical Outcome. Circ Cardiovasc Interv. 2021;14(5):e009863.
14. Cho KH, Han X, Ahn JH, et al.; KAMIR-NIH Investigators. Long-Term Outcomes of Patients With Late Presentation of ST-Segment Elevation Myocardial Infarction. J Am Coll Cardiol. 2021;77(15):1859-70.

CHAPTER 7

Vericiguat—The Fifth Pillar or Default Early Start in Heart Failure: Indian Data

Sanjay Mittal, Abhishek Kumar Tiwari, Aparajita Kumar, Chris Alvis Shaji

INTRODUCTION

Heart failure with reduced ejection fraction (HFrEF) is a leading cause of morbidity and mortality worldwide. Despite decades of therapeutic progress, it remains a major killer: 5-year survival rates for HFrEF are comparable to or worse than those of several common cancers, and recurrent hospitalizations create a relentless cycle of clinical decline, financial burden, and impaired quality of life.[1,2] Globally, over 64 million people live with HF, and its prevalence is expected to rise further due to population aging, improved survival after myocardial infarction, and the continuing epidemic of hypertension and diabetes mellitus.[3]

The last three decades have witnessed a revolution in HFrEF management, culminating in the establishment of the four "pillars" of therapy: Renin–angiotensin system inhibition with ACE inhibitors (ACEIs), ARBs, or angiotensin receptor-neprilysin inhibitors (ARNIs); beta blockers; mineralocorticoid receptor antagonists (MRAs); and sodium–glucose cotransporter-2 inhibitors (SGLT2i).[4,5] Together, these therapies have fundamentally altered the natural history of HFrEF by reducing neurohormonal overactivation, improving survival, and lowering the risk of hospitalization. However, even with maximally tolerated guideline-directed medical therapy (GDMT), patients continue to experience substantial residual risk, which is in no way trivial.[4,5]

This persistent vulnerability has refocused attention on the need to go beyond the established four pillars by identifying novel biological pathways and carefully defining the subgroups of patients who remain at highest risk despite optimal background therapy. The search for such strategies has opened the door for newer therapeutic approaches such as vericiguat.

VERICIGUAT: THE NOVEL PATHWAY—A RAY OF HOPE

Despite the transformative advances of the four therapeutic pillars, residual risk in HFrEF persists, particularly after episodes of clinical deterioration. Vericiguat, the first oral soluble guanylate cyclase (sGC) stimulator, was developed to address this therapeutic gap. Unlike conventional therapies that primarily target neurohormonal and metabolic dysregulation, vericiguat works on the impaired *nitric oxide (NO)–sGC–cyclic guanosine monophosphate (cGMP) pathway*[6-9] (**Box 1**).

In HFrEF, oxidative stress and endothelial dysfunction blunt this pathway, reducing cGMP bioavailability and contributing to vascular stiffness, maladaptive remodeling, and pump failure. By sensitizing sGC to endogenous NO and directly stimulating cGMP production, vericiguat restores signaling, improves vascular tone, enhances myocardial compliance, and attenuates fibrosis.[10]

This mechanistic novelty distinguishes vericiguat from the existing four pillars:

- It does not overlap with adverse effect profiles of other classes.
- It specifically targets a biological deficit unaddressed by conventional therapy (**Figs. 1 and 2**).

BOX 1: Vericiguat in HFrEF—key takeaways.

- *Residual risk remains:* Despite the four foundational pillars (ARNI/ACEI/ARB, beta blocker, MRA, and SGLT2i), patients with HFrEF continue to experience recurrent worsening HF (WHF) and high mortality
- *Mechanism matters:* Vericiguat stimulates soluble guanylate cyclase (sGC), restoring cGMP signaling, targeting endothelial dysfunction, and vascular stiffness—a pathway not addressed by other HF drugs
- *Evidence base:*
  - *SOCRATES trials:* Established safety and biomarker impact
  - *VICTORIA:* First phase III trial in high-risk post-WHF patients; it showed a 10% relative risk reduction (ARR ~4.2 events/100 patient-years, NNT ~24), mainly driven by fewer HF hospitalizations
  - *Post hoc analyses:* Best outcomes in patients with NT-proBNP < 8,000 pg/mL and consistent benefits across renal strata
  - *Indian data:* Real-world case series show feasibility, symptom stabilization, and reduced admissions
- *Patient selection:* Best suited for patients with HFrEF, LVEF <45%, recent WHF event, already on (or attempting) GDMT, with moderately elevated NT-proBNP
- *Safety:* Well tolerated; monitor BP, hemoglobin levels, and renal function; it should be avoided in patients with severe hypotension, pregnancy, or concomitant PDE-5/sGC stimulators
- *Practical use:* Initiate at 2.5 mg once daily and titrate to 10 mg. Simple dosing is safe in CKD down to eGFR 15 mL/min/1.73 m^2
- *Indian context:* Especially relevant in younger, comorbid patients with frequent WHF and limited tolerance to full-dose GDMT; a once-daily regimen is suitable for resource-constrained care models
- *Clinical debate:*
  - *Fifth pillar view:* A core addition for high-risk post-WHF patients
  - *Default early start view:* Used soon after discharge or even earlier in selected "high-risk stable" patients
- *Future needs:* Real-world registries, cost-effectiveness analyses, and pragmatic studies in India

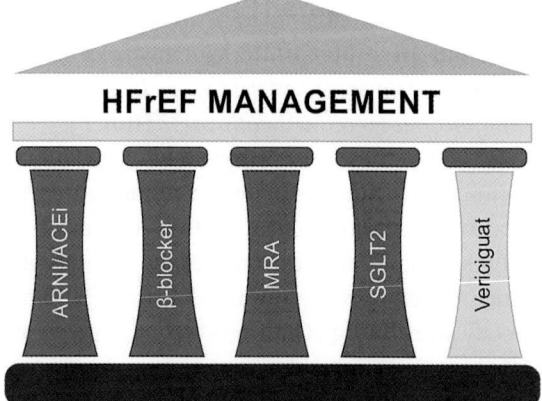

Fig. 1: Core pharmacologic pillars in HFrEF management. *Source:* Adapted from Mauriello A, Ascrizzi A, Roma AS, et al. Effects of Heart Failure Therapies on Atrial Fibrillation: Biological and Clinical Perspectives. Antioxidants. 2024;13(7):806.

The *clinical importance of this pathway was confirmed in the VICTORIA trial*, which established vericiguat as a therapy capable of reducing recurrent hospitalizations in high-risk patients with HFrEF.[12]

IS THE NEW PATHWAY EFFECTIVE? EVIDENCE FROM VICTORIA

Trial Overview

The *VICTORIA trial* was a global, randomized, double-blind, placebo-controlled, phase III study enrolling 5,050 patients with symptomatic chronic HFrEF (LVEF <45%) who had experienced a recent worsening heart failure (WHF) event within 6 months (hospitalization or IV diuretics).[13]

This was a uniquely high-risk group, often underrepresented in previous landmark HF trials. Baseline characteristics reflected the fragility of the cohort:

- *Median age:* 67 years; median LVEF: 29%
- *High comorbidity burden:* ~40% diabetes mellitus, ~70% ischemic etiology, ~45% CKD

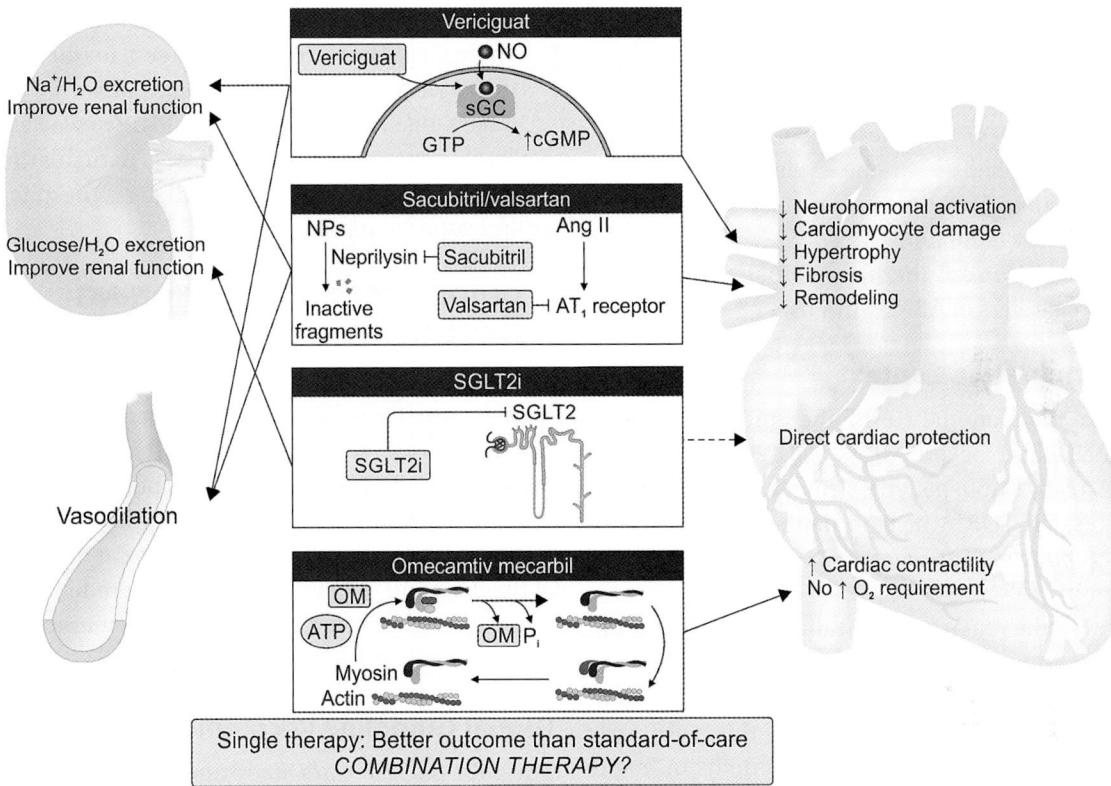

Fig. 2: Novel therapies for heart failure, their mechanisms of action, and final effects.[11] (Ang: angiotensin; ATP: adenosine triphosphate; cGMP: cyclic guanosine monophosphate; GTP: guanosine triphosphate; NO: nitric oxide; NP: natriuretic peptide; OM: omecamtiv mecarbil; sGC: soluble guanylate cyclase; SGLT2i: sodium–glucose cotransporter-2 inhibitors)
Source: Adapted from Aimo et al.[11]

- *Extremely elevated biomarkers:* Median NT-proBNP ~2,800 pg/mL, higher than *PARADIGM-HF* (~1,600)[14] and *DAPA-HF* (~1,400).[15]

Only ~15% of patients were on ARNIs and ~3% on SGLT2 inhibitors, since the trial preceded widespread adoption of these therapies. This makes VICTORIA complementary rather than redundant to evolving quadruple therapy.

Main Findings

Over a median follow-up of 10.8 months, VICTORIA reported:
- Primary endpoint (CV death or first HF hospitalization) in 35.5% (vericiguat) versus 37.8% (placebo); HR 0.90 (95% CI 0.82–0.98, $p = 0.02$).[13]
- *ARR:* 4.2 events per 100 patient-years, yielding NNT ≈24–25/year
- Benefit mainly from reduction in recurrent HF hospitalizations; CV mortality modestly reduced but not significant alone
- ~90% reached target 10 mg dose, showing tolerability
- *Safety:* Mild increases in anemia (7.6% vs. 5.7%) and hypotension (9.1% vs. 7.9%), but no excess syncope or discontinuation; no increase in renal adverse events even in advanced CKD.[16,17]

Subgroup Insights
- *Renal function:* Benefit preserved across eGFR ≥15 mL/min/1.73 m²
- *NT-proBNP:* Greatest benefit <8,000 pg/mL, diminished at extreme levels
- *Timing:* Early initiation post-WHF yielded greater reductions
- *Background therapy:* Consistent benefit regardless of ARNI/MRA use.[13,17]

Comparative Context
Most foundational HFrEF therapies (ACEI/ARB/ARNI, beta blockers, MRAs, SGLT2i) were tested in relatively stable patients with lower annual event rates. VICTORIA instead deliberately studied a *sicker, high-event cohort (>35% annualized event rate)*.

By decreasing hospitalizations, vericiguat helps interrupt the cycle of disease progression, impaired quality of life, and healthcare burden. *Indian experience* also supports this, with early real-world series highlighting benefits in fragile patients.[18]

Critics note the modest relative risk reduction (10%) compared with *PARADIGM-HF (20%)*[14] and *DAPA-HF (25%)*.[15] Yet, because absolute benefit depends on baseline risk, VICTORIA's ARR of 4.2 events/100 patient-years and NNT of ~24/year is clinically meaningful.[13]

Thus, VICTORIA established vericiguat as a therapy with modest relative benefit but substantial absolute benefit in the highest-risk subgroup of HFrEF patients.

Clinical Implications
The significance of VICTORIA extends beyond its numbers:
- It defined *WHF as a vulnerable phase*, where patients face disproportionately high risks of rehospitalization and death.
- It showed benefit *within 10 months*, addressing a critical short-term gap.
- It demonstrated that even in an era of multiple therapies, there remains a need for drugs addressing *residual risk in fragile patients*.

Taken together, vericiguat should be viewed as a *complementary addition to GDMT*, particularly suited for patients who remain at high risk despite optimization of standard therapy.

GUIDELINES AND POSITIONING OF VERICIGUAT

The integration of vericiguat into contemporary heart failure (HF) management has been cautious but progressive since its introduction. While its pivotal trial (VICTORIA) provided robust evidence in a high-risk population, guidelines have taken a conservative stance, reflecting both the novelty of the drug and the modest relative risk reduction compared with earlier transformative therapies such as ARNI and SGLT2 inhibitors.

Global Guideline Recommendations
The *2021 ESC HF Guidelines*[5] and the *2022 AHA/ACC/HFSA Guideline Update*[19] were the first to formally recognize vericiguat. Both positioned the drug with a *class IIb recommendation* ("may be considered") for patients with HFrEF (LVEF <45%) who had experienced a recent episode of WHF despite being on GDMT.

This cautious recommendation represented a milestone: Vericiguat was acknowledged as the first therapy specifically designed and tested in the vulnerable post-worsening HF phase, a period associated with the highest rates of rehospitalization and death.[13,18,20]

In practical terms, a class IIb recommendation reflects a balance between favorable evidence and the need for clinical judgment. Unlike class I therapies, which are mandatory unless contraindicated, class IIb therapies are discretionary and are considered when clinicians identify high-risk features or unmet needs. This is particularly relevant for vericiguat, where the

TABLE 1: Positioning of vericiguat in global and Indian guidelines.

Guideline/consensus	Population criteria	Recommendation class	Key remarks
ESC 2021 guidelines[5]	Symptomatic HFrEF (LVEF <45%) with recent WHF despite GDMT	IIb (may be considered)	First major guideline to recognize vericiguat; conservative due to modest relative benefit and trial specificity
AHA/ACC/HFSA 2022 guidelines[19]	HFrEF with recent WHF despite GDMT	IIb	Aligned with ESC; emphasizes absolute versus relative risk distinction
Indian Expert Consensus 2023[22]	(1) VICTORIA-like patients; (2) high-risk "apparently stable" patients (rising NT-proBNP, escalating diuretics); (3) patients intolerant to maximized GDMT	Consensus-based (expert opinion)	More flexible than global guidelines; positions vericiguat as "fifth pillar" or early add-on
APPROACH-HF Consensus 2025[23]	Implementation of GDMT with real-world Indian challenges	Consensus	Broader framework contextualizing vericiguat as part of tailored GDMT

benefit was most apparent in patients with moderately elevated NT-proBNP and recent WHF, but less pronounced in those with very advanced disease.[21]

Why Guidelines are Conservative?

Several reasons explain why vericiguat did not immediately enter guidelines as a "foundational therapy":

- *Trial population specificity:* VICTORIA[13] enrolled very high-risk patients, unlike the broader ambulatory populations of *PARADIGM-HF*[14] and *DAPA-HF*.[15]
- *Relative risk reduction modesty:* With a hazard ratio of 0.90, vericiguat's relative risk reduction was smaller than ARNI and SGLT2i, though the absolute benefit was meaningful.[13]
- *Unanswered questions:* At the time of guideline drafting, data on long-term outcomes, synergy with quadruple therapy, and applicability in diverse real-world settings were limited.

Thus, guidelines erred on the side of caution, framing vericiguat as a specialty tool rather than a foundational HFrEF therapy.

Clinical Implications of Positioning

- *Targeted therapy, not blanket therapy:* Best suited for HFrEF with recent WHF
- *Complementary, not competing:* Vericiguat complements the four pillars by targeting the NO–sGC–cGMP pathway.[6-9,21]
- *Practical in Indian settings:* Where GDMT optimization is limited by hypotension, renal dysfunction, or cost, vericiguat provides a viable "fifth option".[18,22]
- *Potential for future upgrading:* With accumulating registry and real-world data (e.g., Esteban-Fernández et al.[21]), its positioning may evolve as ARNI and SGLT2i once did[23] **(Table 1)**.

INDIAN AVAILABILITY AND EARLY EXPERIENCE

Regulatory Approval and Market Introduction

Vericiguat was approved for clinical use in India in *February, 2022*, soon after its global approval by the *US FDA* and *European Medicines Agency*. Its entry into the Indian market was timely, as national data from registries such as the *Trivandrum HF Registry* and the *CSI-KHFR* have already highlighted the disproportionate burden of *WHF* in the Indian population.[22,23] The approval positioned vericiguat as the *first-in-class sGC stimulator* available for chronic HFrEF, offering Indian physicians a therapy that is mechanistically distinct from the four foundational pillars.

Indian Guideline Recommendations

Indian Consensus and Adaptations

Recognizing the unique challenges in India, where patients are younger, present later, and have higher rates of comorbidities such as diabetes mellitus and CKD, Indian expert consensus statements proposed a more pragmatic use of vericiguat.[22,23] Unlike global guidelines that restricted its use to narrowly defined post-WHF cohorts, Indian experts suggested a broader application in three scenarios:

1. *True VICTORIA-like patients:* Recent hospitalization or outpatient WHF despite GDMT
2. *High-risk "apparently stable" patients:* Those with recurrent ED visits, rising NT-proBNP levels, or escalating diuretic needs without overt admission
3. *Patients intolerant to GDMT:* Hypotension limiting ARNI, hyperkalemia limiting MRAs, or infections with SGLT2i, where vericiguat could serve as an alternative risk-reducing agent.

This more flexible positioning reflects the reality of Indian practice: Frequent WHF, suboptimal uptake of GDMT, and systemic barriers to intensive monitoring. Both the 2023 Indian Expert Consensus on Worsening HF and the 2025 APPROACH-HF Consensus contextualized vericiguat as either a "fifth pillar" in high-risk patients or as an early add-on when maximizing GDMT is not feasible.[22,23]

Indian Context: Patient Selection, Prescribing, Safety, and Equity

India's HF population is younger, more comorbid, and experiences frequent decompensations, creating a clinical reality in which residual risk remains high despite efforts to deploy the four foundational therapies. These patterns, particularly the clustering of adverse events during the "vulnerable phase" after a worsening HF episode, shape how vericiguat should be positioned in routine practice.[22]

Patient selection: In principle, the best candidates resemble the VICTORIA phenotype: Symptomatic HFrEF with LVEF <45%, a recent worsening HF event [hospitalization or urgent intravenous (IV) diuretics], and background GDMT.[13] However, the *Indian Expert Consensus (2023)* recommended a pragmatic expansion beyond strict trial criteria to include two additional groups frequently encountered in Indian clinics: (1) "Apparently stable," high-risk outpatients with rising natriuretic peptide levels, escalating diuretic requirements, or recurrent ED visits; and (2) patients who cannot tolerate optimal doses of ARNI/ACEI/ARB, beta blocker, MRA, or SGLT2 inhibitor because of hypotension, renal dysfunction, hyperkalemia, or infection risk.[22,23] This approach acknowledges system-level barriers to full GDMT uptake and aims to intercept risk earlier, before overt decompensation occurs.

Practical prescribing: In India, vericiguat is commonly initiated at 2.5 mg once daily with food and uptitrated at roughly 2-week intervals to 10 mg once daily as tolerated, an approach consistent with the pivotal trial and international guidance.[13,18] The drug should not be combined with other sGC stimulators or PDE-5 inhibitors; blood pressure, renal function, and hemoglobin levels are checked during titration.[4] Notably, vericiguat showed acceptable safety down to an eGFR of ~15 mL/min/1.73 m^2, which is relevant given the high burden of CKD in India.[16]

Safety and early experiences in India: Real-world Indian data suggest good tolerability and feasibility of this regimen. In a multicenter case series (2025), >90% of patients reached the 10 mg target dose with few discontinuations; clinicians reported symptomatic stabilization and declines in NT-proBNP despite frequent constraints on laboratory monitoring.[18] These observations echo the trial signal but are noteworthy for having been achieved in busy, resource-limited settings.

Cost, access, and equity: Recurrent HF admissions drive catastrophic expenditure for many families in India; therefore, reducing readmissions is a clinical and public health priority.[22] Vericiguat's once-daily dosing and nonoverlapping mechanism make it a pragmatic add-on for fragile patients in whom full GDMT is difficult to sustain.[4,18] Nevertheless, drug costs and variable insurance coverage remain major obstacles. Wider inclusion in government- or payer-supported HF programs, along with bundled HF clinic models, could improve equitable access.

In summary, within India's high-risk, resource-constrained landscape, vericiguat is emerging not only as a post-worsening HF therapy aligned with VICTORIA[13] and the pooled analyses incorporating VICTOR[24] but also as a practical early add-on for carefully selected high-risk outpatients when implementation of all four pillars is incomplete or poorly tolerated.[22,23]

Real-world Indian Experience

The most detailed early Indian experience was reported by Kaul et al.,[18] who described a multicenter case series of patients with advanced HFrEF. Four representative clinical scenarios were emphasized.

1. *Persistent symptoms despite quadruple therapy:* Vericiguat improves NT-proBNP levels, stabilizes renal function, and reduces rehospitalizations.[18]
2. *Acute decompensation requiring IV diuretics:* Vericiguat initiation facilitated postdischarge stabilization with sustained functional improvement.[18]
3. *Outpatient worsening HF (no admission):* Early initiation avoided hospitalization, with marked symptomatic gains.[18]
4. *Intolerance to GDMT:* In patients unable to tolerate ARNI or MRA, vericiguat provides incremental risk reduction without worsening hypotension or renal dysfunction.[18]

Across these subgroups, >90% of patients tolerated uptitration to the target 10 mg daily dose with low discontinuation rates. Importantly, clinical benefits were observed despite the lack of routine biomarker monitoring in many centers, suggesting that clinical surrogates (diuretic dose, NYHA class, and BP trends) may suffice in resource-constrained environments.[18,22,23]

THE DEBATE: "FIFTH PILLAR" VERSUS "DEFAULT EARLY START"

Despite clear evidence from VICTORIA and subsequent real-world data, the precise role of vericiguat in the therapeutic hierarchy of HFrEF remains unclear. Two distinct narratives have emerged among clinicians and guideline committees, each with important implications for clinical practice.

The "Fifth Pillar" Argument

Proponents of this position argue that vericiguat fulfills the criteria for a mechanistically distinct, evidence-based therapy that reduces morbidity in patients with HFrEF. Similar to the transition from "triple therapy" to "quadruple therapy" with the addition of SGLT2 inhibitors, they view vericiguat as the logical fifth pillar in patients at high residual risk.

The key supporting points include the following:
- *Mechanistic novelty:* Vericiguat stimulates the NO–sGC–cGMP pathway, complementing the

neurohormonal and metabolic mechanisms of the existing four pillars.[6-9]

- *Trial evidence in a high-risk cohort:* VICTORIA demonstrated a significant reduction in the composite endpoint of CV death or HF hospitalization, translating into an absolute risk reduction of 4.2 events per 100 patient-years, with a number needed to treat (NNT) of approximately 24 annually.[13]
- *Nonoverlapping safety profile:* Adverse effects (e.g., anemia, mild hypotension) are modest and distinct from those of ARNI, MRAs, or SGLT2 inhibitors, making vericiguat an additive therapy rather than a competitive substitute.[13,16,17]
- *Guideline endorsements:* Both the ESC 2021 and AHA/ACC/HFSA 2022 guidelines include vericiguat as an option for patients with HFrEF and recent WHF despite GDMT.[5,20,21]

Thus, the fifth pillar framework defines vericiguat as a targeted therapy for patients at the highest risk, that is, those with recent WHF events, moderately elevated NT-proBNP, and incomplete protection despite quadruple therapy.

The "Default Early Start" Argument

However, some experts argue for a broader and earlier application of vericiguat. They emphasize that the very concept of "stable HF" is misleading, as most patients experience silent progression with rising natriuretic peptides, recurrent ED visits, or escalating diuretic requirements long before overt hospitalization.[22,23]

Supporters of this view highlight the following:
- *Early vulnerability:* The postdischarge period after WHF is characterized by extremely high event rates ("vulnerable phase"), with recurrent hospitalizations clustering within the first 3–6 months.[13,22]
- *Opportunity to prevent first readmission:* Initiating vericiguat predischarge or soon after discharge may blunt this high-risk trajectory.[13]
- *Practical Indian context:* In India, where GDMT uptake is often incomplete and follow-up biomarker testing is inconsistent, starting vericiguat early in high-risk "apparently stable" patients may provide protection even before decompensation is fully manifest.[18,22-25]

Critics of this approach, however, caution that vericiguat's benefit was demonstrated in a high-event VICTORIA cohort, and that there is no evidence of benefit in lower-risk or stable patients.[13,26] They argue that widespread early use risks "pill burden" without incremental survival benefit, especially in systems where even the four foundational therapies are underutilized.[22,23]

Reconciling the Two Views: Insights from the VICTOR Trial

The debate between the "fifth pillar" and the "default early start" positions has gained further nuance with the recent publication of the VICTOR trial and its pooled analysis with VICTORIA.[26]

Salient features of VICTOR: This trial deliberately enrolled the lowest-risk HFrEF cohort studied with vericiguat to date—predominantly NYHA class II patients, no HF hospitalization within the preceding year, NT-proBNP levels <6,000 pg/mL, and the highest background use of quadruple therapy of any major trial. Over a median follow-up of 18 months, VICTOR did not meet its primary endpoint of reducing the composite of cardiovascular death or HF hospitalization, largely because of a nonsignificant effect on hospitalization. However, unexpectedly, vericiguat produced a statistically significant reduction in all-cause mortality, cardiovascular mortality, sudden cardiac death, and deaths directly attributed to HF[26] **(Table 2)**.

From a trial-based evidence perspective, this reinforces the conservative guideline stance that positions vericiguat as a "fifth pillar" targeted primarily to patients resembling the VICTORIA population.[13,20,21] VICTORIA enrolled patients at

TABLE 2: Comparison of VICTORIA and VICTOR trials.

Feature	VICTORIA	VICTOR
Population risk profile	*Very high risk:* Recent WHF (hospitalization or IV diuretics), median NT-proBNP ~2,800 pg/mL	*Lower risk:* Stable HFrEF, no hospitalization in prior year, NT-proBNP <6,000 pg/mL
NYHA class	Predominantly III–IV	Predominantly II
Background GDMT	Suboptimal (ARNI ~15%, SGLT2i ~3%)	Best background GDMT to date (majority on quadruple therapy)
Sample size	5,050 patients	~6,000 patients
Follow-up	Median 10.8 months	Median 18 months
Primary endpoint	CV death or first HF hospitalization—met (HR 0.90; $p = 0.02$)	CV death or HF hospitalization—not met (driven by nonsignificant hospitalization effect)
Absolute risk reduction	4.2 events per 100 patient-years	*Neutral for hospitalization; mortality benefit emerged*
Mortality outcomes	Trend to reduction; not statistically significant alone	*Statistically significant reductions in:* All-cause mortality, CV mortality, sudden cardiac death, HF death
Key message	Vericiguat reduces recurrent events in *highest-risk* WHF patients	Even in *stable, lower-risk* patients, vericiguat reduces mortality despite neutral hospitalization outcome

extremely high risk, with recent worsening events and very elevated NT-proBNP, and demonstrated clear reductions in recurrent hospitalizations and composite outcomes. VICTOR, by contrast, showed that in lower-risk, stable patients, hospitalization risk was not reduced, even though mortality benefits were observed.[26] Taken together, the evidence underscores that vericiguat's benefits may vary by baseline risk and timing of initiation.

From a clinical practice perspective, particularly in India and other low- and middle-income countries, the relevance of the VICTOR findings is striking. Many patients are labeled "stable" but in reality are deteriorating—with rising NT-proBNP levels, escalating diuretic requirements, or repeated emergency visits without formal admission.[24,25] These patients are rarely seen until overt decompensation occurs, at which point the opportunity for proactive therapy is lost.[22,23]

Mortality Insights: A 17% Reduction in Heart Failure and Sudden Cardiac Death

One of the most compelling findings emerged from the deeper analyses of cause-specific mortality. Patients receiving vericiguat experienced a 17% reduction in deaths attributed to HF progression and sudden cardiac death compared with those receiving placebo.[13,16,17,26]

This is particularly important because sudden cardiac death remains a major contributor to mortality in HFrEF, even among patients receiving implantable cardioverter-defibrillators (ICDs) and GDMT. Vericiguat's impact on sudden death suggests its ability to stabilize myocardial electrophysiology and improve hemodynamics by restoring the NO–sGC–cGMP pathway.[6-9]

VICTOR trial included lowest risk group HFrEF patients with best background treatment. Yet there was statistically significant mortality benefit including CV mortality, sudden cardiac deaths and even HF-related deaths over and above those treated with background quadruple pillars[26] **(Table 3)**.

BALANCED APPROACH: WHY WORSENING HEART FAILURE MAY BE TOO LATE

One of the most sobering realities in HF care is that therapies lose their effectiveness as the disease progresses. The pathophysiological processes underlying HFrEF is progressive myocardial fibrosis, loss of viable myocytes, microvascular dysfunction, and neurohormonal overdrive. This is cumulative and often irreversible once a certain threshold is reached. By the time patients experience WHF, defined as hospitalization or urgent outpatient IV therapy, the disease has already progressed to a stage where the myocardium is structurally and functionally compromised.

This is evident across all pillars of HF therapy. Large, randomized trials of ACEIs, beta blockers, MRAs, and SGLT2 inhibitors have consistently demonstrated the greatest relative benefit when therapy is initiated earlier in the disease course. Conversely, in patients with advanced HF, characterized by NYHA class IV symptoms, frequent admissions, and markedly elevated natriuretic peptide levels, the impact of these drugs is blunted. Many of these therapies are difficult to tolerate in late-stage HF due to hypotension, renal impairment, or electrolyte disturbances.[9-13,25,26]

The same principle applies to the use of vericiguat. The VICTORIA trial showed that patients with extremely elevated NT-proBNP (>8,000 pg/mL) derived less benefit, suggesting that the therapy is less effective once disease severity reaches an advanced and near-refractory state.[13,27] This raises an important clinical lesson: While WHF events identify a population at very high risk, waiting for such events before intensifying therapy may represent a missed therapeutic opportunity.

From a clinical management perspective, this insight supports a balanced approach:
- Adhere to trial-based indications by prioritizing vericiguat in patients with recent WHF who resemble the VICTORIA population.
- *Recognize the limitations of a purely reactive strategy:* Delaying therapy until after a major worsening event may forfeit opportunities to alter the disease trajectory.
- Adopt a proactive mindset by identifying high-risk "stable" patients—those with rising NT-proBNP levels, worsening renal function, escalating diuretic needs, or repeated emergency visits—and consider earlier initiation of vericiguat.

In India, this argument is even more significant. Hospitalizations often occur late, with limited access to biomarkers, delayed presentation, and systemic barriers to early GDMT optimization.[6-8,22,23,28] By the time a patient is admitted for WHF, the prognosis is already poor, with mortality rates exceeding 20% at 1 year in national registries.[22,23,29] Thus, a purely post-WHF strategy risks underutilization of vericiguat's benefits in the populations that need it most.

Taken together, the balanced approach reframes vericiguat not only as a treatment for patients "after worsening" but also as a therapy that should be considered before the disease becomes too advanced to respond. This principle aligns with the broader evolution of HF care, in which earlier intervention consistently translates into better long-term outcomes.

RESEARCH GAPS: WHAT INDIA SHOULD STUDY NEXT

Although the VICTOR trial did not meet its composite primary endpoint in a lower-risk ambulatory population, its findings of significant reductions in all-cause mortality, cardiovascular

TABLE 3: Comparative data from various trials of the quadruple pillars of HFrEF treatment.

Drug	Trial	Year	Follow-up	No. of patients	Mortality reduction (RRR)	ARR	SCD reduction	ACE/ARBs	ARNI	Beta#	MRAs	SGLT2i
									Background Rx			
ACEI (Enalapril)	SOLVD	1991	41.4 months	2,569	18%	4.5%	NS	NA	–	None	None	None
ARBs (Candesartan)	CHARM Alternative	2003	33.7 months	2,028	17%	3%	–	NA	–	None	None	None
Beta # (Metoprolol Succinate)	MERIT HF	1999	12 months	3,991	34%	3.8%	45%	95%	–	None	None	None
MRAs (Eplerenone)	EMPHASIS HF	2011	21 months	2,737	24%	7.6%	NA	98%	–	87%	None	None
ARNI	PARADIGM HF	2014	27 months	8,442	16%	2.8%	56%	None versus ACEI	–	93.1%	54.2%	None
SGLT2i (Dapagliflozin)	DAPA HF	2019	18.2 months	4,744	17%	2.3%	21%	84%	10.5%	96%	71.5%	NA
sGCi (Vericiguat)	VICTOR	2025	18.5 months	6,105	16%	2.1%	25%	38%	57%	95%	78%	60.1%

death, sudden cardiac death, and HF-related death offer an important complementary perspective to the results of VICTORIA.[26] Taken together, these trials suggest that vericiguat provides mortality benefits even outside the high-risk post-hospitalization population, although the absence of primary endpoint reduction and the costs of lifelong therapy still temper guideline enthusiasm.[11,18]

Therefore, a nuanced interpretation is required. As with other HF therapies, waiting until an overt worsening event may be too late, since advanced HF remains refractory to outcome-modifying therapies.[13,22,23] A balanced approach would be to consider vericiguat in symptomatic HFrEF patients who are not improving despite optimized quadruple therapy, rather than deferring initiation until after a worsening event. In this sense, vericiguat can still be considered the fifth pillar of HFrEF management, but one that may justify earlier initiation in selected high-risk patients.[24,25]

From an Indian perspective, these questions are of added urgency. Registries such as the Trivandrum HF Registry and CSI-KHFR have shown that Indian patients with HFrEF are substantially younger and have disproportionately high rates of diabetes mellitus, CKD, and recurrent hospitalizations.[22-24] In this context, once-daily dosing, favorable tolerability, and mechanistically distinct action of vericiguat are especially appealing for fragile patients already burdened with polypharmacy.[25] Early Indian case series demonstrated that over 90% of patients can be successfully uptitrated to the target dose, with improvements in NT-proBNP, stabilization of renal function, and reduced readmissions, all without excess hypotension or intolerance.[18,22,23]

However, challenges remain. Affordability is a central issue: The average cost of a single HF hospitalization in India (~USD 1,500) can impose catastrophic financial strain,[24] and while reducing rehospitalizations could offset costs at the population level, high upfront drug costs and limited insurance coverage impede widespread access. Real-world pragmatic solutions, such as subsidization, inclusion in government HF programs, or bundling within HF clinic models, may improve equity.[24,25]

To optimize the role of vericiguat in India, future research priorities include:

- Real-world registries evaluate outcomes, tolerability, and adherence in Indian patients.[22-24]
- Cost-effectiveness analyses tailored to the Indian healthcare setting weigh drug costs against avoided hospitalizations.
- Subgroup studies in patients with diabetes mellitus, CKD, and socioeconomically vulnerable populations, where the burden of residual risk is the highest, are needed.
- Pragmatic trials testing simplified clinical algorithms for initiation and monitoring, avoiding overreliance on NT-proBNP testing.
- Exploratory studies have been conducted in HFpEF populations, particularly given the growing burden of metabolic syndrome in India.[17,29]

Such evidence will be crucial in shaping region-specific guidelines and determining whether vericiguat transitions from a narrowly applied "post-worsening rescue therapy" to a proactive cornerstone of Indian HFrEF management.[11,25-29]

CONCLUSION

Heart failure with reduced ejection fraction continues to impose a heavy clinical and socioeconomic burden, particularly in India where patients are younger, more comorbid, and less likely to receive optimized quadruple therapy.[6-8,22,23,28,29] Although the four established drug classes have transformed survival, residual risk persists, especially after worsening HF events.[11,26,27]

Vericiguat addresses this gap through its unique action on the NO–sGC–cGMP pathway. Evidence from VICTORIA and subsequent analyses confirms that it reduces recurrent HF hospitalizations and provides meaningful absolute benefit in the highest-risk patients.[11,13,18,27] The Indian experience, though limited, mirrors these findings and underscores its feasibility, even in resource-constrained environments.[22-24,28,29]

From a global and Indian perspective, vericiguat represents more than just another add-on therapy.
- It introduces a new mechanistic dimension beyond neurohormonal modulation of the heart.
- It offers a pragmatic, once-daily option with good tolerability.
- It may serve as a bridge between evidence and real-world practice in regions where recurrent hospitalizations drive costs and mortality.

The ongoing debate regarding whether vericiguat should be considered as the "fifth pillar" for selected high-risk HFrEF patients or as a default early start in broader populations reflects its clinical promise and the evolving understanding of residual risk. Currently, the most balanced approach is targeted use in recent WHF, high-risk patients, while continuing to optimize GDMT.

Looking forward, with greater real-world adoption, further research in diverse populations, and health-system-level integration, vericiguat has the potential to reshape the management of HFrEF in India and globally. It stands as a candidate not only for incremental benefit but also for a paradigm shift toward quintuple therapy, broadening the therapeutic armamentarium and improving the outlook for millions living with HF.

REFERENCES

1. Rao VN, Diez J, Gustafsson F, et al. Practical patient care considerations with use of vericiguat after worsening heart failure events. J Card Fail. 2023;29(3):389-402.
2. Zhan Y, Li L, Zhou J, et al. Efficacy of vericiguat in patients with chronic heart failure and reduced ejection fraction: a prospective observational study. BMC Cardiovasc Disord. 2025;25:83.
3. Shahim B, Kapelios CJ, Savarese G, et al. Global public health burden of heart failure: an updated review. Card Fail Rev. 2023;9:e11.
4. Vannuccini F, Campora A, Barilli M, et al. Vericiguat in Heart Failure: Characteristics, Scientific Evidence and Potential Clinical Applications. Biomedicines. 2022;10(10):2471.
5. McDonagh TA, Metra M, Adamo M, et al. 2021 ESC Guidelines for the diagnosis and treatment of acute and chronic heart failure. Eur Heart J. 2021;42(36):3599-726.
6. Förstermann U, Sessa WC. Nitric oxide synthases: regulation and function. Eur Heart J. 2012;33:829-37.
7. Tsai EJ, Kass DA. Cyclic GMP signaling in cardiovascular pathophysiology and therapeutics. Pharmacol Ther. 2009;122:216-38.
8. Emdin M, Aimo A, Castiglione V, et aal. Targeting cyclic guanosine monophosphate to treat heart failure: a review. J Am Coll Cardiol. 2020;76:1795-807.
9. Stasch JP, Pacher P, Evgenov OV. Soluble guanylate cyclase as an emerging therapeutic target in cardiopulmonary disease. Circulation. 2011;123:2263-73.
10. Trujillo ME, Ayalasomayajula S, Blaustein RO, et al. Vericiguat, a novel sGC stimulator: Mechanism of action, clinical, and translational science. Clin Transl Sci. 2023;16(12):2458-66.
11. Aimo A, Castiglione V, Vergaro G, et al. The place of vericiguat in the landscape of treatment for heart failure with reduced ejection fraction. Heart Fail Rev. 2022;27:1165-71.
12. Kassis-George H, Verlinden NJ, Fu S, et al. Vericiguat in Heart Failure with a Reduced Ejection Fraction: Patient Selection and Special Considerations. Ther Clin Risk Manag. 2022;18:315-22.
13. Armstrong PW, Pieske B, Anstrom KJ, et al. Vericiguat in patients with heart failure and reduced ejection fraction (VICTORIA). N Engl J Med. 2020;382:1883-93.
14. McMurray JJV, Packer M, Desai AS, et al. Angiotensin–neprilysin inhibition versus

enalapril in heart failure. N Engl J Med. 2014;371: 993-1004.
15. McMurray JJV, Solomon SD, Inzucchi SE, et al. Dapagliflozin in patients with heart failure and reduced ejection fraction. N Engl J Med. 2019; 381:1995-2008.
16. Ezekowitz JA, O'Connor CM, Troughton RW, et al. Safety of vericiguat across the spectrum of kidney function in VICTORIA. Eur J Heart Fail. 2021;23:1231-40.
17. Pieske B, Maggioni AP, Lam CSP, et al. Vericiguat in patients with HFrEF: subgroup analyses of VICTORIA. Eur Heart J. 2021;42:2750-63.
18. Kaul U, Dalal J, Hiremath J, et al. Indian experience with vericiguat: A review based upon case series. J Assoc Physicians India. 2024;72(10):63-8.
19. Heidenreich PA, Bozkurt B, Aguilar D, et al. 2022 AHA/ACC/HFSA Guideline for the Management of Heart Failure: A Report of the American College of Cardiology/American Heart Association Joint Committee on Clinical Practice Guidelines. Circulation. 2022;145:e895-1032.
20. Senni M, Lopez-Sendon J, Cohen-Solal A, et al. Vericiguat and NT-proBNP in patients with heart failure with reduced ejection fraction: analyses from VICTORIA. ESC Heart Fail. 2022; 9(6):3791-803.
21. Esteban-Fernández A, Raposeiras-Roubin S, Cordero A, et al. Clinical profile of an unselected population with heart failure treated with vericiguat in real life: differences with the VICTORIA trial. Front Cardiovasc Med. 2025; 11:1504427.
22. Seth S, Bauersachs J, Mittal S, et al. Expert opinion on the identification and pharmacological management of worsening heart failure: a consensus statement from India. J Pract Cardiovasc Sci. 2023;9(1):1-10.
23. Ponde CK, Mohan JC, Ooman A, et al. An Indian Expert Consensus on patient-profile-based implementation of guideline-directed medical therapy in the management of heart failure with reduced ejection fraction: APPROACH-HF. J Card Fail. 2025:S1071-9164(25)00294-5.
24. Ezekowitz JA, O'Meara E, McDonald M, et al. VICTOR trial and pooled analysis with VICTORIA: outcomes with vericiguat in chronic heart failure. Front Cardiovasc Med. 2025;11:1504427.
25. Butler J, Yang M, Manzi MA, et al. Clinical course of patients with worsening heart failure with reduced ejection fraction. J Am Coll Cardiol. 2019;73:935-44.
26. Kang C, Lamb YN. Vericiguat: A Review in Chronic Heart Failure with Reduced Ejection Fraction. Am J Cardiovasc Drugs. 2022;22:451-9.
27. Greene SJ, Fonarow GC, Vaduganathan M, et al. The vulnerable phase after hospitalization for heart failure. Nat Rev Cardiol. 2015;12:220-9.
28. Greene SJ, Butler J, Albert NM, et al. Medical therapy for heart failure with reduced ejection fraction: the CHAMP-HF registry key insights on vulnerability and optimization. JACC Heart Fail. 2018;6(6):477-89.
29. Armstrong PW, Lam CSP, Anstrom KJ, et al. Effect of vericiguat vs placebo on quality of life in patients with heart failure and preserved ejection fraction: The VITALITY-HFpEF Randomized Clinical Trial. JAMA. 2020;324(15):1512-21.

CHAPTER 8

Antihypertensive Management in 2025: Moving Toward a Single Pill (Triple/Quadruple)

Suman Bhandari, Bhavana Mastebhakti

INTRODUCTION

Hypertension is a serious global health issue and remains a leading modifiable risk factor for cardiovascular disease (CVD). Despite a wide armamentarium of antihypertensive agents, only 33% and 10% people with hypertension achieve BP targets in high-income countries, and in middle- and low-income countries, respectively.[1,2] Uncontrolled hypertension increases the relative risk from two to four times for coronary artery disease (CAD), cerebrovascular accidents (CVA), heart failure (HF), peripheral arterial disease (PAD), renal insufficiency, atrial fibrillation (AF), and cognitive impairment.[3] Long-term prospective studies have shown that monotherapy was ineffective in treating a majority of hypertensive patients, who ultimately needed an average of three drugs for adequate control.[4] Emerging evidence compels the use of monopill low-dose combinations (LDCs) comprising 3 or 4 antihypertensive drugs "hypertension polypills," as an initial therapeutic strategy for hypertension.[5] The rationale for LDC is that most of the BP-lowering effect from an antihypertensive drug is achieved at a fraction of the full therapeutic dose and that the BP lowering effect becomes additive while using different drug classes.[6] Additionally, side effects from antihypertensive agents are dose dependent, and hence, the use of LDCs to achieve the target BP is less likely to cause side effects compared to dose uptitration, which is commonly done when BP targets are not met. By this approach, LDCs can achieve maximum effect while minimizing adverse events. A meta-analysis including 7 trials studied that LDCs reduce the systolic blood pressure (SBP) by an average of 18 mm Hg and 7 mm Hg reduction in SBP compared to placebo and usual care, respectively with a slight increase in dizziness.[7] This chapter will elaborate the pros and cons of LDC regimen as an initial treatment modality in patients newly diagnosed with hypertension along with supportive evidence and guidelines, and whether the benefits outweigh the potential risks.

RATIONALE FOR COMBINATION THERAPY

When the goals of hypertension are not adequately met in hypertensive patients, we can either increase the dose of a particular drug, which the patient is already on, which actually increases the antihypertensive effect minimally, at the cost of greater side effects, or use an LDC, which significantly increases the antihypertensive effects with minimal side effects. The mechanisms responsible for causing high blood pressure are multiple and single drug therapy acts only on one or a maximum of two of these mechanisms, while LDCs act on multiple mechanisms.[7] Two- to fivefold greater antihypertensive effect is obtained by combining two drugs with different mechanisms of action.[7,8] Furthermore, increasing the dose of a single drug alone reduces coronary events by 29% and cerebrovascular events by 40%, while combining two antihypertensive agents in the form of LDCs reduces coronary events by 40% and cerebrovascular events by 54%.[9]

Thus, a greater reduction in blood pressure along with a greater protection from target organ damage (TOD) at the cost of less adverse effects is produced by the use of LDCs than increasing the dose of monotherapy, alone. Also, improved adherence and cost-effectiveness attract the use of the commercially available fixed-dose combinations (FDC). However, their limitation is that they provide less flexibility for dose titration of only one of the drugs from the LDCs.[7,10] The current guidelines recommend the use of LDCs at the beginning of treatment for individuals in whom the SBP/DBP ≥20/10 mm Hg and the probability of achieving the recommended target goals are low. Multiple studies have shown a cardiovascular benefits by using LDCs.[8]

ADVANTAGES AND DISADVANTAGES OF LOW-DOSE COMBINATION VERSUS MONOTHERAPY FOR MANAGEMENT OF HYPERTENSION

The advantages and disadvantages of LDCs compared to monotherapy are enlisted in **Table 1**.

The pros of combination therapy at the start of hypertension treatment include:

- *Rapid and sustained blood pressure lowering:* Hypertension has a multifactorial etiology, and hence, combining different drug classes augments the antihypertensive effect by approximately five times, thereby increasing the control rate of blood pressure. Real-world data on 1,762 adults show an 18.5% earlier target blood pressure achievement in the initial LDC group, corresponding to a 23% risk reduction in cardiovascular events and death.[11] Achieving a rapid control of blood pressure is of utmost priority to provide timely protection in patients with high risk of TOD. Additionally, fewer cardiovascular events were observed after 1 year in hypertensive patients started on LDC compared to those with monotherapy.[12] In another study, sustainable control over a 2-year duration translated into a significant reduction in heart failure (36%) and stroke (21%) risks. Time in the therapeutic range is also inversely related to all-cause mortality (ACM).[13]

- *Nonantihypertensive effects:* In addition to antihypertensive effects, cardiovascular protection is achieved from other mechanisms.[13] In the PETRA study, initial combination

TABLE 1: Low-dose combination (LDC) versus monotherapy for hypertension—advantages and disadvantages.

LDC	Monotherapy
Advantages	
Targets multiple blood pressure pathways	Inability to isolate cause of medication side effects
Simplifies treatment regimen and lowers pill burden	Easier to identify side effects
Reduces clinical inertia and achieves target blood pressure	Indicated in patients with elevated blood pressure/frail and older patients/patients with orthostatic hypotension
Fewer side effects with low dosing of medications	Can be lower in cost than some single pill combinations
Combines first-line medication classes	
Disadvantages	
Some LDCs may be more expensive	Targets a single pathway in blood pressure
Less flexibility in individual medication dosing	Less effective than combination therapy
Inability to isolate cause of medication side effects	Greater risk of clinical inertia

therapy with FDC of perindopril, indapamide, and amlodipine was associated with lower levels of total cholesterol, low-density lipoprotein cholesterol (LDL-c), triglycerides, and fasting plasma glucose. Several other studies including CAFE, J-CORE, ADVANCE, and OLAS, provide evidence on hemodynamic, renal, vascular, and inflammation-induced cardiovascular protection, which are independent from the antihypertensive effect.

- *Low-therapeutic inertia and enhanced patient adherence:* Many physicians are reluctant to prescribe a two-drug combination as first-line therapy. Once patients are initiated on monotherapy, rarely did they receive an additional drug, despite inadequate control. This guideline-practice gap stems from the difference between well-designed randomized controlled trials (RCTs) and the real-world setting. In trials, physicians follow a study protocol strictly and patients must adhere to treatment, whereas, in reality, the compliance of patients with multiple comorbidities rarely exceeds 80%, and physicians are more concerned with the consequences of over-lowering blood pressure.[14] A better strategy to overcome doctor inertia and enhance patient adherence is combination therapy in the form of an LDC pills, which have a flat dose-response and sharp dose adverse effect curve, providing a rapid blood pressure control with limited adverse effects.

- *Homologous blood pressure lowering and good safety profile:* As LDCs exhibit simultaneous effects on multiple mechanisms, they tend to achieve therapeutic goals regardless of baseline blood pressure and other comorbidities. The currently available LDC pill offers flexible dosing of individual components, allowing for easy drug-dose titration and enhancing therapeutic target achievement.

The cons of combination therapy at the start of hypertension treatment include:

- *Elevated blood pressure or stage 1 hypertension with low cardiovascular risk:* For stage 1 hypertensives with high cardiovascular risk, the guidelines recommend an LDC regimen at the outset for timely and prolonged protection. One concern is the over-reduction of blood flow to vital organs as, even in high-risk patients, the lowest possible blood pressure is not necessarily the optimal target. A post-hoc analysis of the ONTARGET study proved a J-curve response in blood pressure level. Specifically, mean SBP less than 120 mm Hg during treatment is associated with increased adverse cardiovascular outcomes, except myocardial infarction and stroke. However, in high-risk young patients, the net clinical benefit of cardiovascular protection favors the use of an LDC from the beginning.

- *Patients 80 years and above:* The elderly often suffer from impairment in hemodynamic autoregulation, leading to a higher risk of hypotensive episodes and subsequent falls. Femoral neck fracture is common and associated with higher mortality compared to the general population of the same age.[14] The SPRINT trial, which included 2,600 patients aged 75 or above, concluded that intensive BP control was associated with greater serious adverse events relating to hypotension and possibly syncope, but not falls.[15,16] The preferred algorithm in elderly is "start slow, go slow", as cerebral autoregulation is impaired in this group, leading to cognitive decline, which gets exacerbated by overtreatment of hypertension. This should be done taking into account patient's comorbidities, polypharmacy, frailty, fall risk, cognitive status and life expectancy, with careful monitoring of patient response.

- *Pseudoresistance:* Pseudoresistance occurs in a patient who claims to have no response, whereas in actuality, the patient is not fully compliant to the prescription. Some dislike long-term treatment and choose SOS (when and as needed) approach, others take smaller or infrequent dosing in fear of hypotension. As a result, pills keep on increasing on the prescription and patients are mistakenly labeled "resistant".
- *Dose confusion and polypharmacy:* Due to a large number of comorbidities involving high pill burden, double-dosing and missed dosing are frequently encountered. These either lead to profound hypotension or rebound hypertension. LDC pill although more economical than free forms, still it is less affordable than monotherapy. Physicians should encourage patients on the cost-effectiveness of combination therapy.

WHAT DO THE GUIDELINES SAY?
ESC 2024: Class 1 Recommendation

Low-dose double combination therapy with first-line antihypertensive agents which include angiotensin-converting enzyme inhibitors (ACEI)/angiotensin receptor blockers (ARB), calcium channel blockers (CCB), and diuretics. If BP is not controlled after 1–3 months of therapy, then low-dose triple combination therapy with first-line antihypertensive agents is recommended.

Monotherapy is indicated in the following conditions:
- Age ≥85 years
- *Elevated BP:* 120/70–139/89 mm Hg
- Moderate-to-severe frailty
- Symptomatic orthostatic hypotension

AHA 2025: Class 1 Recommendation

In adults with stage 2 hypertension, i.e., SBP ≥140 mm Hg and DBP ≥90 mm Hg, initiation of therapy with two first-line agents from different classes, in the form of SPC, is recommended.

EVIDENCE IN SUPPORT OF LOW-DOSE COMBINATION THERAPY

Table 2 enlists RCTs comparing triple or quadruple LDCs with placebo, monotherapy, and usual care for management. The QUADRO trial also demonstrated that adding a β-blocker, bisoprolol, to a combination of three first-line BP-lowering drugs in the form of a quadruple SPC was more effective at reducing BP than taking the same three drugs in separate pills in patients with resistant hypertension.[17]

These studies reveal that low-dose triple or quadruple combination therapies are safe and effective initial antihypertensive agents and that these effects were sustained at 6–12 months.[5] Although LDC therapy was associated with higher rates of giddiness, the need for treatment withdrawal due to adverse effects was similar between LDC pill therapy, monotherapy or usual care, and placebo.

These studies unveiled a new concept of "autotitration", that is, a much larger BP reduction is achieved with the same initial dose of LDC among individuals with a higher baseline BP, compared to individuals with only mildly elevated BP.[18] Three or four different drug classes combined as LDCs exhibit enhanced BP-reducing effect with a small increase in the rate of adverse events as the BP-lowering effects of different drug classes are synergistic and most of these drugs produce therapeutic effects at low doses, and the adverse effects are directly proportional to the doses of the individual drug components.[6]

These studies reveal that starting with LDC therapy compared to an initial monotherapy achieves 1.5 times higher rates of target BP.[6] LDC proved to be superior with 80% of patients achieving target BP compared to 65% of patients achieving target BP in the usual care

TABLE 2: Randomized controlled trials (RCTs) comparing low-dose combinations (LDCs) with placebo, monotherapy, and usual care of management.

Trial	Year	No. of patients	LDC pill	Comparator	Baseline BP (mm Hg)	Duration of follow-up
TRIUMPH[22]	2018	700	Telmisartan 20 mg, amlodipine 2.5 mg, and chlorthalidone 6.25 mg	Usual care	154/90	6 months
QUARTET[23]	2021	591	Irbesartan 37.5 mg, amlodipine 1.25 mg, indapamide 0.625 mg, and bisoprolol 2.5 mg	Irbesartan 150 mg	152/88	12 months
Mahmud and Feely[24]	2007	108	Amlodipine 1.25 mg, atenolol 12.5 mg, bendroflumethiazide 0.625 mg, and captopril 12.5 mg	Amlodipine 5 mg, atenolol 50 mg, bendroflumethiazide 2.5 mg, or captopril 100 mg	160/96	4 weeks
Hong et al.[25]	2020	238	Losartan 25 mg, amlodipine 5 mg, and chlorthalicone 6.25 mg	Amlodipine 5 or 10 mg, losartan 100 mg, and placebo	154/91	8 weeks
Chow et al.[26]	2017	21	• Irbesartan 37.5 mg, amlodipine 1.25 mg, hydrochlorothiazide 6.25 mg, and atenolol 12.5 mg	Placebo	154/90	4 weeks
Sung et al.[27]	2022	176	Telmisartan 20 mg, amlodipine 2.5 mg, and chlorthalidone 6.25 mg	Amlodipine 5 or 10 mg, losartan 100 mg and placebo	151/92	4 weeks
Wald et al.[28]	2012	86	Amlodipine 2.5 mg, losartan 25 mg, hydrochlorothiazide 6.25 mg, and simvastatin 40 mg	Placebo	143/86	12 weeks

TABLE 3: Trends in selecting a combination therapy for hypertension.

Risk factors, hypertension-mediated organ damage (HMOD), cardiovascular disease (CVD), and chronic kidney disease (CKD)	BP (in mm Hg)			
	High-normal 130–139/80–89	Grade 1 140–159/90–99	Grade 2 160–179/100–109	Grade 3 ≥180/110
No risk factors	No therapy	Monotherapy or dual LDC	Dual LDC	Triple LDC
1 or 2 risk factors	No therapy	Dual LDC	Dual/triple LDC	Triple LDC
≥3 risk factors	Monotherapy or dual	Dual LDC	Dual/triple LDC	Triple LDC
HMOD, CKD grade 3, and diabetes mellitus	Dual LDC	Dual LDC	Dual/triple LDC	Triple LDC
Established CVD, CKD ≥4	Dual LDC	Dual LDC	Dual/triple LDC	Triple LDC

arm that involved clinician-guided treatment uptitration.[6] These findings suggest that initiating antihypertensive treatment with monotherapy or the usual physician-guided treatment intensification do not catch up with the upfront use of LDC therapy. Therefore, initial therapy with LDCs rapidly transits the patients from uncontrolled BP range to the target BP range, which is strongly associated with lesser risk of cardiovascular adverse events.[19]

Irrespective of whether LDCs were used as an initial therapy in treatment naïve patients or among those on monotherapy at baseline, the magnitude of BP reduction by LDC was similar. The findings in these studies also shed light on a previously described aspect called the Wilder's principle[20,21]—the pretreatment BP value determines post-treatment BP-lowering response. Each 10 mm Hg increase in pretreatment SBP was associated with a 6 mm Hg difference in the mean SBP post-treatment between LDC and placebo, with LDC showing an enhanced BP-lowering effect, i.e., Wald et al. reported that for each 10 mm Hg pretreatment increase in SBP, an increase in SBP reduction by 1 mm Hg and 2–3 mm Hg was observed for monotherapy and for dual and triple therapy.[21] The clinical significance attributed is that LDCs are more effective at high BP levels, compared to lower pretreatment BP levels, where they are relatively less potent.

TRENDS IN SELECTING A COMBINATION THERAPY FOR HYPERTENSION

Table 3 provides a general overview for selecting monotherapy/dual therapy or triple LDC therapy in hypertensive patients.[29]

CONCLUSION

In conclusion, initiation of antihypertensive treatment with triple or quadruple LDC therapies, comprising less than standard doses of each drug, is safe, effective, sustainable, and well tolerated. LDCs effectively achieve target BP in approximately two-thirds of patients at first follow-up visit and have shown to be superior to placebo, monotherapy and usual care that involves physician-guided uptitration of antihypertensive agents. Also, BP reduction with LDCs is proportional to pretreatment BP, with greater BP-lowering effects witnessed in patients with higher grades of hypertension compared to lower grades of hypertension.

REFERENCES

1. Mills KT, Bundy JD, Kelly TN, et al. Global Disparities of Hypertension Prevalence and Control: A Systematic Analysis of Population-Based Studies From 90 Countries. Circulation. 2016;134(6):441-50.
2. Chow CK, Teo KK, Rangarajan S, et al. Prevalence, awareness, treatment, and control of hypertension in rural and urban communities in high-, middle-, and low-income countries. JAMA. 2013;310(9):959-68.
3. Oparil S, Acelajado MC, Bakris GL, et al. Hypertension. Nat Rev Dis Primer. 2018;4:18014.
4. Pimenta E, Oparil S. Fixed combinations in the management of hypertension: patient perspectives and rationale for development and utility of the olmesartan-amlodipine combination. Vasc Health Risk Manag. 2008;4(3):653-64.
5. Wang N, Rueter P, Atkins E, et al. Efficacy and Safety of Low-Dose Triple and Quadruple Combination Pills vs Monotherapy, Usual Care, or Placebo for the Initial Management of Hypertension: A Systematic Review and Meta-analysis. JAMA Cardiol. 2023;8(6):606-11.
6. Law MR, Wald NJ, Morris JK, et al. Value of low dose combination treatment with blood pressure lowering drugs: analysis of 354 randomised trials. BMJ. 2003;326(7404):1427.
7. Burnier M. Antihypertensive Combination Treatment: State of the Art. Curr Hypertens Rep. 2015;17(7):51.
8. Wald DS, Law M, Morris JK, et al. Combination therapy versus monotherapy in reducing blood pressure: meta-analysis on 11,000 participants from 42 trials. Am J Med. 2009;122(3):290-300.
9. Rubio-Guerra AF, Castro-Serna D, Barrera CIE, et al. Current concepts in combination therapy for the treatment of hypertension: combined calcium channel blockers and RAAS inhibitors. Integr Blood Press Control. 2009;2:55-62.
10. Bakris GL. Combined therapy with a calcium channel blocker and an angiotensin II type 1 receptor blocker. J Clin Hypertens Greenwich Conn. 2008;10(1 Suppl 1):27-32.
11. Gradman AH, Parisé H, Lefebvre P, et al. Initial combination therapy reduces the risk of cardiovascular events in hypertensive patients: a matched cohort study. Hypertension. 2013;61(2):309-18.
12. Egan BM, Bandyopadhyay D, Shaftman SR, et al. Initial monotherapy and combination therapy and hypertension control the first year. Hypertension. 2012;59(6):1124-31.
13. Doumas M, Tsioufis C, Fletcher R, et al. Time in Therapeutic Range, as a Determinant of All-Cause Mortality in Patients With Hypertension. J Am Heart Assoc. 2017;6(11):e007131.
14. Mancia G, Rea F, Corrao G, et al. Two-Drug Combinations as First-Step Antihypertensive Treatment. Circ Res. 2019;124(7):1113-23.
15. Goldacre MJ, Roberts SE, Yeates D. Mortality after admission to hospital with fractured neck of femur: database study. BMJ. 2002;325(7369):868-9.
16. Corrao G, Mazzola P, Monzio Compagnoni M, et al. Antihypertensive Medications, Loop Diuretics, and Risk of Hip Fracture in the Elderly: A Population-Based Cohort Study of 81,617 Italian Patients Newly Treated Between 2005 and 2009. Drugs Aging. 2015;32(11):927-36.
17. European Society of Cardiology. A single tablet with 4 blood pressure-lowering drugs can be more effective than taking 3 drugs in separate pills. [online] Available from https://www.escardio.org/The-ESC/Press-Office/Press-releases/A-single-tablet-with-4-blood-pressure-lowering-drugs-can-be-more-effective-than-taking-3-drugs-in-separate-pills [Last accessed November, 2025].
18. Wang N, Rueter P, Salam A, et al. Low-Dose Combinations With 3 or 4 Blood Pressure-Lowering Medications for the Treatment of Hypertension. JACC Adv. 2025;4(7):101883.
19. Gnanenthiran SR, Wang N, Di Tanna GL, et al. Association of Low-Dose Triple Combination Therapy vs Usual Care With Time at Target Blood Pressure: A Secondary Analysis of the TRIUMPH Randomized Clinical Trial. JAMA Cardiol. 2022;7(6):645-50.
20. Messerli FH, Bangalore S, Schmieder RE. Wilder's principle: pre-treatment value determines post-treatment response. Eur Heart J. 2015;36(9):576-9.
21. Law MR, Morris JK, Wald NJ. Use of blood pressure lowering drugs in the prevention of cardiovascular disease: meta-analysis of 147 randomised trials

in the context of expectations from prospective epidemiological studies. BMJ. 2009;338:b1665.
22. Webster R, Salam A, de Silva HA, et al. Fixed Low-Dose Triple Combination Antihypertensive Medication vs Usual Care for Blood Pressure Control in Patients With Mild to Moderate Hypertension in Sri Lanka: A Randomized Clinical Trial. JAMA. 2018;320(6):566-79.
23. Chow CK, Atkins ER, Hillis GS, et al. Initial treatment with a single pill containing quadruple combination of quarter doses of blood pressure medicines versus standard dose monotherapy in patients with hypertension (QUARTET): a phase 3, randomised, double-blind, active-controlled trial. Lancet Lond Engl. 2021;398(10305):1043-52.
24. Mahmud A, Feely J. Low-dose quadruple antihypertensive combination: more efficacious than individual agents--a preliminary report. Hypertension. 2007;49(2):272-5.
25. Hong SJ, Sung KC, Lim SW, et al. Low-Dose Triple Antihypertensive Combination Therapy in Patients with Hypertension: A Randomized, Double-Blind, Phase II Study. Drug Des Devel Ther. 2020;14:5735-46.
26. Chow CK, Thakkar J, Bennett A, et al. Quarter-dose quadruple combination therapy for initial treatment of hypertension: placebo-controlled, crossover, randomised trial and systematic review. Lancet. 2017;389(10073):1035-42.
27. Sung KC, Sung JH, Cho EJ, et al. Efficacy and safety of low-dose antihypertensive combination of amlodipine, telmisartan, and chlorthalidone: A randomized, double-blind, parallel, phase II trial. J Clin Hypertens. 2022;24(10):1298-309.
28. Wald DS, Morris JK, Wald NJ. Randomized Polypill Crossover Trial in People Aged 50 and Over. PLOS ONE. 2012;7(7):e41297.
29. Rosas-Peralta M, Mancia G, Camafort M, et al. Single pill combination therapy for hypertension: New evidence and new challenges: Combination Therapy for Hypertension. Trends Cardiovasc Med. 2025;S1050-1738(25)00082-9.

Cuffless Blood Pressure Measurement Devices: How Accurate and Feasible?

CHAPTER 9

Akhilesh Kumar, Suman Bhandari

INTRODUCTION

Hypertension is a leading global health issue, affecting over a billion individuals and serving as a major risk factor for cardiovascular disease, stroke, and early mortality. Despite advancements in antihypertensive therapies and diagnostic methods, effective BP control remains a challenge worldwide. One contributing factor is the limitation of current BP monitoring techniques, which often fail to provide continuous or patient-friendly assessment.

Traditional BP measurement relies on cuff-based devices, such as office-based sphygmomanometers and ambulatory blood pressure monitoring (ABPM). ABPM, considered the clinical gold standard for out-of-office assessment, provides valuable data on circadian BP variability and nocturnal hypertension. However, the discomfort caused by repeated cuff inflations, limited mobility, and unsuitability for long-term use reduce patient compliance and the ability to monitor BP during daily activities or sleep. To overcome these challenges, significant interest has developed in cuffless blood pressure monitoring technologies, which estimate BP using physiological signals such as photoplethysmography (PPG), electrocardiography (ECG), tonometry, and bioimpedance. These methods, often supported by advanced machine learning algorithms, offer the potential for noninvasive, continuous, and user-friendly BP tracking, enabling better integration into daily life and proactive hypertension management.

Despite promising innovations, clinical adoption of cuffless BP devices is limited due to concerns about accuracy, calibration requirements, sensitivity to motion and physiological variability, and the lack of standardized validation protocols. Additionally, regulatory hurdles remain a significant barrier. This chapter aims to summarize the current state of cuffless BP monitoring technologies, outlining their principles, applications, limitations, and future role in the management of hypertension.

CUFFLESS BLOOD PRESSURE TECHNOLOGIES

Cuffless BP technologies are categorized as requiring individual user cuff calibration or not. Those requiring user calibration need each individual user to firstly take a self-measurement of BP using a classic upper-arm cuff-BP device, which is entered into the monitor before use. This calibration procedure is usually repeated periodically (e.g., every day, few weeks, or months). Some cuffless devices are calibrated by entering simple demographic data (e.g., age, sex, and body size), which are well known to correlate with BP, yet these are less reliable. Other technologies do not require calibration by user. Main technologies are summarized in **Table 1** and **Figure 1**.

CUFFLESS BLOOD PRESSURE DEVICES

The Food and Drug Administration (FDA) has granted approval to various cuffless blood pressure monitoring devices that utilize techniques such as pulse arrival time (PAT), pulse compression

TABLE 1: Cuffless blood pressure technologies.

Technique	Definition	Example (device or study)
Pulse transit time (PTT)/ pulse arrival time (PAT)	PTT is the time taken by the pulse wave to travel between two arterial sites, typically from the heart (ECG R-wave) to a peripheral site (PPG sensor). BP is inversely related to PTT. PAT includes preejection period, so it is slightly longer[1]	Biobeat (wearable chest sensor), Samsung Galaxy Watch (PAT-based, calibrated with cuff)
Photoplethysmography (PPG)	An optical method that detects blood volume changes in the microvascular bed using infrared or green light; BP is estimated from waveform features such as slope, amplitude, and area[2]	Fitbit Sense, Apple Watch (under research; BP estimation from PPG), Aktiia Bracelet
Applanation tonometry	A pressure sensor flattens a superficial artery (e.g., radial) against bone to measure waveform pressure without occluding it; requires steady positioning[3]	AtCor Medical's SphygmoCor device (clinical-grade tonometer)
Ultrasound-based measurement	Uses Doppler ultrasound to measure blood velocity or arterial wall displacement; changes correlate with BP; mostly used in research or specialized settings[4]	Uscom BP+, SonoPatch (research prototype)
Bioimpedance (electrical impedance plethysmography)	Measures impedance changes in tissue as blood volume changes during each cardiac cycle; used to estimate BP indirectly[5]	Zio patch (ECG, bioimpedance), Impli's embedded biosensors (under development)
Machine learning algorithms	AI models trained on ECG, PPG, accelerometer data, age, gender, etc. to estimate BP; works in background with multiple inputs[6]	BPro+ Watch, Valencell's BP technology, Omron HeartGuide (uses hybrid ML + PPG model)
Ballistocardiography (BCG)	Measures tiny movements of the body caused by cardiac ejection of blood; typically embedded in beds, chairs, or smart scales[7]	Withings Body Cardio Scale, Emfit QS sleep sensor

method (PCM), and arterial tonometry. The earliest approved model was based on tonometry, which estimates blood pressure by sensing arterial pressure directly from the radial artery. However, locating the precise measurement point on the artery remains a significant challenge. To address this, devices often use a sensor array placed on the forearm to identify the highest pressure reading, which corresponds to the arterial site. The Accurate 24 system, for example, employs ultrasound imaging to accurately locate the radial artery. For overnight blood pressure monitoring, the ViSi system is commonly used. This system requires calibration with a traditional cuff-based sphygmomanometer before and after data collection to ensure reliable readings. CareTaker's VitalStream monitor features a finger sensor and interface, where light pressure (around 2–3 mm Hg) is applied to the finger to reduce motion artifacts and enable continuous BP measurement.

Biobeat introduced the first smartwatch-style cuffless BP monitor, alongside a patch-based version. However, the smartwatch format is particularly susceptible to movement-related errors and is less suited for prolonged monitoring. In addition, a smart shirt version was developed, which records both ECG and PPG signals. For accurate measurements, this wearable must fit snugly against the body. Recent cuffless devices are summarized in **Table 2** and **Figures 2A to K**.

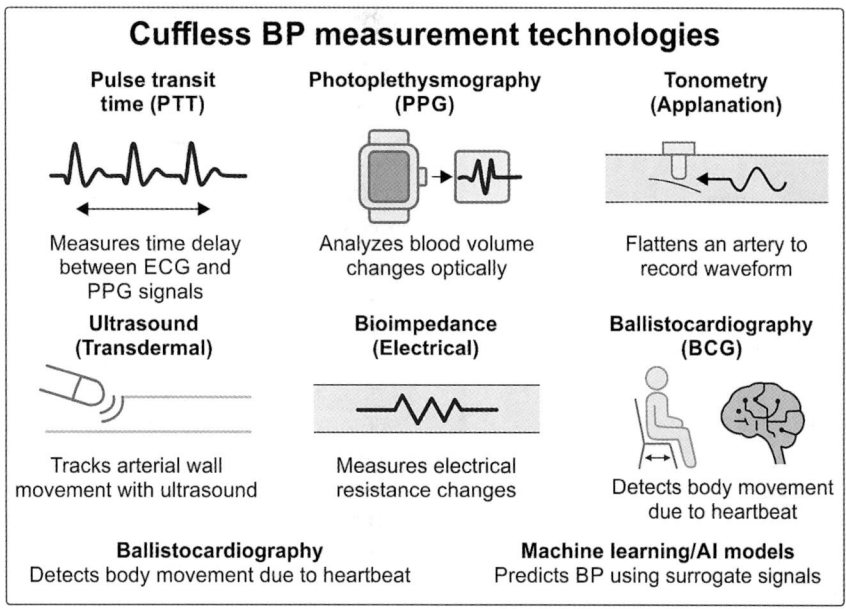

Fig. 1: Different measurement techniques.

TABLE 2: Cuffless BP devices.

Device name	Requires cuff calibration?	BP measurement method	Regulatory status	Notes
Biobeat[8] BB-613 Wrist Watch	✗ No	PPG-based (wrist/patch)	✗ FDA 510(k), CE	True cuffless BP; clinically validated
Valencell PPG Sensor[9]	✗ No	PPG-only (finger sensor)	– Research phase	Calibration-free; strong performance in trials
Leman e-Checkup[10]	✗ No	Camera + pulse waveform	– Not yet approved	ISO-compliant trial data, not yet commercial
Samsung Galaxy Watch[11] (4/5)	✓ Yes	PPG-based with app calibration	✗ Not FDA-approved	Requires recalibration every 4 weeks
Huawei Watch GT Series[12]	✓ Yes	PPG-based estimation	✗ No regulatory approval	Manual calibration with cuff required
Aktiia Bracelet[13]	✓ Yes	PPG (optical sensors)	✓ CE-marked (Europe)	Requires cuff calibration every few weeks
Checkme (Viatom)[14]	✓ Yes	ECG + PPG (PTT-based)	✓ FDA 510(k)	Periodic cuff calibration required
Maisense Freescan[15]	✓ Yes	ECG + PPG	✓ CE-certified	Validated via ANSI/AAMI/ISO 81060-2
ViSi Mobile Sensor[16]	✓ Yes	PAT based on ECG-r PPG	✓ FDA 510(k)	PAT with ECG lead on chest and PPG on wrist
BPro[17]	✓ Yes	Applanation tonometry	✓ FDA 510(k)	Applanation tonometry at wrist
Apple Watch[18]	✓ (External cuff needed)	No built-in BP measurement	✓ If paired with FDA cuff	Tracks BP via bluetooth cuffs like QardioArm, Omron Evolv

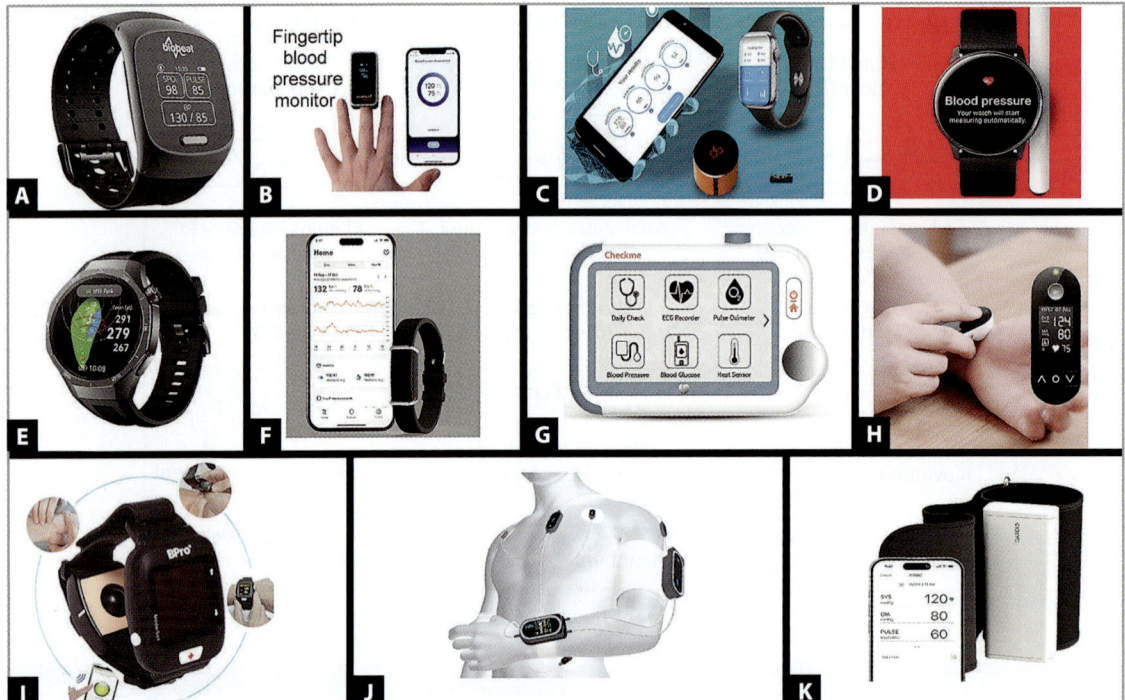

Figs. 2A to K: Cuffless BP measurement devices: (A) Biobeat; (B) Valencell; (C) Leman e-Checkup; (D) Samsung Galaxy Watch; (E) Huawei Watch GT Series; (F) Aktiia bracelet; (G) Checkme (Viatom); (H) Maisense Freescan; (I) BPro; (J) ViSi Mobile Sensor; and (K) QardioArm for Apple Watch.

■ VALIDATION

The US FDA utilizes the 510(k) clearance process to determine whether a new medical device is substantially equivalent to one already available on the US market. This process does not represent formal approval of the device, nor does it verify its clinical accuracy.

The first among these was the ViSi Mobile System[19] by Sotera Wireless (soterawireless.com), which received clearance in 2012 [510(k) number K112478]. It provides continuous BP monitoring through a combination of ECG and PPG signals, gathered via multiple chest electrodes and a wrist sensor—eliminating the need for a finger strap. The CareTaker device[20] from CareTaker Medical, LLC (caretakermedical.net), cleared in 2017 (K163255), monitors BP continuously using pulse wave analysis (PWA) from the finger, in conjunction with a wrist strap.

In 2018, the BPro system developed by Med Tach Inc. (medtach.com) received clearance (K173028). It employs applanation tonometry at the wrist and requires a finger strap to ensure proper sensor contact. The Biobeat monitor,[21] developed by Biobeat Technologies Ltd. (biobeat.com), gained clearance in 2019 (K190792). It continuously estimates BP through PPG-based measurements, using a wrist-worn or chest-mounted sensor, and does not need a finger strap. Notably, all of these devices depend on initial calibration with a standard cuff-based brachial BP measurement to ensure their accuracy before clinical or personal use. The Institute of Electrical and Electronics Engineers validation standards recommend using a cutoff of <7 mm Hg for the mean absolute difference between test and reference devices.[22]

A systematic review and meta-analysis from 2022 evaluated validation protocols of 15 cuffless devices; 12 of the 16 studies included in the analysis reported mean absolute difference data.[1] Results revealed no statistically significant differences between the wearable cuffless and reference devices, with a pooled mean difference of 3.42 mm Hg SBP (95% CI: −2.17–9.01 mm Hg) and 1.16 mm Hg DBP (95% CI: −1.26–3.58 mm Hg).[23] Although these data are promising, the use of cuffless devices risks the underestimation or overestimation of BP due to the marked heterogeneity in the devices being tested. These limitations must be overcome before cuffless devices can be recommended for clinical use.

In 2022, the International Organization for Standardization published a validation protocol (ISO 81060-3:2022) for "continuous noninvasive sphygmomanometers" that could be used for cuffless BP devices that continuously measure BP but may not be appropriate for outpatient use. In 2023, the European Society of Hypertension Working Group on BP Monitoring and Cardiovascular Variability recommended procedures for validating intermittent cuffless BP devices.[24] Scarce data exist on using these protocols to test cuffless BP devices.

■ CURRENT STATUS

Continued studies are needed in the realm of accurate wearable and cuffless devices to provide near-accurate blood pressure. At present, cuffless blood pressure monitoring remains an exciting but evolving field. A wide range of devices, from wristbands and rings to chest patches and smartphone-based sensors, have demonstrated feasibility in estimating blood pressure using approaches such as PWA, PAT, and multimodal signal integration. Some have even achieved

TABLE 3: ACC/AHA 2025 Recommendation

Recommendation	Class	Level
In adults, the use of cuffless BP devices is not recommended for the diagnosis or management of high BP	III	C-LD

regulatory clearance, highlighting progress toward clinical translation. Yet, their accuracy is still constrained by the need for individual calibration, susceptibility to physiological variability, and the absence of universally accepted validation standards. Consequently, while these technologies cannot yet replace cuff-based methods in routine clinical decision-making, they are steadily advancing toward greater reliability and usability. Continued efforts to refine calibration-free approaches, establish robust validation protocols, and demonstrate real-world clinical value will be critical in determining whether cuffless monitoring can fulfil its promise of transforming hypertension detection and management.

AS per 2025 AHA/ACC Joint Committee on Clinical Practice Guidelines for hypertension, in adults, cuffless blood pressure devices should *not* be used for diagnosing or managing hypertension **(Table 3)**.[22]

■ CONCLUSION

While cuffless blood pressure monitoring devices hold immense promise for enhancing accessibility, comfort, and continuous cardiovascular assessment, their clinical accuracy and reliability remain under scrutiny. Until robust validation standards are established and calibration-free solutions mature, these devices should be viewed as complementary tools rather than replacements for conventional cuff-based methods. Continued innovation, coupled with rigorous clinical evaluation, will ultimately determine whether cuffless technologies can transition from experimental promise to a trusted component of routine hypertension care.

■ REFERENCES

1. Finnegan E, Davidson S, Harford M, et al. Pulse arrival time as a surrogate of blood pressure. Sci Rep. 2021;11:22767.
2. Park J, Seok HS, Kim SS, et al. Photoplethysmogram Analysis and Applications: An Integrative Review. Front Physiol. 2022;12:808451.
3. Zhang Q, Zhang N, Kang L, et al. Technology Development for Simultaneous Wearable Monitoring of Cerebral Hemodynamics and Blood Pressure. IEEE J Biomed Health Inform. 2019;23(5):1952-63.
4. Meusel M, Wegerich P, Bode B, et al. Measurement of Blood Pressure by Ultrasound-The Applicability of Devices, Algorithms and a View in Local Hemodynamics. Diagnostics (Basel). 2021;11(12):2255.
5. Horinaka S, Sakuma M, Yonezawa Y, et al. Usefulness of Blood Flow Measurement Device Using Bioelectrical Impedance Plethysmography in Lower-Extremity Artery Disease. Circ Rep. 2025;7(2):113-21.
6. Erick Martinez-Ríos, Luis Montesinos, Mariel Alfaro-Ponce, et al. A review of machine learning in hypertension detection and blood pressure estimation based on clinical and physiological data. Biomed Signal Process Control. 2021; 68:102813.
7. Etemadi M, Inan OT. Wearable ballistocardiogram and seismocardiogram systems for health and performance. J Appl Physiol (1985). 2018;124(2): 452-61.
8. Nachman D, Gepner Y, Goldstein N, et al. Comparing blood pressure measurements between a photoplethysmography-based and a standard cuff-based manometry device. Sci Rep. 2020;10:16116.
9. Valencell Inc. (2021). Valencell Launched the World's First Calibration-Free Blood Pressure Sensor System for Hearables and Wearables Powered by Ambiq Edge AI. [online] Available from https://ambiq.com/news/valencell-launched-the-worlds-first-calibration-free-blood-pressure-sensor-system-for-hearables-and-wearables-powered-by-ambiq-micro-edge-ai/ [Last accessed November, 2025].
10. Steinman J, Barszczyk A, Sun HS, et al. Smartphones and Video Cameras: Future Methods for Blood Pressure Measurement. Front Digit Health. 2021;3:770096.
11. Samsung Electronics. How to calibrate blood pressure on Samsung Watch. [online] Available from https://www.samsung.com/uk/support/apps-services/how-do-i-recalibrate-the-galaxy-watch/ [Last accessed November, 2025].
12. Huawei Consumer. Blood pressure on Watch GT 4. [online] Available from https://consumer.huawei.com/en/community/details/Blood-pressure-on-watch-gt-4/topicId_197957/ [Last accessed November, 2025].
13. Shcherbina A, Mattsson C, Wuerzner G, et al. Validation of the cuffless optical Aktiia bracelet for blood pressure measurement according to ISO 81060-2. J Hypertens. 2021;39(Suppl 1):e372.
14. US Food and Drug Administration. (2025). 510(k) Premarket Notification: Checkme Pro Health Monitor (K193348). [online] Available from https://www.accessdata.fda.gov/scripts/cdrh/cfdocs/cfpmn/pmn.cfm?ID=K193348 [Last accessed November, 2025].
15. Chuang SY, Chen CH, Cheng HM, et al. Clinical validation of a novel cuffless blood pressure monitoring device (Freescan) using photoplethysmography. J Hypertens. 2017; 35(5):981-8.
16. US Food and Drug Administration. (2012). 510(k) Premarket Notification: ViSi Mobile Monitoring System (K112064). [online] Available from https://www.accessdata.fda.gov/cdrh_docs/pdf11/K112064.pdf [Last accessed November, 2025].
17. Williams B, Lacy PS, Yan P, et al. Development and validation of the BPro continuous ambulatory blood pressure monitor. J Hypertens. 2011; 29(12):2381-9.
18. Mazoteras-Pardo V, et al. QardioArm Upper Arm Blood Pressure Monitor Against Omron M3 Upper Arm Blood Pressure Monitor in Patients With Chronic Kidney Disease: A Validation Study According to the European Society of Hypertension International Protocol Revision 2010. J Med Internet Res. 2019 Dec

2;21(12):e14686. doi: 10.2196/14686. PMID: 31789600; PMCID: PMC6915457
19. Sotera Wireless, Inc. (2013). 510(k) Premarket Notification: ViSi Mobile Monitoring System (K130709). [online] Available from https://www.accessdata.fda.gov/cdrh_docs/pdf13/K130709.pdf [Last accessed November, 2025].
20. CareTaker Medical, LLC. (2017). 510(k) Premarket Notification: CareTaker cardiovascular monitoring device (K163255). [online] Available from https://www.accessdata.fda.gov/cdrh_docs/pdf16/K163255.pdf [Last accessed November, 2025].
21. US Food and Drug Administration. (2025). 510(k) Premarket Notification: BB-613WP and BB-613-BPM. [online] Available from https://www.accessdata.fda.gov/cdrh_docs/pdf24/K241066.pdf [Last accessed November, 2025].
22. Jones DW, Ferdinand KC, Taler SJ, et al. 2025 AHA/ACC/AANP/AAPA/ABC/ACCP/ACPM/AGS/AMA/ASPC/NMA/PCNA/SGIM guideline for the prevention, detection, evaluation and management of high blood pressure in adults: A report of the American College of Cardiology/American Heart Association Joint Committee on Clinical Practice Guidelines. Circulation. 2025;152(11):e114-e218.
23. Islam SMS, Chow CK, Daryabeygikhotbehsara R, et al. Wearable cuffless blood pressure monitoring devices: a systematic review and meta-analysis. Eur Heart J Digit Health. 2022;3(2):323-37.
24. Hu JR, Martin G, Iyengar S, et al. Validating cuffless continuous blood pressure monitoring devices. Cardiovasc Digit Health J. 2023;4(1):9-20.

CHAPTER 10

Dual Antiplatelet Therapy: Newer Direction in 2025

Mrinal Kanti Das

■ INTRODUCTION

Coronary artery disease (CAD) is a leading cause of global morbidity and mortality. The central role of platelet aggregation in acute coronary syndromes (ACS) and stent thrombosis mandates effective antiplatelet protection. For over a decade, the standard of care has been dual antiplatelet therapy (DAPT). However, the balance between preventing ischemic events (e.g., stent thrombosis, MI, and stroke) and avoiding bleeding complications has been a constant clinical challenge.[1,2] The disease may be affected by atherosclerotic plaque formation leading to coronary artery stenosis or obstruction with symptoms, a condition known as chronic coronary syndrome (CCS). But under the influence of various risk and stress factors, the arteries may get occluded via the mechanism of thrombogenesis. Platelets play an important role in the latter phenomenon where their activation and aggregation result in clot formation. Initially, it is white thrombus devoid of any red corpuscles which when attracted toward the activated and aggregated platelets form the red thrombus bound by the fibrin. With the onset of thrombogenesis, the various manifestations appear in the form of ACS, either as unstable angina, non-ST elevation myocardial infarction (NSTEMI) or ST elevation myocardial infarction (STEMI) depending the area of luminal obstruction. **Figure 1** depicts the various mechanisms of platelet activity and their interventions. DAPT, combining aspirin with a P2Y$_{12}$ inhibitor, remains a cornerstone in managing CAD, including ACS and chronic CAD. Though the journey started long time back, but since 2020, multiple landmark trials have refined DAPT strategies, focusing on personalized duration, newer antiplatelet agents, and balancing ischemic versus bleeding risks. The year 2025 represents a maturation of the shift from empirical, duration-focused protocols to dynamic, patient-tailored algorithms powered by better risk scores, genetic testing, and new drug options.[3] This review summarizes the various thoughts from the different key trials, which should stand as the platform for the new directions in 2025 and subsequent years.

■ STANDARD ANTITHROMBOTIC THERAPY AFTER PERCUTANEOUS CORONARY INTERVENTION

The goal of antithrombotic therapy after percutaneous coronary intervention (PCI) is to prevent both *stent thrombosis* and *atherothrombotic events* (like a heart attack or stroke), while minimizing the risk of bleeding.[1,2] The standard therapy is *DAPT*, which combines aspirin with a P2Y12 inhibitor.

- *Aspirin:* Irreversibly inhibits cyclooxygenase (COX-1), preventing the formation of thromboxane A2, a potent platelet activator.
- *P2Y12 inhibitors:* Block the P2Y12 receptor on platelets, preventing their activation and aggregation. The three main inhibitors are:
  1. *Clopidogrel:* A less potent P2Y12 inhibitor
  2. *Ticagrelor:* A more potent, reversible P2Y12 inhibitor
  3. *Prasugrel:* A more potent, irreversible P2Y12 inhibitor.

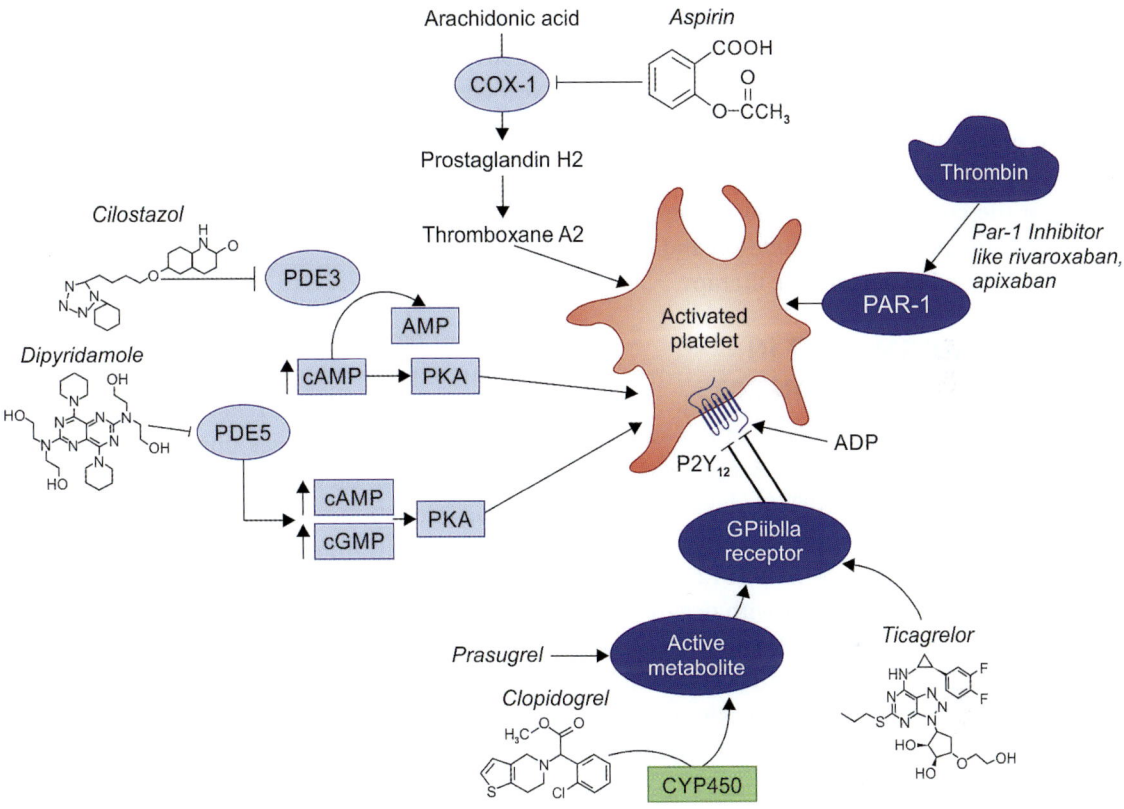

Fig. 1: Mechanisms of antiplatelet activity.

The choice and duration of DAPT depend on the patient's clinical presentation (acute vs. CCS) and their individual risk profile for both ischemic events and bleeding.

ESC AND ACC GUIDELINES FOR DUAL ANTIPLATELET THERAPY DURATION[3,4]

- *Acute coronary syndrome:*
  - *Standard recommendation:* DAPT (aspirin plus a potent P2Y12 inhibitor like ticagrelor or prasugrel) is recommended for 12 months.
  - *Rationale:* Patients with ACS have a higher risk of stent thrombosis and recurrent ischemic events, justifying a longer and more potent antiplatelet regimen.
  - *High bleeding risk (HBR):* In patients with an HBR, a shorter DAPT duration (e.g., 3–6 months) followed by P2Y12 inhibitor monotherapy can be considered.
- *Chronic coronary syndrome:*
  - *Standard recommendation:* DAPT (aspirin plus clopidogrel) is typically recommended for 6 months.
  - *Rationale:* The risk of stent thrombosis is lower in stable patients, allowing for a shorter duration to reduce bleeding risk.
  - *High ischemic risk:* In select patients with high ischemic risk and low bleeding risk, DAPT may be extended beyond 6 months.

THE JOURNEY FROM CLOPIDOGREL TO PRASUGREL/TICAGRELOR

The journey began with the move from clopidogrel to more potent P2Y12 inhibitors (prasugrel and ticagrelor), which significantly reduced ischemic events at the cost of increased bleeding.[5,6] This established the potency-risk trade-off and set the stage for the need to personalize therapy.

THE PARADIGM SHIFT IN ABBREVIATED DAPT IN 2025

A major trend solidified by 2025 is the strategy of shorter-duration DAPT (1–3 months) and ultra-short duration of DAPT (4 days followed by SAPT initially ticagrelor followed by clopidogrel) with subsequent P2Y12 inhibitor monotherapy (most commonly with ticagrelor or clopidogrel) in patients at HBR. Landmark trials such as TWILIGHT, TICO, and STOPDAPT-2 demonstrated that this strategy significantly reduces major bleeding without a significant increase in ischemic events, especially in patients with high-risk clinical features or complex PCI who received newer-generation drug-eluting stents (DES).[7-9] The recent and latest trials including *DUAL-ACS, NEO-MINDSET, TARGET FIRST and TAILORED-CHIP*[10-13] are constantly evolving the antiplatelet and antithrombotic strategy, and challenging and refining established practices.

Early withdrawal of aspirin following successful PCI for ACS and in low-risk patients following an acute myocardial infarction (MI) was the focus of two separate hot line trials presented at ESC Congress 2025. A third trial provided insights into early escalation and late de-escalation of antiplatelet therapy after complex PCI.

DUAL-ACS trial: Findings from the *trial* presented suggest that 3 months of DAPT following an acute MI has the potential for better survival and lower bleeding rates compared with 12 months of DAPT.

Researchers randomized approximately 5,000 patients from Scotland, England, and New Zealand to either 3 months or 12 months of DAPT. The real-world population of patients had experienced a type 1 MI within 12 weeks and had been treated with stents, bypass grafting, or medical therapy alone.

After a 15-month follow-up period, the primary endpoint of all-cause mortality occurred in 2.7% of patients assigned to 3-month DAPT compared with 3.4% of patients assigned to 12-month DAPT. No difference in cardiovascular death or nonfatal MI was observed. Fatal and nonfatal major bleeding occurred in 3.2% of patients in the 3-month DAPT group and 4.0% of patients in the 12-month DAPT group.

This all-comer real-world trial recruited only 30% of the planned participants and was unable to address the primary question definitively. However, there was no evidence that DAPT given for 12 months conferred any additional benefit. Indeed, the trends for lower mortality and bleeding risk with 3 months of DAPT are consistent with prior meta-analyses and suggest that limiting DAPT duration to 3 months may be safer in a real-world contemporary population.

In the *NEO-MINDSET trial (Ultra short DAPT trial)*, researchers in Brazil randomized patients with ACS who had undergone successful PCI, approximately 3,410 patients in the intention-to-treat population (1,712 in the monotherapy group and 1,698 in the DAPT group) within the first 4 days of hospitalization following a successful PCI to either stop treatment with aspirin and receive potent P2Y12 inhibitor monotherapy (ticagrelor or prasugrel) or to receive DAPT that included aspirin and a potent P2Y12 inhibitor for 12 months.

At 12 months, the primary endpoint of death from any cause, MI, stroke or urgent revascularization had occurred in 119 patients in the monotherapy group and in 93 patients in the DAPT group ($p = 0.11$ for noninferiority). Researchers also noted that major or clinically relevant nonmajor bleeding occurred in 33 patients assigned to monotherapy versus 82 patients assigned to DAPT. Stent thrombosis occurred in 12 patients in the monotherapy group and in 4 in the DAPT group.

Trial with P2Y12 inhibitor monotherapy early (*within 4 days of PCI*) and continuing for 12 months in ACS patients *failed to demonstrate noninferiority* of P2Y12 inhibitor monotherapy versus DAPT for death and ischemic events. This reinforces the importance of an initial, more intensive period of DAPT in high-risk ACS patients. Results suggested that the excess ischemic risk with monotherapy occurred in the first 30 days, with comparable outcomes thereafter. Bleeding appeared to be lower at both 30 days and 12 months with monotherapy versus DAPT.

In *TARGET-FIRST, P2Y12-inhibitor monotherapy was noninferior to continued DAPT* with respect to the occurrence of adverse cardiovascular and cerebrovascular events among low-risk patients with acute MI who had undergone early complete revascularization and had completed *1 month of DAPT* without complications. It also resulted in lower incidence of bleeding events.

Nearly 2,000 patients from 40 centers in Europe were randomized to receive P2Y12-inhibitor monotherapy or to continue DAPT for 11 months. A primary-outcome event occurred in 20 patients (2.1%) in the P2Y12-inhibitor monotherapy group and in 21 patients (2.2%) in the DAPT group ($p = 0.02$ for noninferiority). Major bleeding occurred in 2.6% of the patients assigned to P2Y12-inhibitor monotherapy group compared with 5.6% of those assigned to DAPT ($p = 0.002$ for superiority). The incidence of stent thrombosis and serious adverse events appeared to be similar in the two groups, researchers said.

It was noted that no previous randomized trials assessed early aspirin discontinuation in acute MI patients who achieve early, complete revascularization with modern stents. The present trial results reflect the benefits of modern stents, high procedural success and optimal medical therapy, making early aspirin discontinuation feasible in this selected population.

The *TAILORED-CHIP trial* found early escalation and late de-escalation of antiplatelet therapy is *not beneficial in patients with high-risk anatomical or clinical characteristics undergoing complex PCI.*

South Korean workers randomized approximately 2,000 patients to standard DAPT (clopidogrel plus aspirin for 12 months) or a tailored antiplatelet strategy consisting of early escalation (low-dose ticagrelor at 60 mg twice daily plus aspirin for 6 months) followed by late de-escalation (clopidogrel monotherapy for 6 months).

Overall findings showed no significant difference in the incidence of major ischemic events at 12 months with tailored therapy compared with standard DAPT. However, the incidence of clinically relevant bleeding was significantly higher with tailored therapy, according to study investigators who suggested that a tailored strategy in patients undergoing complex high-risk PCI does not provide a net clinical benefit, as they observed an increase in bleeding complications without a significant reduction in ischemic events. This challenges the notion that "more is better" even in carefully selected patients at high ischemic risk.

Key suggestions for 2025 were abbreviated DAPT (1–3 months) → P2Y12 inhibitor monotherapy as the default strategy for a large majority of patients undergoing PCI, particularly those meeting HBR criteria. The present guideline, however, still recommends 12-month default strategy.

PRECISION MEDICINE: GENOTYPE-GUIDED DE-ESCALATION

A pivotal newer direction is the use of point-of-care genetic testing to identify patients with loss-of-function (LOF) alleles of the *CYP2C19* gene, which confers reduced clopidogrel efficacy. For patients diagnosed with ACS, trials such as *POPular Genetics and TAILOR-PCI* have shown that a genotype-guided strategy—where CYP2C19 LOF carriers are prescribed ticagrelor/prasugrel, while noncarriers are de-escalated to clopidogrel—results in non-inferior ischemic outcomes with significantly lower bleeding rates compared to uniform potent DAPT.[14,15]

CYP2C19-guided DAPT (avoiding clopidogrel in poor metabolizers) reduced cardiovascular events as per *POPular Genetics study*.

PRECISE-DAPT & DAPT Score (for validation) showed better risk stratification for bleeding/thrombosis, aiding in DAPT duration decisions.[16,17]

Key suggestions for 2025: CYP2C19 genotyping in ACS patients should become a standard of care in many centers to guide the initial selection of P2Y12 inhibitor, optimizing the efficacy-safety profile.

THE "ESCALATION" STRATEGY: CILOSTAZOL-BASED TRIPLE THERAPY

While de-escalation dominates, there remains a small, select group of patients at exceptionally high ischemic risk (e.g., complex left main PCI, prior stent thrombosis on DAPT, and diabetes with diffuse disease) and low bleeding risk. For these patients, intensification beyond standard DAPT is considered. The registry data of 2020 showed the addition of cilostazol, a phosphodiesterase III inhibitor, to create triple antiplatelet therapy (TAPT) may be a strategy supported by some meta-analyses to reduce repeat revascularization, though its effect on hard endpoints like mortality is less clear, and its use is limited by side effects (headache and tachycardia).[18]

Key suggestion for 2025 that is TAPT with cilostazol is a niche but not practiced widely and may be considered option for the highest-risk ischemic patients where every tool for prevention is warranted.

ARTIFICIAL INTELLIGENCE INTEGRATION AND THE ROLE OF RISK SCORES

The decision-making process in 2025 is increasingly data driven. Validated risk scores like the DAPT Score (ischemic risk) and PRECISE-DAPT (bleeding risk) are integrated directly into electronic health records.[16,17] Furthermore, artificial intelligence (AI) algorithms are being piloted to analyze vast datasets—including clinical, angiographic, and genetic information—to provide personalized predictions *of* individual patient risk, suggesting optimal DAPT type and duration **(Table 1)**.

Key suggestion for 2025 is automated risk score calculation, and emerging AI clinical decision support tools may be essential for cardiologists to objectify and personalize DAPT plans. However, it must be remembered that use of *AI should be supported by clinical judgment as there is* no replacement for bedside evaluation.

TABLE 1: Clinical trials validating artificial intelligence (AI) in dual antiplatelet therapy (DAPT).

Trial	AI Model	Key finding
AI-ACS (2023)	PREDICT-DAPT[19]	30% fewer major bleeds versus standard care
DAPT-AI (2024)	OPTIMACS[20]	22% lower MACCE (CV death/MI/stroke)

LOOKING BEYOND 2025: NOVEL AGENTS AND CONCEPTS BASED ON NEW TRIAL FINDINGS

Reversible P2Y12 Inhibitors

Agents like *selatogrel* offer ultra-rapid onset and offset, potentially ideal for patient-administered therapy for suspected ACS onset. It is $P2Y_{12}$ inhibitor given subcutaneously. In *SOLID-TIMI 53* (2025) in prehospital ACS, selatogrel showed rapid platelet inhibition, potentially replacing oral loading in emergency settings.

In *ACS patients for bridging therapy,* cangrelor in PCI patients reduced periprocedural MI without excess major bleeding as per *CHAMPION-PHOENIX* (2024 extended follow-up) trial.[21]

Factor XI inhibitors though not antiplatelet agents, but the trials (e.g., PACIFIC-AMI) show promise for simultaneously reducing ischemic events without increasing bleeding. Their potential combination with antiplatelet therapy could redefine "dual pathway" inhibition.

Bioresorbable scaffolds should come back as technology improves. Fully bioresorbable stents that eliminate the permanent metallic nidus for thrombosis could eventually obviate the need for prolonged DAPT.

BALANCING ANTIPLATELET AND ANTICOAGULANT THERAPY

A major challenge arises when a patient undergoing PCI also requires chronic oral anticoagulation (OAC), most commonly for *atrial fibrillation (AF)*. The combination of antiplatelet and anticoagulant agents significantly increases the risk of bleeding.

Traditional Strategy: Triple Therapy

The historical approach was *triple therapy* (aspirin + P2Y12 inhibitor + OAC). This was often associated with high rates of major bleeding. Current guidelines and trial data have led to a de-escalation strategy.

Current Recommendations for Double Therapy

Based on landmark trials such as *PIONEER AF-PCI, RE-DUAL PCI*, and *AUGUSTUS*, the current standard of care is to use *double therapy* (a P2Y12 inhibitor plus OAC) for a limited duration, avoiding aspirin.[22-24]

Initiation: For patients requiring an OAC who undergo PCI, a short course of triple therapy (e.g., for the duration of the hospital stay, up to 1 week) may be considered, particularly if the ischemic risk is very high. However, the default strategy is to initiate *dual anti-thrombotic therapy (DAT)* with an OAC (preferably a nonvitamin K oral anticoagulant, NOAC) and a P2Y12 inhibitor (usually clopidogrel).

Duration of Double Therapy

- *ACC/ESC guidelines:* For most patients, DAT with an OAC and a P2Y12 inhibitor is recommended for 6 months, followed by OAC monotherapy.
- *High ischemic risk:* In patients with very high ischemic risk, DAT may be extended up to 12 months.
- *Long-term:* After the initial period, OAC monotherapy is the long-term regimen to prevent thromboembolism from AF.

Aspirin use with OAC in AQUATIC Trial (ESC 2025)[25]*:* The AQUATIC trial provided crucial data for patients on OAC who are more than 6 months out from PCI. The trial found that adding aspirin to an OAC regimen *worsened clinical outcomes*, driven by a higher risk of cardiovascular death, and also increased major bleeding. This strongly supports the practice of dropping aspirin in patients on chronic OAC, especially after the initial high-risk period following PCI has passed.

SOME SPECIAL THOUGHTS FOCUSING ASIAN, ESPECIALLY EAST ASIAN POPULATIONS, MORE PRONE TO BLEEDING RISKS WITH DAPT[26]

East Asian patients (e.g., Japanese, Korean, and Chinese) have a *higher bleeding risk* compared to Western populations when treated with standard-dose DAPT. This is due to a combination of *genetic, physiological, and clinical factors*: (A) Genetic factors like (i) CYP2C19 polymorphism. 50–60% of East Asians are clopidogrel poor/intermediate metabolizers (vs. 30% in Caucasians), leading to higher active drug levels and bleeding risk. However, East Asians also have higher on-treatment platelet reactivity paradoxically, requiring careful dosing. (ii) *ABCB1* gene variants affect clopidogrel absorption, increasing variability in response. (B) Lower body weight and altered drug metabolism, where East Asians have lower average BMI, leading to higher drug exposure per kg. *Prasugrel/ticagrelor:* Standard doses (e.g., prasugrel 10 mg) may be excessive; studies support reduced doses (e.g., prasugrel 3.75 mg in Japan). (C) Higher prevalence of intracranial hemorrhage (ICH) with East Asians having a 2–3× higher risk of hemorrhagic stroke versus Western populations, making potent P2Y$_{12}$ inhibitors riskier. Gastrointestinal (GI) bleeding is also more common due to higher *H. pylori* infection rates and NSAID use. (D) Differences in platelet biology in some studies suggesting lower baseline platelet reactivity in East Asians, making them more sensitive to antiplatelet effects.

Variation in bleeding risk: While East Asians share general trends, there are subtle differences between countries. These are shown in **Table 2**.

Balance bleeding risk in East Asian ACS patients with the rationale of reducing bleeding while maintaining ischemic protection.

- To use lower doses of potent P2Y$_{12}$ inhibitors. Prasugrel: 3.75 mg/day (Japan/Korea) instead of 10 mg and ticagrelor: 90 mg once daily (instead of 90 mg BID) under study.
- To shorten DAPT duration. HBR patients: 1–3 months DAPT → P2Y$_{12}$ inhibitor monotherapy (e.g., clopidogrel). Non-HBR ACS: 6 months (per HOST-REDUCE-POLYTECH-ACS).
- To follow de-escalation strategies → Step 1 to start with ticagrelor/prasugrel in ACS → Step 2 to switch to clopidogrel after 1–3 months if stable.
- To use risk scores for personalization like PRECISE-DAPT (for bleeding) and DAPT Score (for ischemia) help guide duration and CYP2C19 testing for identifying clopidogrel responders in stable CAD.
- To use proton pump inhibitor (PPI) cotherapy should be mandatory in high GI bleeding risk (e.g., prior ulcer, *H. pylori*+) pantoprazole being preferred (least interaction with clopidogrel).

TABLE 2: Variation in bleeding risk among East Asian populations.

Country	Key differences in bleeding risk	Proposed adjustments in patients
Japan	• Highest ICH risk • Very low BMI (~23 kg/m²)	• Prasugrel 3.75 mg (not 10 mg) • 1–3 months DAPT for HBR
Korea	• Intermediate ICH risk • More clopidogrel use	• Favor clopidogrel in HBR • 6-month DAPT for ACS (HOST-REDUCE)
China	• High GI bleeding • Less prasugrel/ticagrelor use	• CYP2C19 testing common • De-escalation strategies

TABLE 3: Alternative strategies without genotyping.

Scenario	Suggested approach
ACS (high bleeding risk)	3-month DAPT → clopidogrel (despite resistance risk)
ACS (non-HBR)	Ticagrelor 90 mg BID (if affordable) or double-dose clopidogrel (150 mg/day)
Stable CAD post-PCI	Clopidogrel 75 mg + aspirin (consider 6-month DAPT)
Diabetes + CAD	Favor ticagrelor (if no budget constraints)

- To avoid triple therapy (DAPT + anticoagulants) → If AF + PCI, to use clopidogrel + DOAC (as per AUGUSTUS trial strategy).

Dual antiplatelet therapy in South Asians (India, Pakistan, Bangladesh, and Sri Lanka): Clopidogrel resistance and practical strategies.

South Asians have high clopidogrel resistance rates (30–50%) due to: CYP2C19 2/3 variants (higher than Caucasians, lower than East Asians), diabetes/metabolic syndrome (upregulates platelet reactivity), and poor adherence (cost, access issues).

Suggested recommendations are: (i) CYP2C19 testing (wherever available), to test if high thrombotic risk (e.g., prior stent thrombosis and diabetes) and if poor metabolizer (PM) → To switch to ticagrelor (prasugrel less available). (ii) Alternative strategies without genotyping could be as shown in **Table 3**. (iii) Double-dose clopidogrel (150 mg) in resistant patients.

Adjunctive therapies are: Mandatory PPI in high GI bleeding risk (spicy diet, *H. pylori*), pantoprazole being preferred and to avoid triple therapy (DAPT + anticoagulant). Instead, to use clopidogrel + DOAC, if there is AF.

CONCLUSION

The management of DAPT in CAD in 2025 is defined by nuance and personalization. It is pure act of balancing. The dogma of prolonged, potent DAPT for all has been successfully challenged. The contemporary approach is to start smart and adapt quickly. It is proposed to:

- Stratify using clinical, genetic, and algorithmic tools.
- Initiate with potent P2Y12 inhibitors in ACS.
- De-escalate early based on genotype or routinely to P2Y12 monotherapy in HBR patients after a short course of DAPT.
- Escalate rarely and only in the most extreme ischemic-risk scenarios.
- Re-assess continuously throughout the treatment period.

This patient-centric paradigm maximizes the benefit of preventing thrombotic complications while robustly mitigating the risk of bleeding, ultimately improving long-term net clinical outcomes for patients with CAD.

REFERENCES

1. Natsuaki M, Morimoto T, Shiomi H, et al. Effects of acute coronary syndrome and stable coronary artery disease on bleeding and ischemic risk after percutaneous coronary intervention. Circ J. 2021;85:1928-41.
2. Giustino G, Mehran R, Dangas GD, et al. Characterization of the average daily ischemic and bleeding risk after primary PCI for STEMI. J Am Coll Cardiol. 2017;70:1846-57.
3. Rao SV, O'Donoghue ML, Ruel M, et al. 2025 ACC/AHA/ACEP/NAEMSP/SCAI guideline for the management of patients with acute coronary syndromes: a report of the American College of Cardiology/American Heart Association Joint Committee on Clinical Practice Guidelines. Circulation. 2025;151(13):e771-862.
4. Byrne RA, Rossello X, Coughlan JJ, et al.; ESC Scientific Document Group. 2023 ESC Guidelines for the management of acute coronary syndromes. Eur Heart J. 2023;44;3720-826.
5. Wiviott SD, Braunwald E, McCabe CH, et al. Prasugrel versus clopidogrel in patients with acute coronary syndromes. N Engl J Med. 2007;357(20):2001-15.
6. Wallentin L, Becker RC, Budaj A, et al. Ticagrelor versus clopidogrel in patients with acute coronary syndromes. N Engl J Med. 2009;361(11):1045-57.

7. Mehran R, Baber U, Sharma SK, et al. Ticagrelor with or without aspirin in high-risk patients after PCI. N Engl J Med. 2019;381(21):2032-42.
8. Lee YJ, Kim SY, Cho YH, et al. Ticagrelor monotherapy after 3-month dual antiplatelet therapy in acute coronary syndrome by high bleeding risk: the subanalysis from the TICO Trial. Korean Circulation Journal, 52, Article: e19. https://doi.org/10.4070/KCJ.2021.0321
9. Watanabe H, Domei T, Morimoto T, et al. Effect of 1-month dual antiplatelet therapy followed by clopidogrel vs 12-month dual antiplatelet therapy on cardiovascular and bleeding events in patients receiving PCI: The STOPDAPT-2 randomized clinical trial. JAMA. 2022;327(17):1651-61.
10. The DUAL-ACS trial: Duration of DAPT in ACS' presented during HOT LINE 6 on 31 August 2025 at 09:09 to 09:19 in Madrid (Main Auditorium).
11. Guimarães PO, Franken M, Tavares CAM, et al.; For the NEO-MINDSET Trial Investigators. Early withdrawal of aspirin after PCI in acute coronary syndromes. NEJM. 2025. DOI: 10.1056/NEJMoa2507980
12. Tarantini G, Honton B, Paradies V, et al.; For the TARGET-FIRST Investigators. Early discontinuation of Aspirin after PCI in low-risk acute myocardial infarction. N Engl J Med. 2025 Aug 31. doi: 10.1056/NEJMoa2508808
13. Duk-Woo Park. TAILORED-CHIP: Tailored antiplatelet therapy for complex high-risk PCI. Reported from ESC Congress 2025 presented by at the ESC Congress 2025 in Madrid.
14. Claassens DMF, Vos GJA, Bergmeijer TO, et al. A genotype-guided strategy for oral $P2Y_{12}$ inhibitors in primary PCI. N Engl J Med. 2019; 381(17):1621-31.
15. Pereira NL, Farkouh ME, So D, et al. Effect of genotype-guided oral P2Y12 inhibitor selection vs conventional clopidogrel therapy on ischemic outcomes after percutaneous coronary intervention: The TAILOR-PCI randomized clinical trial. JAMA. 2020;324(8):761-71.
16. Costa F, van Klaveren D, James S, et al. Derivation and validation of the predicting bleeding complications in patients undergoing stent implantation and subsequent dual antiplatelet therapy (PRECISE-DAPT) score: a pooled analysis of individual-patient datasets from clinical trials. Lancet. 2017;389(10073):1025-34.
17. Yeh RW, Secemsky EA, Kereiakes DJ, et al. Development and validation of a prediction rule for benefit and harm of dual antiplatelet therapy beyond 1 year after percutaneous coronary intervention. JAMA. 2016;315(16):1735-49.
18. Chen J, Meng H, Xu L, Liu J et al. Efficacy and safety of cilostazol based triple antiplatelet treatment versus dual antiplatelet treatment in patients undergoing coronary stent implantation: an updated meta-analysis of the randomized controlled trials. J Thromb Thrombolysis. 2015; 39(1):23-34. doi: 10.1007/s11239-014-1090-5
19. Yang Yi, Yan Y, Zhou Z, et al. Accurate prediction of bleeding risk after coronary artery bypass grafting with dual antiplatelet therapy: A machine learning model vs. the PRECISE-DAPT score. Int J Cardiol. 2025:421:132925, doi.org/10.1016/j.ijcard.2024.132925
20. Li F, Rasmi L, Xiang Y, et al. Dynamic prognosis prediction for patients on DAPT after drug-eluting stent implantation: model development and validation. J Am Heart Assoc. 2024;13(3):e029900. https://doi.org/10.1161/JAHA. 123.029900
21. Abtan J, Steg PG, Stone GW, et al. Efficacy and safety of cangrelor in preventing periprocedural complications in patients with stable angina and acute coronary syndromes undergoing percutaneous coronary intervention: The CHAMPION PHOENIX trial. JACC Cardiovasc Interv. 2016;9(18):1905-13.
22. Özdemir M. PIONEER AF-PCI trial. Turk Kardiyol Dern Ars. 2017;45(Suppl 4):10-14.
23. Cannon CP, Bhatt DL, Oldgren J, et al; For the RE-DUAL PCI Steering Committee and Investigators. Dual Antithrombotic Therapy with Dabigatran after PCI in Atrial Fibrillation. N Engl J Med. 2017;377:1513-24.
24. Lopes RD, Heizer G, Aronson R, et al.; for the AUGUSTUS Investigators. Antithrombotic therapy after acute coronary syndrome or PCI in atrial fibrillation. N Engl J Med. 2019;380:1509-24.
25. Lemesle G, Didier R, Steg PG, et al. For the AQUATIC Trial Investigators. Aspirin in patients with chronic coronary syndrome receiving oral anticoagulation. N Engl J Med. 2025;393(16):1578-88.
26. Gong Y, Jeong YH, Wang TD, et al. Position Statement on Antiplatelet Therapy for East Asians with Coronary Artery Disease 2025 Update. JACC Asia. 2025;5(7):821-46.

CHAPTER 11

High Bleeding Risk: Making Antiplatelet Safe

Vaibhav Bandil, Suman Bhandari

INTRODUCTION

In patients with coronary artery disease (CAD), percutaneous coronary intervention (PCI) procedures are the mainstay of treatment for acute coronary syndrome (ACS) and chronic coronary syndrome (CCS).[1] Optimal PCI outcomes depend on adjunct medication, particularly antithrombotic treatment.[2,3] Patients undergoing PCI may experience acute and long-term ischemic events.[4]

Over the past 40 years, PCI patients' antiplatelet regimens have evolved. Refinement in stent technologies has led to safer (i.e., less thrombogenic) stent platforms, the development of new antiplatelet drugs, and an understanding of the prognostic implications of bleeding, the most feared adverse effect of antiplatelet therapies.[2,5]

Numerous studies have also identified persons at risk of ischemic and bleeding complications.[2] These characteristics, along with an understanding of how antiplatelet drugs affect people differently, have enabled customized therapy regimens to optimize efficacy and safety.[6]

RATIONALE FOR THE USE OF ANTIPLATELET THERAPY IN PATIENTS UNDERGOING PERCUTANEOUS CORONARY INTERVENTION

Arterial thrombus formation is a dynamic and intricate pathological process that is initiated by contact activation on a foreign surface or within an injured blood vessel wall.[7] The initial tethering of platelets is mediated by the interaction between the complex glycoprotein (GP) Ib-IX-V and Von Willebrand factor, as well as by collagen receptors present on the platelet surface, such as glycoprotein VI (GPVI) **(Fig. 1)**.[7-9] Platelets are essential for thrombus formation. The development of atherosclerosis and the occurrence of thrombotic complications following plaque destabilization are significantly influenced by the interaction between platelets, the hemostatic system, and inflammatory pathways.[10-16]

Antiplatelet therapy mitigates thrombotic-related periprocedural myocardial injury that is linked to blood vessel wall trauma, including dissections, plaque ruptures, embolization, and side branch occlusions. In addition, it reduces the likelihood of stent thrombosis (ST), which is more prevalent during the acute or subacute phase of PCI **(Fig. 2)**.[17-19]

Dual antiplatelet therapy (DAPT) is standard for PCI patients.[1,20-23] All patients should take aspirin (160–325 mg orally or 250–500 mg intravenously, followed by 75–100 mg once daily). The DAPT regimen, including the *P2Y12* inhibitor, depends on the clinical situation (ACS or CCS) and patient thrombotic and bleeding risk. **Figure 3** shows the European Society of Cardiology (ESC) guidelines.

BLEEDING RISK ASSESSMENT

The Academic Research Consortium for High Bleeding Risk (ARC-HBR) recently proposed a consensus definition of HBR, which includes 14

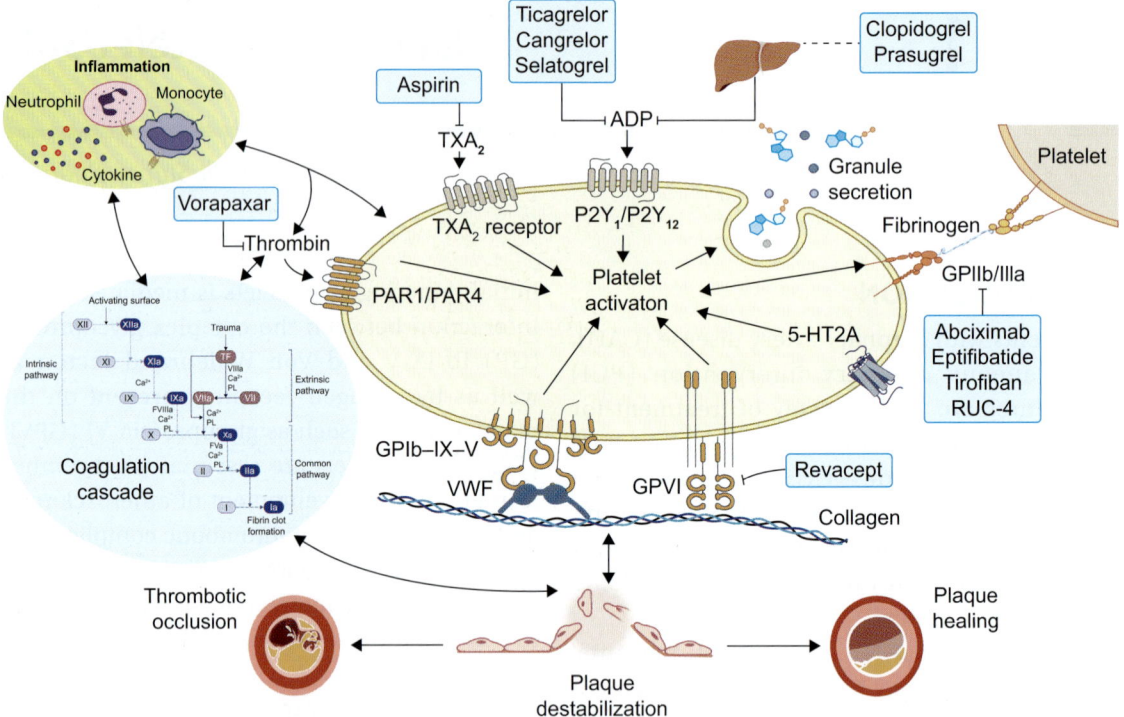

Fig. 1: Interplay between platelets, coagulation and inflammation in atherothrombosis, and sites of action of antiplatelet agents.
Note: Destabilization of plaque, resulting from rupture or erosion, triggers the activation of platelets and coagulation factors, alongside subsequent inflammatory responses. This process can culminate in thrombotic occlusion of the coronary artery, which is associated with acute coronary syndromes, or in plaque healing, which may promote plaque progression and stable coronary artery disease. Platelet tethering occurs through the interaction of the glycoprotein complex Ib-IX-V with Von Willebrand factor, as well as through other collagen receptors on the platelet surface, including GPVI. Thrombin serves as a critical intermediary between platelet activation and the coagulation cascade. The mechanisms of action of common antiplatelet agents are outlined: aspirin inhibits thromboxane A2 (TXA2), while clopidogrel, prasugrel, ticagrelor, and cangrelor act as inhibitors of the ADP *P2Y12* receptor. Clopidogrel and prasugrel necessitate hepatic activation. Vorapaxar functions as a thrombin-receptor inhibitor (protease-activated receptor, PAR-1), while abciximab, eptifibatide, tirofiban, and RUC-4 serve as GPIIb/IIIa receptor inhibitors. Revacept acts as a competitive antagonist of collagen-GPVI signaling. Yellow represents subcutaneous or intramuscular administration. (ADP: adenosine diphosphate; GP: glycoprotein; PAR-1: platelet protease-activated receptor-1; TXA2: thromboxane A2; vWF von Willebrand factor; 5HT2A: serotonergic receptor)

main and 6 minor criteria **(Table 1)**.[24] A HBR is indicated by the presence of at least one main and two minor criteria. This definition has been validated by retrospective studies; however, prospective studies that stratify patients to specific antiplatelet regimens using ARC-HBR criteria are justified.[25]

STRATEGIES FOCUSED ON REDUCING BLEEDING EVENTS

The introduction of low-thrombogenic stent platforms and the fact that thrombotic risk is highest in the first month after PCI and decreases thereafter, while bleeding risk remains stable and has prompted bleeding event reduction studies.

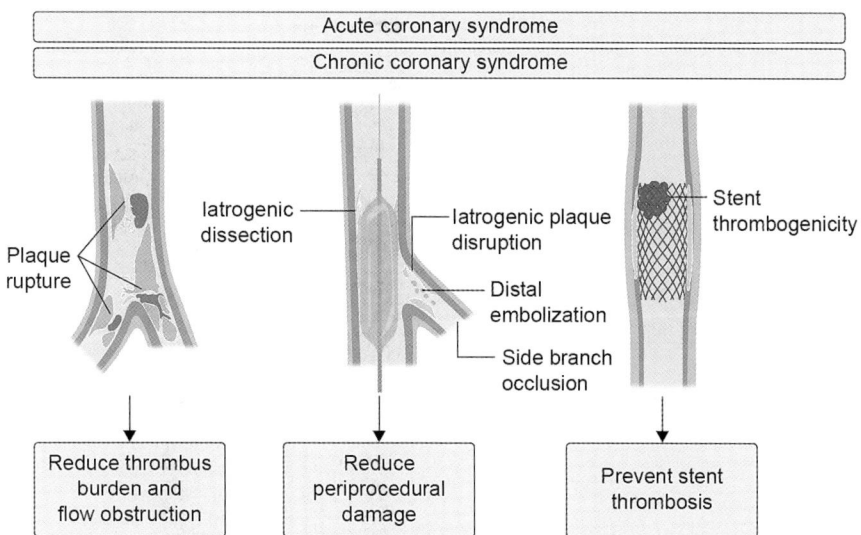

Fig. 2: Rationale for the use of antiplatelet therapy during percutaneous coronary intervention (PCI).
Note: In patients undergoing PCI in the setting of chronic coronary syndrome (CCS), antiplatelet therapy reduces the occurrence of intraprocedural or very early stent thrombosis (right), periprocedural damage caused by iatrogenic dissections, plaque disruption, distal embolization or side branch occlusion (middle). During acute coronary syndrome, antiplatelet therapy also plays a role in reducing thrombus burden and flow obstruction (left). (PCI: percutaneous coronary intervention)

Both major and small bleeding affect prognosis. Major bleeding has prognostic implications (i.e., mortality) equivalent to or greater than a major ischemic event, but mild bleeding can cause an abrupt termination of antiplatelet medication, thus causing higher ischemia events.[26] Next, we examine the main bleeding-reduction techniques tested in RCTs to improve the bleeding-ischemic risk trade-off over time. DAPT shortening, *P2Y12* monotherapy, and inhibitor de-escalation are these techniques. Most were not meant to reduce major adverse cardiovascular events (MACE). In this situation, meta-analyses increase statistical power to define the impact on hard ischemic endpoints.

SHORT DUAL ANTIPLATELET THERAPY IN HIGH BLEEDING RISK

The latest generation of stents features an enhanced thrombotic risk profile due to the incorporation of inert fluoropolymers and reduced strut thickness. Additionally, there is an increased recognition of the adverse outcomes linked to bleeding following PCI, leading to a contemporary focus on reducing bleeding events. Historically, patients with HBR received bare metal stents (BMS) accompanied by 1 month of DAPT to ensure sufficient thrombotic protection. Improvements in drug-eluting stents (DES) prompted a re-evaluation of this paradigm, as evidenced by three randomized controlled trials that compared BMS to DES with 1 month of DAPT in patients with the HBR.[27-29] The LEADERS FREE trial (2015) evaluated the BioFreedom biolimus-coated stent (Biosensors) against a BMS in a cohort of 2,466 patients with HBR following PCI, of whom 42% had ACS. Participants were randomized to receive 1 month of DAPT with aspirin and clopidogrel, followed by aspirin alone, or to continue DAPT for 12 months.[27] At 1 year, the BioFreedom stent demonstrated superior

		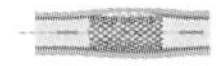 Before PCI	During PCI	After PCI
Stable		Aspirin — I A Clopidogrel — IIb C (high probability of PCI)	Clopidogrel — I A Prasugrel or ticagrelor over Clopidogrel (high ischemic risk) — IIb C	DAPT for 6 months — I A Extended DAPT (high ischemic and low bleeding risk) — IIa A 3-month DAPT→aspirin (high bleeding risk) — IIa A 1-month DAPT→aspirin (high bleeding risk) — IIb C
NSTE-ACS		Aspirin — I A Routine P2Y$_{12}$ inhibitor — III A	Prasugrel — I A Ticagrelor — I A Clopidogrel — I C Prasugrel over ticagrelor — IIa B	DAPT for 12 months — I A Extended DAPT or DPI (high ischemic risk) — IIa A 1-month DAPT→clopidogrel (very high bleeding risk) — IIa B 3-month DAPT→aspirin (high bleeding risk) — IIa B 3-month DAPT with ticagrelor→ticagrelor — IIa B Extended DAPT or DPI (moderate ischemic risk) — IIb A Guided de-escalation — IIb A
STE-ACS		Aspirin — I B Potent P2Y$_{12}$ inhibitor — I A		DAPT for 12 months — I A 6-month DAPT→aspirin (high bleeding risk) — IIa B Extended DAPT or DPI (high ischemic/low bleeding risk) — IIb B Guided de-escalation — IIb A

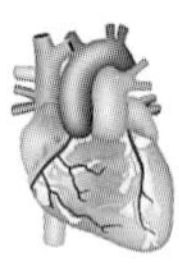

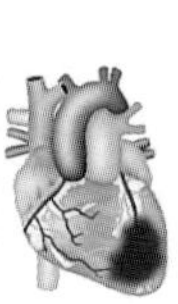

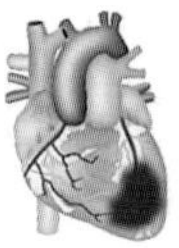

Fig. 3: Current guidelines of the European Society of Cardiology recommendations for oral antiplatelet agents among patients undergoing PCI. (DAPT: dual antiplatelet therapy; DPI: dual pathway inhibition; NSTE-ACS: non-ST-elevation acute coronary syndrome; PCI: percutaneous coronary intervention; STE-ACS: ST segment-elevation acute coronary syndrome)

performance compared to BMS concerning the primary endpoint of composite cardiac death, myocardial infarction (MI), or ST (9.4 vs. 12.9%; $p = 0.005$ for superiority). A prespecified subgroup analysis involving 828 patients with HBR (63% ACS) from the ZEUS trial (2015) revealed comparable results. The zotarolimus-eluting Endeavor Sprint stent (Medtronic) exhibited significantly lower rates of MACE (22.6 vs. 29.0%; $p = 0.03$) and ST (6.2 vs. 2.6%; $p = 0.02$) at 1 year following 30 days of DAPT, in comparison to BMS.[28] The SENIOR trial (2018) assessed 1,200 elderly patients (≥75 years), with half diagnosed with ACS. It demonstrated that the Synergy bioabsorbable polymer DES (Boston Scientific), following 30 days of DAPT, resulted in significantly lower rates of MACE (12 vs. 16%; $p = 0.02$) at 1 year compared to BMS[29] **(Fig. 4)**.

Several studies have aimed to assess the efficacy of very short (1 month) duration DAPT in the HBR population **(Table 2)**. As of now, six trials have been published, all indicating noninferiority and/or superiority concerning ischemic and bleeding outcomes with 1 month of DAPT.[30-35] Significant variability exists in the design of these studies, including the implementation of a blanking period, the evaluation for noninferiority versus superiority, and the selection of a comparator arm, which has included randomized and historical controls, as well as performance goals. Additionally, while the ACS population was adequately represented in these trials, patients

TABLE 1: Major and minor criteria for HBR at the time of PCI.

Major	Minor
	Age ≥75 years
Anticipated use of long-term oral anticoagulation*	
End-stage CKD (eGFR < 30 mL/min)	Moderate CKD (eGFR: 30–59 mL/min)
Hemoglobin <11 g/dL	Hemoglobin 11–12.9 g/dL for men and 11–11.9 g/dL for women
Spontaneous bleeding requiring hospitalization or transfusion in the past 6 months or at any time, if recurrent	Spontaneous bleeding requiring hospitalization or transfusion within the past 12 months not meeting the major criterion
Moderate or severe baseline thrombocytopenia† (platelet count < 100 × 10⁹/L)	
Chronic bleeding diathesis	
Liver cirrhosis with portal hypertension	
	Long-term use of oral NSAIDs or steroids
Active malignancy‡ (excluding nonmelanoma skin cancer) within the past 12 months	
Previous spontaneous ICH (at any time) Previous traumatic ICH within the past 12 months Presence of a bAVM Moderate or severe ischemic stroke§ within the past 6 months	Any ischemic stroke at any time not meeting the major criterion
Nondeferrable major surgery on DAPT	
Recent major surgery or major trauma within 30 days before PCI	

*This excludes vascular protection doses.
†Baseline thrombocytopenia is defined as thrombocytopenia before PCI.
‡Active malignancy is defined as diagnosis within 12 months and/or ongoing requirement for treatment (including surgery, chemotherapy, or radiotherapy).
§National Institutes of Health Stroke Scale score ≥5.
(bAVM: brain arteriovenous malformation; CKD: chronic kidney disease; DAPT: dual antiplatelet therapy; eGFR: estimated glomerular filtration rate; HBR: high bleeding risk; ICH: intracranial hemorrhage; NSAID: nonsteroidal anti-inflammatory drug; PCI: percutaneous coronary intervention)

with STEMI were under-represented, comprising 0–7% of total participants in all trials except for the MASTER DAPT trial, where they accounted for 12%. In conclusion, while the populations in the HBR study did not exhibit particularly complex coronary disease, a recent subanalysis of the MASTER DAPT trial indicated that individuals with complex coronary disease and HBR experienced no significant differences in NACE or MACE. Additionally, there was a notable reduction in bleeding following the cessation of either aspirin or *P2Y12i* at 1 month.[36] At least seven ongoing trials are assessing 1-month DAPT therapy in HBR populations. This includes the COMPARE STEMI ONE trial, which aims to enrol 1,608 STEMI patients to compare 30–45 days of

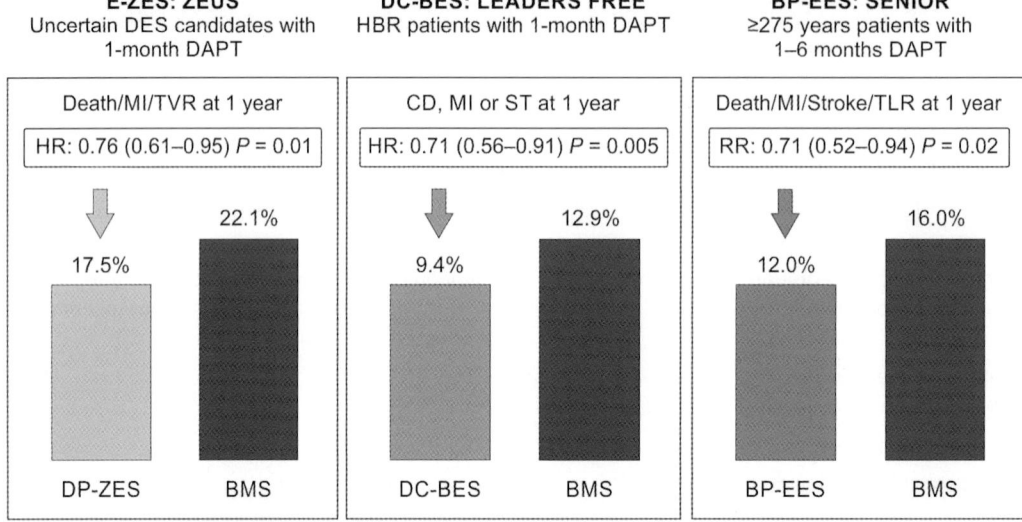

Fig. 4: Trials of drug-eluting stents versus bare metal stents (BMS) with 1-month dual antiplatelet therapy (DAPT).

DAPT followed by prasugrel monotherapy against the currently recommended 12 months of DAPT (NCT05491200) **(Table 2)**.

Many of these trials were published since 2020, following the release of most DAPT guidelines, and have not been integrated into current recommendations. Additionally, much of the data concerning HBR populations originates from earlier trials that included HBR cohorts and primarily assessed a more conservative 3-month DAPT duration. The current AHA/ACC guidelines offer 2b recommendations for the HBR population, suggesting the consideration of DAPT discontinuation at 3 months and 6 months post-PCI for SIHD and ACS populations, respectively.[37] The ESC guidelines provide 2a recommendations for discontinuing DAPT at 3 months in both SIHD and ACS contexts for patients with HBR, and a 2a recommendation to consider stopping DAPT after 1 month when the bleeding risk is assessed as very high. At present, XIENCE (Abbott Vascular) and Resolute Onyx (Medtronic) stents are approved by the Food and Drug Administration (FDA) for 1-month DAPT in patients classified as having HBR.

Emphasizing the substantial overlap between patients at high risk for bleeding and those at high risk for ischemia is essential. This complexity necessitates clinical decisions regarding the duration of DAPT to be individualized based on specific patient risk factors. The development of various risk-stratifying tools has emerged to support decision-making, including the DAPT, PARIS (Patterns of Nonadherence to Antiplatelet Regimen in Stented Patients), PARIS-DAPT, and Predicting Bleeding Complications in Patients Undergoing Stent Implantation and Subsequent Dual Antiplatelet Therapy (PRECISE-DAPT) scores, with the PRECISE-DAPT score being recommended in the ESC guidelines.[38] Given the limitations and absence of consensus among these risk scores, the Academic Research Consortium for HBR established a consensus document aimed at improving the identification and classification of factors associated with HBR in patients undergoing PCI.[24] This detailed enumeration of clinical features is categorized into major and minor criteria and was validated in a cohort of approximately 10,000 patients post-PCI. Classification as HBR (defined as at least 1

TABLE 2: Summary of recent and ongoing 1-month DAPT trials in patients at HBR.

Trial (y)[a]	N[b]	ACS % (STEMI %) of total population	Comparison	DES	Design	DAPT duration study (control)	P2Y₁₂i	Monotherapy	Primary outcome	Timepoint	Primary outcome	P value
LEADERS FREE II (2020)	1,148	44% (3%)	DCS vs. BMS[c]	BioFreedom	Superiority	1 m (1 m)	C preferred	A preferred	CV death, MI TLR MACE	1 year	9.3 vs. 12.4% 7.2 vs. 9.2%	$P = 0.015$ $P = 0.034$
Onyx ONE Global (2020)	1,996	51% (5–6%)	ZES vs. DCS	Resolute Onyx vs. BioFreedom	Noninferiority	1 m (1 m)	87% C, 11% T, <1% P	51% A, 41% P2Y₁₂i		1 year	17.1 vs. 16.9%	$P = 0.01$
Onyx ONE Clear (2020)	1,506	49% (4%)	ZES vs. OPC	Resolute Onyx	Noninferiority	1 m (12 m)	C preferred	A or P2Y₁₂i	CV Death, MI	1 year	7.0 vs. OPC 9.7%	$P < 0.001$
XIENCE 28 (2021)	1,605	34% (0%)	EES vs. EES[c]	XIENCE	Noninferiority	1 m (6 m)	86% C, 13% T, 1% P	91% A, 6% P2Y₁₂i	All-cause death, MI	6 months or 12 months	3.5 vs. 4.3%	$P = 0.0005$
MASTER DAPT (2021)	4,434	59% (12%)	SES vs. SES	Ultimaster	Noninferiority Noninferiority Superiority	1 m (>3 m)	80% C, 17% T, 3% P	31% A, 71% P2Y₁₂i (56% C)	NACE MACCE Bleeding	1 year 1 year 1 year	7.5 vs. 7.7% 6.1 vs. 5.9% 6.5 vs. 9.4%	$P < 0.001$ $P = 0.001$ $P < 0.001$
POEM (2022)	4.43	41% (7%)	EES vs. OPC	Synergy	Noninferiority	1 m (1 m)	88% C, 10% T, <1% P	A preferred	MACE	1 year	4.82 vs. OPC 9.4%	$P < 0.001$
EluNIR HBR (2021) (NCT03877848)	316	SIHD + ACS	RES vs OPC	EluNIR	Noninferiority	1 m SIHD, 3 m ACS	—	—	MACE	1 year	—	
Bioflow-DAPT (2023) (NCT04137510)	1,949	SIHD + ACS	SES vs. ZES	Orsiro vs. Resolute Onyx	Noninferiority	1 m	—	—	MACE	1 year		

Contd...

Contd...

Trial (y)[a]	N[b]	ACS % (STEMI %) of total population	Comparison	DES	Design	DAPT duration study (control)	P2Y$_{12}$i	Monotherapy	Primary outcome	Timepoint	Primary outcome P value
COMPARE 60/80 HBR (2023) (NCT04500912)	736	SIHD + ACS	SES vs. SES	Supraflex Cruz vs. Ultimaster Tansei	—	1 m	—	—	NACE	1 year	
TARGET SAFE (2023) (NCT03287167)	1,720	SIHD + ACS	SES vs. SES	Firehawk	Noninferiority	1 m (6 m)	—	—	NACE	1 year	
ZEVS-HBR (2025) (NCT05240781)	280	SIHD + ACS	SES vs. ZES	Ultimaster vs. Resolute Onyx	Noninferiority	1 m or 3 m (high ischemic risk)	—	P2Y$_{12}$i preferred A or C	TLF	1 year	
C-MODE (2025) (NCT05320926)	3,744	SIHD only	ZES vs. ZES	Resolute Onyx	Superiority	1 m (HBR arm)	C	—	NACE	1 year	
COMPARE STEMI ONE (2026) (NCT05491200)	1,608	STEMI only	—	—	Noninferiority	30–45 d (12 m)	P	P2Y$_{12}$i preferred	NACE	1 year	

[A: aspirin; ACS: acute coronary syndromes; BMS: bare metal stent; C: clopidogrel; CV: cardiovascular; DAPT: dual antiplatelet therapy; DCS: drug-coated stent; DES: drug-eluting stent; EES: everolimus-eluting stent; HBR: high bleeding risk; MACCE: major adverse cardiac or cerebral events (a composite of death from any cause; myocardial infarction; or stroke); MACE: major adverse cardiac events; MI: myocardial infarction; NACE: net adverse clinical events (a composite of death from any cause; myocardial infarction; stroke; or major bleeding); OPC: objective performance criteria; P: prasugrel; P2Y12i: P2Ypurinoceptor-12 inhibitor; RES: ridaforolimus-eluting stent; SES, sirolimus-eluting stent; SIHD: stable ischemic heart disease; STEMI: ST-segment elevation myocardial infarction; T: ticagrelor; TLF: target lesion failure; TLR: target lesion revascularization; ZES: zotarolimus-eluting stent]

[a]For ongoing trials, the year represents the planned completion date.
[b]For ongoing trials, N represents planned enrollment.
[c]Historical cohort

major or 2 minor criteria) was linked to nearly a threefold increase in bleeding risk compared to non-HBR patients, as well as an elevated 1-year mortality rate (4.7 vs. 0.6%) and MI (4.2 vs. 2.0%).[39] The findings indicated a stepwise escalation in bleeding risk correlated with the frequency of meeting the Academic Research Consortium for HBR definition. Specifically, patients meeting the criteria once exhibited a twofold increased risk of bleeding, while those meeting the criteria four times showed a 12-fold increased risk. Current risk stratification tools primarily emphasize bleeding; however, recent evidence indicates that bleeding may be prioritized over ischemic risk, except in extreme cases, when patients exhibit both moderate-to-high bleeding and ischemic risk factors.[40]

4D-ACUTE CORONARY SYNDROME RANDOMIZED TRIAL (2025)

The study aimed to assess the safety and efficacy of a 1-month prasugrel-based DAPT regimen, followed by reduced-dose monotherapy, in ACS patients undergoing drug-coated stent (DCS) placement.

In a multicenter, randomized, open-label trial, 656 patients with the ACS (mean age: 60.9 ± 9.7 years; 82.6% male) receiving DAPT (DCS) were assigned to either 1-month DAPT with aspirin 100 mg and prasugrel 10 mg (or 5 mg for patients aged ≥75 years or weighing <60 kg) followed by prasugrel 5 mg monotherapy (1M-DAPT) or 12-month DAPT with aspirin and prasugrel 5 mg (12M-DAPT). The main endpoint was the 12-month net adverse clinical events (NACE), which included a composite of death, nonfatal MI, stroke, ischemia-driven target vessel revascularization, and Bleeding Academic Research Consortium Type 2–5 bleeding.

NACE was observed in 4.9% of the 1M-DAPT group and 8.8% of the 12M-DAPT group, satisfying the criteria for both noninferiority [noninferiority margin: 2.0%; absolute difference: –3.9%; 95% confidence interval (CI) for absolute difference: –6.7% to –0.2%; $p = 0.014$) and superiority {hazard ratio (HR) 0.51; 95% CI: 0.27–0.95; $p = 0.034$]. Bleeding events were observed in 1.2% of the 1M-DAPT group compared to 5.2% in the 12M-DAPT group (HR: 0.23; $p = 0.009$). Major bleeding occurred in 0.6% of the 1M-DAPT group versus 4.6% in the 12M-DAPT group (HR: 0.13; $p = 0.007$). The ischemic outcomes were comparable.

In patients with ACS treated with dual antiplatelet therapy, a 1-month prasugrel-based regimen followed by prasugrel 5 mg monotherapy resulted in a 49% reduction in NACE, primarily due to a 77% decrease in bleeding incidents, while maintaining ischemic safety[41] **(Figs. 5A to C)**.

DUAL ANTIPLATE THERAPY IN ATRIAL FIBRILLATION

Patients necessitating simultaneous oral anticoagulation (OAC) and antiplatelet therapy following PCI represent a distinct HBR subgroup. Initially, both OAC and DAPT were considered essential to mitigate the severe complications of stroke, thromboembolism, and ST in patients undergoing triple therapy. Triple therapy is associated with a significant bleeding risk, reaching up to 16% annually.[42] The prevalence of atrial fibrillation in 5–8% of the PCI population necessitates urgent measures to reduce excess bleeding complications.[43]

Currently, five randomized controlled trials have assessed antiplatelet therapies in the atrial fibrillation population necessitating OAC. The WOEST trial (2013) involved 573 patients on warfarin undergoing PCI, with 27% classified as ACS. Participants were randomized to receive either clopidogrel (dual therapy) or a combination of aspirin and clopidogrel (triple therapy). At 1 year, dual therapy significantly decreased bleeding rates (19.4% compared to 44.4%; $p < 0.0001$) and MACE (11% compared to

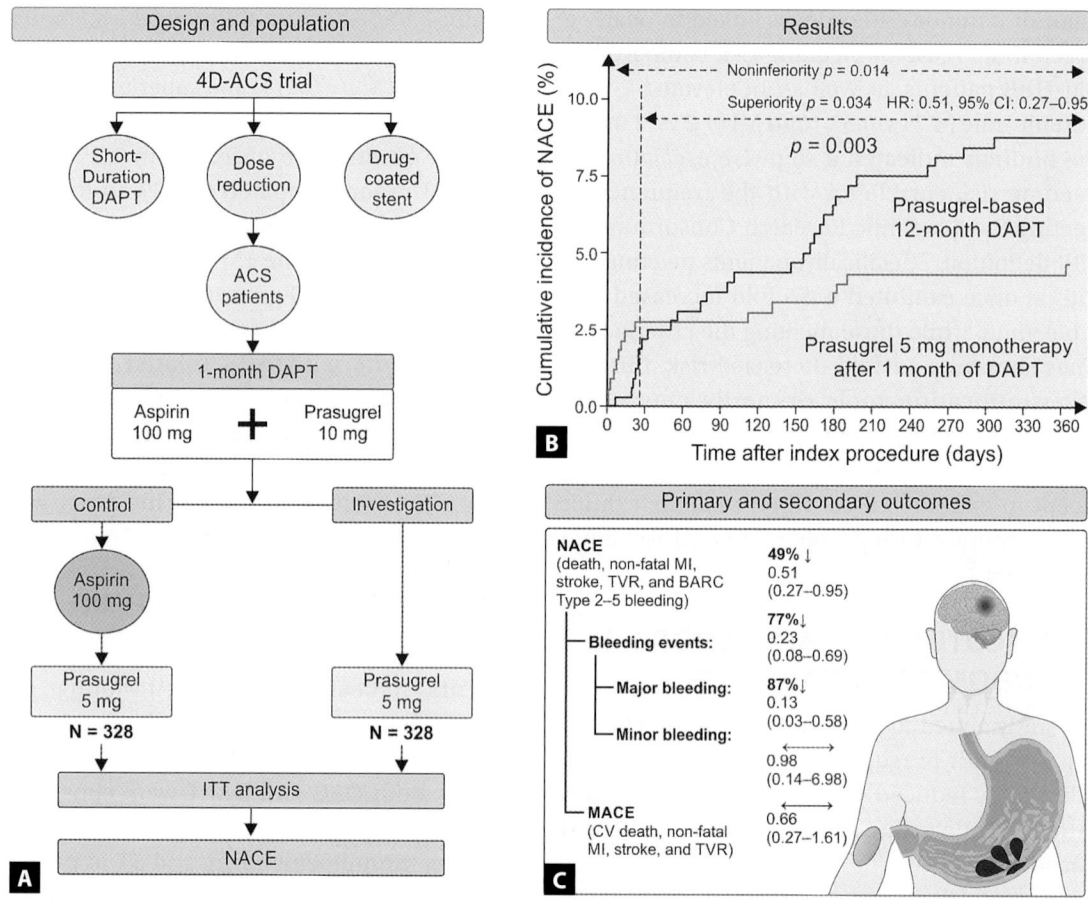

Figs. 5A to C: Summary of the 4D-acute coronary syndrome (ACS) trial.

18%; $p = 0.025$), while also showing a numerical reduction in ST (1.4% compared to 3.2%).[44] The PIONEER-AF study (2016) assessed 2,124 patients with atrial fibrillation undergoing PCI (51% ACS) through a randomized design in a 1:1:1 allocation to one of three treatment groups. (1) Rivaroxaban (15 mg/d) combined with a *P2Y12* inhibitor for 12 months, (2) very-low-dose rivaroxaban (2.5 mg twice daily) in conjunction with dual antiplatelet therapy (DAPT) for 1, 6, or 12 months, or (3) standard treatment involving a dose-adjusted vitamin K antagonist (once daily) alongside DAPT for 1, 6, or 12 months, with clopidogrel as the primary *P2Y12* inhibitor in 93–96% of cases.[43] Rivaroxaban demonstrated superior efficacy compared to warfarin regarding the primary outcome of clinically significant bleeding, with rates of 17, 18, and 27% for groups 1, 2, and 3, respectively. There were no significant differences observed in MACE or ST. The RE-DUAL PCI (2017) trial demonstrated that dual therapy involving dabigatran with clopidogrel or ticagrelor resulted in reduced bleeding rates, with no significant differences observed in MACE or ST when compared to triple therapy (warfarin, a P2Y12 inhibitor, and 1–3 months of aspirin) among 2,725 patients, of whom 50% had ACS.[45] The ENTRUST-AF PCI trial (edoxaban; 2019) and the AUGUSTUS trial (apixaban; 2019) showed noninferior and superior bleeding

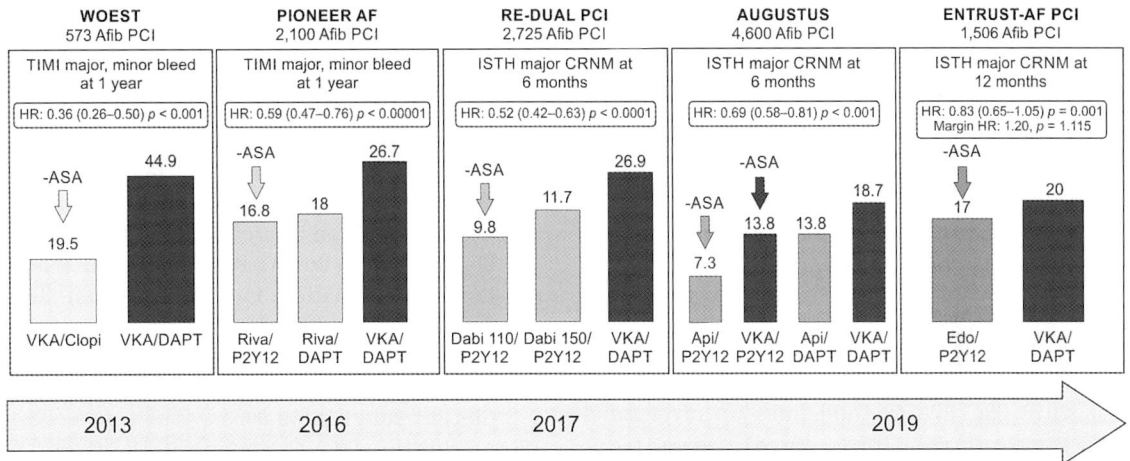

Fig. 6: Major trials of dual versus triple therapy in atrial fibrillation following percutaneous coronary intervention.

outcomes, respectively, for DOACs compared to warfarin when using dual therapy instead of triple therapy. There was no difference in ischemic outcomes among 1,506 patients (52% ACS) in the ENTRUST-AF PCI trial and 4,614 patients (61% ACS, 37% with PCI, and 24% without PCI) in the AUGUSTUS trial **(Fig. 6)**.[46,47] A comprehensive meta-analysis involving 10,234 patients assessed the safety and efficacy of double versus triple antithrombotic therapy (with over 90% receiving clopidogrel). This analysis, which included the four previously mentioned DOAC trials, revealed significantly lower rates of major and clinically relevant nonmajor bleeding [rate ratio (RR), 0.66; 95% CI: 0.56–0.78; $p < 0.0001$) without notable differences in all-cause mortality, cardiovascular mortality, or trial-defined MACE among patients receiving dual therapy.[48] Interestingly, individuals undergoing dual therapy exhibited a borderline significant increase in the rate of MI (3.6% compared to 3.0%; $p = 0.07$), primarily influenced by the RE-DUAL PCI cohort, as well as a significantly elevated incidence of ST (1.0% vs. 0.6%; $p = 0.04$), driven by both the RE-DUAL PCI and AUGUSTUS populations. This meta-analysis indicates that the signal for harm associated with dual therapy was primarily observed in individuals who were at very low and low risk for bleeding, yet had predominantly high ischemic risk. Consequently, there is a continuing discussion regarding the necessity and duration of a short course of triple therapy in populations characterized by high ischemic risk and low bleeding risk. Current trials are assessing 7 and 30 days of triple therapy (NCT04436978) as well as the application of more potent *P2Y12* inhibitors (NCT04695106).

CONCLUSION

Antiplatelet therapy is the mainstay of care for CAD patients receiving PCI in order to prevent both local and systemic ischemic sequelae. Over the past few decades, a variety of antiplatelet regimens using *P2Y12* inhibitors and aspirin have been developed and put into clinical practice. A more thorough understanding of the patient's ischemic and bleeding-risk profile, as well as their sensitivity to antiplatelet medications, has helped to select the best course of treatment for each patient. It is important to modify the length and intensity of aspirin and *P2Y12* inhibiting medication to lower the risk of ischemic complications and hemorrhage. Among the tactics used to lower the risk of bleeding include de-escalation, DAPT duration reduction, and *P2Y12* inhibitor monotherapy. An integrated strategy that incorporates procedural features, definitions, and scores to define ischemic and bleeding risk, and tools to evaluate medication response is the most promising method for a customized choice of antiplatelet drugs among patients having PCI.

■ REFERENCES

1. Neumann FJ, Sousa-Uva M, Ahlsson A, et al. 2018 ESC/EACTS Guidelines on myocardial revascularization. EuroIntervention. 2019;14(14):1435-534.
2. Cao D, Chandiramani R, Chiarito M, et al. Evolution of antithrombotic therapy in patients undergoing percutaneous coronary intervention: a 40-year journey. Eur Heart J. 2020;42:339-51.
3. Capodanno D, Alfonso F, Levine GN, et al. ACC/AHA Versus ESC Guidelines on Dual Antiplatelet Therapy: JACC Guideline Comparison. J Am Coll Cardiol. 2018;72:2915-31.
4. Prasad A, Herrmann J. Myocardial infarction due to percutaneous coronary intervention. N Engl J Med. 2011;364:453-64.
5. Moon JY, Franchi F, Rollini F, et al. Evolution of Coronary Stent Technology and Implications for Duration of Dual Antiplatelet Therapy. Prog Cardiovasc Dis. 2018;60:478-90.
6. Sibbing D, Aradi D, Alexopoulos D, et al. Updated Expert Consensus Statement on Platelet Function and Genetic Testing for Guiding P2Y12 Receptor Inhibitor Treatment in Percutaneous Coronary Intervention. JACC Cardiovasc Interv. 2019;12:1521-37.
7. Lippi G, Franchini M, Targher G. Arterial thrombus formation in cardiovascular disease. Nat Rev Cardiol. 2011;8:502-12.
8. Cosemans JM, Schols SE, Stefanini L, et al. Key role of glycoprotein Ib/V/IX and von Willebrand factor in platelet activation-dependent fibrin formation at low shear flow. Blood. 2011;117:651-60.
9. Angiolillo DJ, Ueno M, Goto S. Basic principles of platelet biology and clinical implications. Circ J. 2010;74:597-607.
10. Borissoff JI, Spronk HMH, ten Cate H. The hemostatic system as a modulator of atherosclerosis. N Engl J Med. 2011;364:1746-60.
11. Stark K, Massberg S. Interplay between inflammation and thrombosis in cardiovascular pathology. Nat Rev Cardiol. 2021;18:666-82.
12. Libby P. Inflammation in atherosclerosis. Arterioscler Thromb Vasc Biol. 2012;32:2045-51.
13. Biasucci LM, La Rosa G, Pedicino D, et al. Where Does Inflammation Fit? Curr Cardiol Rep. 2017;19:84.
14. Libby P, Pasterkamp G, Crea F, et al. Reassessing the Mechanisms of Acute Coronary Syndromes. Circ Res. 2019;124:150-60.
15. Angiolillo DJ, Capodanno D, Goto S. Platelet thrombin receptor antagonism and atherothrombosis. Eur Heart J. 2010;31:17-28.
16. Foley JH, Conway EM. Cross Talk Pathways Between Coagulation and Inflammation. Circ Res. 2016;118:1392-408.
17. Cavender MA, Bhatt DL, Stone GW, dural Myocardial Infarction With Cangrelor as Assessed by Multiple Definitions: Findings From CHAMPION PHOENIX (Cangrelor Versus Standard Therapy to Achieve Optimal Management of Platelet Inhibition). Circulation. 2016;134:723-33.
18. Bhatt DL, Stone GW, Mahaffey KW, et al.; CHAMPION PHOENIX Investigators. Effect of platelet inhibition with cangrelor during PCI on ischemic events. N Engl J Med. 2013;368:1303-13.
19. Galli M, Migliaro S, Rodolico D, et al. Intracoronary bolus of glycoprotein IIb/IIIa inhibitor as bridging or adjunctive strategy to oral P2Y12 inhibitor load in the modern setting of STEMI. Minerva Cardiol Angiol. 2022;70(6):697-705.
20. Knuuti J, Wijns W, Saraste A, et al.; ESC Scientific Document Group. 2019 ESC Guidelines for the diagnosis and management of chronic coronary syndromes. Eur Heart J. 2020;41:407-77.
21. Collet JP, Thiele H, Barbato E, et al.; ESC Scientific Document Group. 2020 ESC Guidelines for the management of acute coronary syndromes in patients presenting without persistent ST-segment elevation. Eur Heart J. 2021;42:1289-367.
22. Ibanez B, James S, Agewall S, et al.; ESC Scientific Document Group. 2017 ESC Guidelines for the management of acute myocardial infarction in

patients presenting with ST-segment elevation: The Task Force for the management of acute myocardial infarction in patients presenting with ST-segment elevation of the European Society of Cardiology (ESC). Eur Heart J. 2018;39:119-77.

23. Levine GN, Bates ER, Bittl JA, et al. 2016 ACC/AHA Guideline Focused Update on Duration of Dual Antiplatelet Therapy in Patients With Coronary Artery Disease: A Report of the American College of Cardiology/American Heart Association Task Force on Clinical Practice Guidelines: An Update of the 2011 ACCF/AHA/SCAI Guideline for Percutaneous Coronary Intervention, 2011 ACCF/AHA Guideline for Coronary Artery Bypass Graft Surgery, 2012 ACC/AHA/ACP/AATS/PCNA/SCAI/STS Guideline for the Diagnosis and Management of Patients With Stable Ischemic Heart Disease, 2013 ACCF/AHA Guideline for the Management of ST-Elevation Myocardial Infarction, 2014 AHA/ACC Guideline for the Management of Patients With Non-ST-Elevation Acute Coronary Syndromes, and 2014 ACC/AHA Guideline on Perioperative Cardiovascular Evaluation and Management of Patients Undergoing Noncardiac Surgery. Circulation. 2016;134:e123-55.

24. Urban P, Mehran R, Colleran R, et al. Defining high bleeding risk in patients undergoing percutaneous coronary intervention. Circulation. 2019;140(3):240-61.

25. Gargiulo G, Esposito G. Consolidating the value of the standardised ARC-HBR definition. EuroIntervention. 2021;16:1126-8.

26. Buccheri S, Capodanno D, James S, et al. Bleeding after antiplatelet therapy for the treatment of acute coronary syndromes: a review of the evidence and evolving paradigms. Expert Opin Drug Saf. 2019;18:1171-89.

27. Urban P, Meredith IT, Abizaid A, et al. Polymer-free drug-coated coronary stents in patients at high bleeding risk. N Engl J Med. 2015;373(21):2038-47.

28. Ariotti S, Adamo M, Costa F, et al. Is bare-metal stent implantation still justifiable in high bleeding risk patients undergoing percutaneous coronary intervention?: A pre-specified analysis from the ZEUS trial. JACC Cardiovasc Interv. 2016;9(5):426-36.

29. Varenne O, Cook S, Sideris G, et al. Drug-eluting stents in elderly patients with coronary artery disease (SENIOR): a randomised single-blind trial. Lancet. 2018;391(10115):41-50.

30. Kandzari DE, Kirtane AJ, Windecker S, et al. One-month dual antiplatelet therapy following percutaneous coronary intervention with zotarolimus-eluting stents in high-bleeding-risk patients. Circ Cardiovasc Interv. 2020;13(11), e009565.

31. Windecker S, Latib A, Kedhi E, et al. Polymer-based or polymer-free stents in patients at high bleeding risk. N Engl J Med. 2020;382(13):1208-18.

32. Mehran R, Cao D, Angiolillo DJ, et al. 3- or 1-month DAPT in patients at high bleeding risk undergoing everolimus-eluting stent implantation. JACC Cardiovasc Interv. 2021;14(17):1870-83.

33. Valgimigli M, Frigoli E, Heg D, et al. Dual antiplatelet therapy after PCI in patients at high bleeding risk. N Engl J Med. 2021;385(18):1643-55.

34. Pivato CA, Reimers B, Testa L, et al. One-month dual antiplatelet therapy after bioresorbable polymer everolimus-eluting stents in high bleeding risk patients. J Am Heart Assoc. 2022;11(6):e023454.

35. Krucoff MW, Urban P, Tanguay JF, et al. Global approach to high bleeding risk patients with polymer-free drug-coated coronary stents: the LF II study. Circ Cardiovasc Interv. 2020;13(4):c008603.

36. Valgimigli M, Smits PC, Frigoli E, et al. Duration of antiplatelet therapy after complex percutaneous coronary intervention in patients at high bleeding risk: a Master DAPT trial sub-analysis. Eur Heart J. 2022;43(33):3100-14.

37. Writing Committee Members; Lawton JS, Tamis-Holland JE, et al. 2021 ACC/AHA/SCAI Guideline for Coronary Artery Revascularization: A Report of the American College of Cardiology/American Heart Association Joint Committee on Clinical Practice Guidelines. J Am Coll Cardiol. 2022;79(2):e21-e129.

38. Valgimigli M, Bueno H, Byrne RA, et al. 2017 ESC focused update on dual antiplatelet therapy in coronary artery disease developed in collaboration with EACTS: the Task Force for dual antiplatelet therapy in coronary artery disease of the European Society of Cardiology (ESC) and

of the European Association for Cardio-Thoracic Surgery (EACTS). Eur Heart J. 2018;39(3):213-60.

39. Cao D, Mehran R, Dangas G, et al. Validation of the Academic Research Consortium high bleeding risk definition in contemporary PCI patients. J Am Coll Cardiol. 2020;75(21):2711-22.

40. Costa F, Van Klaveren D, Feres F, et al. Dual antiplatelet therapy duration based on ischemic and bleeding risks after coronary stenting. J Am Coll Cardiol. 2019;73(7):741-54.

41. Jang Y, Park SD, Lee JP, et al. One-Month Dual Antiplatelet Therapy Followed by Prasugrel Monotherapy at a Reduced Dose: The 4D-ACS Randomised Trial. EuroIntervention. 2025;21(14):e796-e809.

42. Hansen ML, Sørensen R, Clausen MT, et al. Risk of bleeding with single, dual, or triple therapy with warfarin, aspirin, and clopidogrel in patients with atrial fibrillation. Arch Intern Med. 2010;170(16):1433-41.

43. Gibson CM, Mehran R, Bode C, et al. Prevention of bleeding in patients with atrial fibrillation undergoing PCI. N Engl J Med. 2016;375(25):2423-34.

44. Dewilde WJ, Oirbans T, Verheugt FW, et al. Use of clopidogrel with or without aspirin in patients taking oral anticoagulant therapy and undergoing percutaneous coronary intervention: an open-label, randomised, controlled trial. Lancet. 2013;381(9872):1107-15.

45. Cannon CP, Bhatt DL, Oldgren J, et al. Dual antithrombotic therapy with dabigatran after PCI in atrial fibrillation. N Engl J Med. 2017;377(16):1513-24.

46. Lopes RD, Heizer G, Aronson R, et al. Antithrombotic therapy after acute coronary syndrome or PCI in atrial fibrillation. N Engl J Med. 2019;380(16):1509-24.

47. Vranckx P, Valgimigli M, Eckardt L, et al. Edoxaban-based versus vitamin K antagonist-based antithrombotic regimen after successful coronary stenting in patients with atrial fibrillation (ENTRUST-AF PCI): a randomised, open-label, phase 3b trial. Lancet. 2019;394(10206):1335-43.

48. Gargiulo G, Goette A, Tijssen J, et al. Safety and efficacy outcomes of double vs. triple antithrombotic therapy in patients with atrial fibrillation following percutaneous coronary intervention: a systematic review and meta-analysis of non-vitamin K antagonist oral anticoagulant-based randomized clinical trials. Eur Heart J. 2019;40(46):3757-67.

CHAPTER 12

Infective Endocarditis: What is the Management in 2025?

Vibhav Sharma, Satyavir Yadav

INTRODUCTION

Infective endocarditis (IE) is defined as an infection of the endocardial surface of the heart, involving native or prosthetic valves, the mural endocardium, atrial or ventricular septal defects, or intracardiac devices. This chapter reviews the contemporary management of IE with emphasis on recent advances. A particular focus is placed on changes in epidemiology, developments in diagnostic and therapeutic approaches, the evolution of diagnostic criteria from the original Duke's criteria, the application of novel molecular and imaging modalities, the role of outpatient antibiotic therapy, and other updates.

EPIDEMIOLOGY

The annual incidence of IE was fewer than 10 cases per 100,000 person-years prior to 2000, but rose to 13.8 cases per 100,000 person-years in 2019, representing a 40% increase,[1] with comparable figures reported in our country. The disease now occurs more frequently in older, non-rheumatic populations, with a male predominance. Staphylococci and enterococci have become more common than viridans streptococci.[2] *Staphylococcus aureus* is currently the leading pathogen, particularly in healthcare-associated and injection drug use-related IE in developed countries, whereas streptococci remain predominant in developing regions. Rheumatic heart disease continues to be the principal predisposing factor in developing countries, while degenerative valvular and congenital heart disease are more common in developed nations. Despite advances in care, the overall mortality remains high at approximately 30% **(Table 1)**.

Comparison of two major registries, the earlier ICE-PCS and the more recent EURO-ENDO, demonstrates several notable epidemiological changes.

DIAGNOSIS

Diagnosis of infective endocarditis requires integration of clinical assessment, microbiological evidence, and multimodality imaging.

Clinical Features

The presentation of IE has evolved significantly compared with traditional descriptions. Key changes in signs and symptoms are summarized in **Table 2**.

Laboratory Findings

Laboratory abnormalities in IE include anemia, variable white cell count changes (leukocytosis or leukopenia), the presence of immature granulocytes, and elevated inflammatory markers such as C-reactive protein, procalcitonin, and erythrocyte sedimentation rate. Biochemical indices of organ dysfunction—such as elevated serum lactate, creatinine, bilirubin, thrombocytopenia, and cardiac biomarkers (troponins and natriuretic peptides)—reflect sepsis-related burden. However, none of these parameters is specific enough to confirm the diagnosis of IE.

TABLE 1: Change in epidemiology over time.

	ICE registry (ICE-PCS, 2000–2005; n ≈ 2,800)[3]	EURO-ENDO registry (2016–2018; n ≈ 3,100)[4]
Age	Median ~58 years	Older population
Valve	NVE ~72%; PVE ~28%	NVE ~57%; PVE ~30%; CIED ~10%
Healthcare association	~25%	~33%
Predominant organisms	S. aureus (~31%); viridans streptococci (17%) and enterococci (11%)	Staphylococci ~44% (including S. aureus); enterococci ~16%; oral streptococci ~12%
Valves most affected	Mitral (≈41%) Aortic (≈38%)	Predominantly, aortic and mitral but right-sided/device IE proportion higher than ICE
Heart failure	About one-third	Frequent
Neurological events	Stroke in ~17%; other systemic emboli ~23%	Embolic complications ~21%, often associated with vegetation burden and S. aureus
Paravalvular extension	Abscess detected in ~14%	Abscess or peri-annular extension noted; independently predicted adverse outcomes
Use of advanced imaging	Not routinely applied	PET/CT or WBC SPECT used in ~17%; especially valuable for prosthetic valve IE
Surgery during index admission	Nearly half underwent surgery (≈48%)	Surgical indication present in majority; actual surgery performed in ~51%
In-hospital mortality	~18%	~17% overall

TABLE 2: Change in clinical presentation of infective endocarditis.

Clinical feature	ICE-PCS registry (2000–2005; n ≈ 2,800)	EURO-ENDO registry (2016–2018; n ≈ 3,100)
Fever	~96%	~75%–80%
General constitutional symptoms (fatigue, weight loss, malaise, and night sweats)	~33%	~25%
Heart murmur	New or changing murmur in ~48%.	~32%
Peripheral embolic phenomena (Janeway lesions, splinter hemorrhages, Osler nodes, and Roth spots)	<10% overall	<5%
Splenomegaly	~11%	<5%
Silent or atypical presentation	Minority (~5–10%) presented without fever, particularly elderly or immunocompromised	Higher proportion of afebrile/atypical cases, again reflecting older age, comorbidities, and prosthetic/device IE

Blood Culture

Blood culture remains the cornerstone of microbiological diagnosis. Ideally, three sets should be obtained from peripheral veins at 30-minute intervals before starting antibiotics, with ~10 mL of blood in each, incubated under aerobic and anaerobic conditions. Nearly all cultures should be positive because of persistent bacteremia, while a single positive culture requires cautious interpretation.

Matrix-Assisted Laser Desorption/Ionization-Time of Flight Mass Spectrometry (MALDI-TOF MS) provides rapid identification by analyzing microbial protein "fingerprints." This technique allows species identification from positive cultures within 24–48 hours but is less reliable for fastidious organisms and does not provide minimum inhibitory concentration (MIC) data.

Blood Culture–Negative Infective Endocarditis

The most frequent cause of blood culture-negative infective endocarditis (BCNIE) is prior antibiotic exposure. Other etiologies include fungi and fastidious or obligate intracellular organisms that require specialized media and prolonged incubation. Modern microbiological techniques have substantially improved diagnostic yield. A structured approach begins with targeted blood cultures for likely pathogens; if negative, systematic serological testing is advised for *Coxiella burnetii*, *Bartonella* spp., *Aspergillus*, *Legionella pneumophila*, *Brucella*, and *Mycoplasma pneumoniae*. Additional investigations may include rheumatoid factor, antiphospholipid antibodies (anticardiolipin IgG, anti-β2-glycoprotein-1 IgG/IgM), antinuclear antibodies, and in select cases anti-pork antibodies, as hypersensitivity to porcine bioprosthetic valves can mimic IE. The choice of serological testing should be individualized according to patient profile (e.g., *Aspergillus* in immunocompromised hosts), regional epidemiology, and known test limitations. For patients undergoing surgery, excised tissue or prosthetic material should always be examined by culture, histopathology, and molecular assays such as 16S/18S rRNA sequencing to enhance diagnostic accuracy **(Table 3)**.

Imaging Modalities in Infective Endocarditis

Echocardiography

- *Transthoracic echocardiography (TTE):* First-line imaging tool
- *Transoesophageal echocardiography (TEE):* Recommended when TTE is inconclusive, negative despite strong suspicion, or positive but complications need evaluation.

Cardiac Computed Tomography

- Higher accuracy than TEE for perivalvular or prosthetic complications (abscesses, pseudoaneurysms, and fistulae)
- Echocardiography remains superior for small vegetations (<10 mm), leaflet perforations, and intracardiac fistulae.

Computed Tomography Beyond the Heart

- *Systemic complications:* Whole-body/brain CT can detect extracardiac emboli or mycotic aneurysms.
- *Neurological involvement:* Less sensitive than MRI but preferred in emergency settings for detecting ischemic or hemorrhagic events
- *Source detection:* May identify extracardiac foci such as occult malignancy, but does not replace targeted tests (e.g., colonoscopy).

Magnetic Resonance Imaging

- Brain MRI is more sensitive than CT for neurological complications; 60–80% of

TABLE 3: Current diagnostic techniques in infective endocarditis.

Method	Sample used	Application	Limitations	Key references
Broad-range 16S/18S rRNA PCR	Blood, valve tissue	Detects bacterial or fungal DNA	Risk of contamination; limited sensitivity for rare pathogens	5,6
Pathogen-specific PCR	Blood, valve tissue	Targets fastidious organisms (*Bartonella*, *T. whipplei*, and fungi)	Restricted to selected microbes	5,7
Fluorescence in situ hybridization (FISH) + PCR	Prosthetic valve tissue	Enhances detection when cultures are negative, especially in prosthetic valve IE	Needs advanced laboratory facilities	8
Next-generation sequencing (NGS)	Plasma microbial cell-free DNA, valve tissue	Unbiased, broad pathogen detection; useful in BCNIE	High cost; limited routine availability	9,10
MALDI-TOF mass spectrometry	Positive blood cultures, excised valve tissue	Rapid species-level identification within hours	Does not provide susceptibility; database dependent	11
Serology	Serum	Identifies *Coxiella burnetii*, *Bartonella*, *Brucella*, etc.	Cross-reactivity; cannot confirm active infection alone	5,12
Histopathology with immunohistochemistry	Resected valve or embolic tissue	Detects microorganisms and helps differentiate infectious vs. autoimmune/neoplastic lesions	Requires tissue; may miss organisms if unevenly distributed	5,13

patients show CNS lesions (often silent and ischemic).
- Severe complications (hemorrhage, abscess, and mycotic aneurysm) occur in <10%.
- Routine brain MRI may provide additional minor Duke criteria, reclassifying ~25% of inconclusive cases.
- Cerebral microbleeds (seen in 50–60%) lack correlation with ischemia and are not Duke criteria.
- Magnetic resonance imaging is the reference standard for spondylodiscitis/vertebral osteomyelitis, with 90–95% accuracy.

Nuclear Imaging (PET/CT, SPECT/CT)
- *Prosthetic valve Infective endocarditis:*
  - *[18F]FDG-PET/CT:* Sensitivity ~86%, specificity ~84%.
  - *White blood cells SPECT/CT:* Sensitivity 64–90%, specificity 36–100%; best for periprosthetic abscesses.
  - 99mTc-HMPAO-SPECT/CT reduces "possible IE" misclassification by ~30%.
- *Native valve IE (NVE):* Lower sensitivity (~31%) but very high specificity (~98%).
- *Whole-body PET/CT:* Valuable for detecting septic emboli, metastatic infection, or portals of entry.

- *Treatment monitoring:* FDG-PET/CT may help track persistence or resolution of infection.

Evolution of Diagnostic Criteria

The diagnostic framework for infective endocarditis has progressed from the *2000 Modified Duke criteria* to the *2015 ESC modification*, and most recently the *2023 ESC update*, with refinements reflecting advances in imaging (including CT, MRI, PET/CT, and SPECT/CT) and microbiological diagnostics **(Table 4)**.

Note: The Duke–ISCVID 2023 updates,[25] published in Clinical Infectious Diseases (2023), represent a joint revision of the Duke criteria by the International Society for Cardiovascular Infectious Diseases (ISCVID). This marked the first major update since 2000, aiming to enhance both sensitivity and specificity by integrating advances in microbiology and imaging. Key modifications include broader recognition of typical microorganisms, such as *Enterococcus faecalis* and *Staphylococcus lugdunensis*; the inclusion of advanced imaging modalities—FDG-PET/CT, cardiac CT, and WBC-SPECT/CT—as major diagnostic criteria; and a more structured set of minor criteria, encompassing embolic phenomena and metastatic infections. These revisions were designed for global applicability, not restricted to Europe. The ESC 2023 criteria incorporate many of the Duke–ISCVID updates and extend them further by embedding the diagnostic approach within a comprehensive clinical guideline framework. The table below presents the ESC 2023 diagnostic criteria for infective endocarditis, reflecting all the aforementioned updates **(Table 5)**.

■ TREATMENT
Principles of Treatment

- Bactericidal agents are more effective than bacteriostatic drugs in the management of infective endocarditis.
- Aminoglycosides are often used in combination with other antibiotics to exploit their synergistic activity.
- *Tolerant bacteria:* These organisms remain susceptible to the administered antibiotics but can evade drug-induced killing by entering a dormant state and may resume growth later. This tolerance may result from specific genetic mutations or the presence of exopolysaccharides in biofilms. In such cases, prolonged courses of bactericidal drug combinations are recommended.
- In patients requiring surgical intervention, the antibiotic regimen should follow the protocol for native valve endocarditis rather than prosthetic valve endocarditis, and the duration of therapy should be calculated from the day of the first negative blood culture, rather than from the day of surgery.
- A recent retrospective cohort study published in 2021[26] evaluated 180 patients with staphylococcal prosthetic valve endocarditis [*S. aureus* and coagulase-negative staphylococci (CONS)]. The study compared outcomes in patients who received rifampicin versus those who did not, finding no significant difference in 1-year mortality or relapse. Although larger randomized controlled trials are warranted, rifampicin remains recommended in susceptible cases of prosthetic valve endocarditis. Rifampicin should be initiated 3–5 days after starting the primary antibiotic regimen due to its antagonistic activity against actively replicating bacteria.
- Robust evidence comparing different antibiotic regimens for infective endocarditis remains limited.
- The POET trial, a multicenter, randomized, non-blinded study published by Iversen et al. in 2019,[27] enrolled 400 clinically stable patients with left-sided native or prosthetic

TABLE 4: Evolution of the current diagnostic criteria.

Aspect	2000 (Modified Duke criteria)	2015 ESC criteria	2023 ESC criteria
Overall framework	Clinical + microbiological + echocardiographic, sensitivity ~80%[14]	Included multimodality imaging to overcome limitations of Duke, especially in prosthetic/device-related IE	Refined and updated criteria; introduced structured diagnostic algorithms, microbiological upgrades, molecular biology, and new classification system
Limitations	Reduced accuracy in PVE, CIED, CHD, aortic grafts. Up to 30% of cases inconclusive with echo alone[15-17]	Improved yield but required ≥3 months post-surgery before nuclear imaging considered reliable	PET/CT uptake accepted as major criterion even early post-operative if focal/heterogeneous uptake present[18-20] as opposed to mild, diffuse homogeneous post-operative changes
Microbiological criteria	"Typical" organisms defined (e.g., S. aureus, viridans streptococci). E. faecalis not considered typical	No major microbiological changes from 2000	E. faecalis now recognized as a typical pathogen, improving sensitivity (70% → 96%)[21]
Echocardiography	Mainstay	Complemented with CT, MRI, and nuclear imaging	First-line, but clearly integrated into diagnostic algorithms alongside CT, PET/CT, MRI for specific clinical contexts
CT/MRI	Not part of diagnostic framework.	Cardiac/whole-body CT and cerebral MRI added for complications and embolic events	Explicitly incorporated in diagnostic algorithms (native valve IE, PVE, CIED)
PET/CT and WBC SPECT/CT	Not included	Introduced as supportive evidence; uptake considered diagnostic for PVE only after 3 months	Now a major criterion: Focal or heterogeneous uptake diagnostic of PVE even in early post-op period (if interpreted correctly)
Minor criteria	Predisposing condition, fever, vascular and immunological phenomena, microbiology not meeting major criteria	Similar, but broader recognition of embolic complications	Expanded: Distant lesions (e.g., cerebral emboli, spondylodiscitis) formally included[22,23]
Molecular methods	Not included	Not included	16S/18S rRNA PCR on valve/embolic tissue included; high specificity (90–100%)[24]
Classification	• Definite, possible, or rejected IE • Applied once	Retained Duke-based classification with modifications	New classification system: Diagnosis should be re-evaluated during hospital stay and follow-up by endocarditis team.
Diagnostic algorithms	Not available	Not structured; emphasis on multimodality imaging	Clear algorithms for NVE, PVE, and CIED
Key innovation	Foundation criteria integrating clinical + echo + microbiology	First integration of multimodality imaging into IE diagnosis	Major refinement: new microbiological/imaging thresholds, inclusion of molecular methods, structured algorithms, and dynamic classification

TABLE 5: ESC 2023 diagnostic criteria for infective endocarditis.

Category	Definition

Major criteria	• *Microbiological evidence:*
	  – *Blood cultures positive for typical organisms (from two separate cultures)*: Oral streptococci, *Streptococcus gallolyticus*, HACEK group, *Staphylococcus aureus*, *Enterococcus faecalis*.
	  – *Persistent bacteremia with organisms consistent with IE*:
	    - ≥2 positive cultures drawn >12 hours apart, *or*
	    - All of three or the majority of ≥4 cultures positive (with first and last sample ≥1 hours apart)
	  – Single positive culture for *Coxiella burnetii* or phase I IgG antibody titer >1:800
	• *Imaging evidence:* Anatomic or metabolic lesions typical of IE detected by:
	  – Echocardiography (TTE/TOE)
	  – Cardiac CT
	  – [^18F]FDG PET/CT
	  – WBC SPECT/CT

Minor criteria	• *Predisposition:* High/intermediate risk cardiac condition or injection drug use • *Fever:* >38°C • *Vascular/embolic events:* Systemic/pulmonary emboli, infarcts, abscesses, mycotic aneurysms, osteoarticular infection (e.g., spondylodiscitis), intracranial hemorrhage or ischemia, Janeway lesions, conjunctival hemorrhages • *Immunological phenomena:* Glomerulonephritis, Osler nodes, Roth spots, positive rheumatoid factor • *Microbiology not meeting major criteria:* Positive culture not fulfilling major thresholds, or positive serology for an organism known to cause IE
Classification of IE	• *Definite IE:* Two major criteria *or* one major + ≥3 minor criteria *or* five minor criteria • *Possible IE:* One major + 1–2 minor criteria *or* 3–4 minor criteria • *Rejected IE:* Criteria not met for "definite" *or* "possible" IE, with *or* without an alternative confirmed diagnosis

valve endocarditis caused by *S. aureus*, CONS, *Enterococcus faecalis*, or *Streptococcus* spp. Participants were randomized to receive either intravenous or oral antibiotics and followed for 6 months. Oral therapy was found to be non-inferior to intravenous therapy regarding a composite outcome of mortality, embolic events, unplanned surgery, or relapse. This non-inferiority was maintained during extended follow-up of 5 years. Patients received dual oral antibiotics tailored to pathogen susceptibility. However, the trial excluded MRSA cases and is applicable only to the pathogens studied. Notably, only about 20% of screened patients were eligible for randomization, indicating that in real-world practice, only a subset of patients may be suitable for oral therapy. The specific antibiotic regimens used in the study are detailed below **(Table 6)**.

On clinical suspicion of IE, ≥3 blood cultures (from different sites, ≥30 minutes apart) should be sent immediately. If patient is hemodynamically unstable, empirical antibiotics may be started immediately after sending cultures.

Empiric Therapy (Table 7)

Following the isolation of microorganisms, the antibiotic regimen should be modified accordingly.

TABLE 6: Antibiotic regimen used in the POET trial.

Microorganism	Oral regimen	Remarks
Streptococcus spp.	Amoxicillin + moxifloxacin *or* Amoxicillin + linezolid	Amoxicillin at 1 g q6h. Moxifloxacin for broad gram-positive coverage
Enterococcus faecalis	Amoxicillin + moxifloxacin *or* Amoxicillin + linezolid	If fluoroquinolone resistance or contraindication → linezolid was used
MSSA (*Staphylococcus aureus*)	Dicloxacillin + rifampin *or* Moxifloxacin + rifampin	
Coagulase-negative staphylococci	Dicloxacillin + rifampin *or* Moxifloxacin + rifampin	

TABLE 7: Empirical antibiotic regimen for infective endocarditis.

	Regimen of choice (iv)	Duration	Remarks
Community-acquired NVE or late PVE (≥12 months post-surgery)	Ampicillin *plus* ceftriaxone *or* (flu)cloxacillin *plus* gentamicin	Switch once culture reports are available	Cover streptococci, MSSA, enterococci
Early PVE (<12 months) *or* healthcare-associated IE	Vancomycin *plus* gentamicin *plus* rifampin	As above	Aims to cover MRSA, CONS, enterococci; consider non-HACEK GNB risk
β-lactam allergy (community NVE/late PVE)	Cefazolin (if not anaphylaxis-type) *or* vancomycin, *plus* gentamicin	As above	

Specific Therapy

Treatment of oral Streptococci including Streptococcus gallolyticus: Oral streptococci: includes viridans group (*mitis, sanguinis, anginosus, salivarius, downei,* and *mutans*) and *Streptococcus gallolyticus* (formerly *S. bovis*). Following table summarizes the recommended antibiotic regimens. After 10–14 days of iv antibiotics, outpatient iv antibiotic therapy (OPAT) or oral antibiotics may be considered **(Table 8)**.

Staphylococcus aureus and coagulase-negative staphylococci (CONS): Staphylococcus aureus typically causes a fulminant course of endocarditis, whereas CONS generally presents with a subacute form. The recommended antibiotic regimens for staphylococcal infective endocarditis are outlined in the table that follows. For methicillin-sensitive *S. aureus* (MSSA), β-lactams remain superior to vancomycin. Prosthetic valve endocarditis (PVE) due to *S. aureus* carries high mortality and often requires early surgical intervention. In a prospective cohort study involving 94 patients with staphylococcal PVE,[28] adjunctive gentamicin showed no clear benefit; however, in the absence of randomized trials, current guidelines still advise its short-term use.

Methicillin-resistant S. aureus (MRSA): Treatment options include vancomycin, daptomycin, ceftaroline, and dalbavancin. Increasingly, strains with reduced susceptibility or resistance to vancomycin have been reported globally.

TABLE 8: Treatment of Streptococcal endocarditis.

	Clinical setting	Antibiotic	Duration (weeks)	If β-lactam allergy
Penicillin-susceptible oral streptococci and *S. gallolyticus* group	NVE/PVE	Penicillin G 12–18 MU/day IV (4–6 divided doses or continuous infusion) or Amoxicillin 100–200 mg/kg/day IV (4–6 divided doses) or Ceftriaxone 2 g/day IV	4/6	Vancomycin 30 mg/kg/day IV in two divided doses
	Non-complicated NVE (fast-track option)	Same as above *plus* Gentamicin 3 mg/kg/day IV *or* IM (once daily)	2	–
Penicillin-resistant *or* increased-exposure group	NVE	Same as above *plus* Gentamicin	4	Vancomycin
	PVE	Same as above *plus* Gentamicin	6	Vancomycin *plus* Gentamicin 3 mg/kg/day

Streptococcus pneumonia IE is treated along similar lines.
IE due to group A, B, C, or G streptococci, including the *Streptococcus anginosus* group (*S. constellatus, S. anginosus,* and *S. intermedius*) is relatively rare.
Group A streptococci are uniformly susceptible to beta-lactams. Group B streptococci, previously seen in peripartum, is now seen in all age and both sexes. Groups B, C, and G streptococci and *S. anginosus* predispose to intracardiac abscesses. Antibiotic regimen is similar to other streptococci.
Nutritionally variant streptococci—*Abiotrophia* and *Granulicatella* induce large vegetations. Treated with penicillin G, ceftriaxone or vancomycin. Gentamicin is added for initial 2 weeks in PVE.

Daptomycin, a lipopeptide antibiotic approved for *S. aureus* bacteremia and right-sided IE, demonstrates greater efficacy in cases with vancomycin resistance.

Other alternatives: Potential regimens include combinations such as fosfomycin with imipenem, ceftaroline, quinupristin–dalfopristin (with or without β-lactams), β-lactams with oxazolidinones (e.g., linezolid), β-lactams with vancomycin, as well as high-dose trimethoprim-sulfamethoxazole or clindamycin **(Table 9)**.

Enterococcal Infective Endocarditis

The majority of enterococcal IE cases are caused by *Enterococcus faecalis*, whereas *E. faecium* and other species account for <10%. These organisms often require *prolonged synergistic bactericidal therapy*. Resistance mechanisms are frequent and clinically relevant:

- *High-level aminoglycoside resistance (HLAR):* Observed in up to 75% of isolates, leading to loss of synergy with aminoglycosides.
- *β-lactam resistance:* It can result from either altered penicillin-binding proteins (PBPs) or β-lactamase production.
- *Vancomycin resistance:* Most often associated with *E. faecium*, and less commonly with *E. faecalis*.

For *E. faecalis* endocarditis, recent evidence indicates that the combination of *ampicillin* +

TABLE 9: Treatment of staphylococcal endocarditis.

	Regimen of choice	Duration (weeks)	Remarks
MSSA NVE	(Flu)cloxacillin 12 g/day iv in 4–6 divided doses or Cefazolin 6 g/day in three divided doses (IV)	4–6	• *If immediate penicillin allergy*: Cefazolin • *If severe β-lactam allergy:* Consider *daptomycin* ± ceftaroline or fosfomycin • Daptomycin – 10 mg/kg/day iv in one dose • Ceftaroline – 1,800 mg/day iv in three divided doses • Fosfomycin – 8–12 g/day iv in four doses
MSSA PVE	(Flu)cloxacillin *or* cefazolin + *rifampin* (≥6 weeks) + *gentamicin* (first 2 weeks) Rifampicin 900 mg/day oral or iv in three divided doses	≥6	*If penicillin allergy:* Cefazolin + rifampin + gentamicin
MRSA NVE	Vancomycin (IV)	4–6	*If intolerance/poor response:* Consider *daptomycin* ± anti-staph β-lactam
MRSA PVE	Vancomycin + *rifampin* (≥6 weeks) + *gentamicin* (first 2 weeks)	≥6	—

ceftriaxone is as effective as *ampicillin + gentamicin*, but with a significantly *lower risk of nephrotoxicity*. Importantly, this benefit is restricted to *E. faecalis* and does not extend to *E. faecium* or other enterococci[29] **(Table 10)**.

HACEK Group

The *HACEK organisms* [*Haemophilus, Aggregatibacter* (formerly *Actinobacillus*), *Cardiobacterium, Eikenella*, and *Kingella*] are fastidious gram-negative bacteria. Standard therapy is *ceftriaxone 4 g/day IV for 6 weeks*.

Blood Culture–Negative Infective Endocarditis (Table 11)

- *Brucella:* Doxycycline 200 mg/day + cotrimoxazole 960 mg every 12 hours + rifampin 300–600 mg/day, orally for 3–6 months. *Treatment goal*: Antibody titer <1:60.
- *Tropheryma whipplei:* Doxycycline 200 mg/day + Hydroxychloroquine 200–600 mg/day, orally for ≥18 months.
- *Mycoplasma:* Levofloxacin 500 mg every 12 hours, IV or oral, for ≥6 months.
- *Legionella:* Levofloxacin 500 mg every 12 hours, IV or oral, for ≥6 weeks; or clarithromycin 500 mg every 12 hours IV for 2 weeks, then oral for 4 weeks, plus rifampin 300–1200 mg/day.
- *Bartonella:* Doxycycline 100 mg every 12 hours for 4 weeks + gentamicin for 2 weeks.
- *Coxiella burnetii (Q fever):* Doxycycline 200 mg/day + hydroxychloroquine 200–600 mg/day for ≥18 months. *Treatment success*: Antiphase I IgG <1:400 and IgA/IgM <1:50.

Step-down/Outpatient Therapy

Transition to *OPAT (outpatient parenteral antibiotic therapy)* or *partial oral therapy* can be considered based on predefined objective criteria **(Table 11)**. Selection of oral agents should be based on susceptibility testing (please refer ESC 2023 IE guidelines online supplementary **Table S9**).[30]

TABLE 10: Treatment of enterococcal endocarditis.

	Regimen of choice	Duration (weeks)	Remarks
Non-HLAR enterococcus (usually E. faecalis), NVE/PVE HLAR – high level aminoglycoside resistance	Ampicillin or Amoxicillin plus Ceftriaxone	6	Alternative: ampicillin/amoxicillin + gentamicin (gentamicin for 2 weeks if NVE)
HLAR enterococcus (NVE or PVE)	Ampicillin or Amoxicillin plus Ceftriaxone	6	
β-lactam-resistant enterococcus (e.g., E. faecium)	Vancomycin plus Gentamicin	6 (Genta for 2 weeks)	
VRE (vancomycin-resistant)	High-dose daptomycin plus a β-lactam (ampicillin, ertapenem, or ceftaroline) or Fosfomycin	≥6	

TABLE 11: Criteria for transitioning to outpatient antibiotic therapy (compiled from ESC 2023 IE guidelines).[30]

Step	Criteria
Step 1: Confirm diagnosis and initial phase completed	■ IE diagnosis confirmed ■ Minimum 10 days of in-hospital IV therapy completed (longer if unstable at onset)
Step 2: Clinical stability check	☑ A febrile for ≥48–72 hours ☑ Hemodynamically stable ☑ No signs of ongoing sepsis or decompensated heart failure
Step 3: Microbiological control	☑ Blood cultures negative for ≥48–72 hours ☑ Pathogen identified, antibiotic susceptibility known
Step 4: Cardiac and complication status	☑ No urgent indication for surgery ☑ No uncontrolled perivalvular abscess or conduction block progression ☑ No recent (<2 weeks) major CNS event with unstable neurological status
Step 5: Exclusion of high-risk IE types	⊘ Early PVE (<60 days post-surgery) ⊘ Fungal IE ⊘ IE with multidrug-resistant organisms ⊘ infected CIED in situ
Step 6: OPAT infrastructure and patient factors	☑ Reliable venous access ☑ OPAT team with infectious disease + cardiology input ☑ Weekly laboratories: CBC, renal, liver, CRP ☑ Home support system + transport ☑ Patient understands treatment plan and signs of complication
Eligibility decision	If ALL boxes in Steps 1–6 are ☑ → Eligible for OPAT → Discharge with structured OPAT plan, weekly review, and rapid readmission pathway. If ANY box in Steps 1–5 is ⊘ → Continue inpatient care.

Role of Dalbavancin in Infective Endocarditis

Dalbavancin[31,32] is a long-acting lipoglycopeptide active against *Staphylococcus aureus* (MSSA/MRSA), *Streptococcus spp.*, and *E. faecalis*. Its ~14-day half-life allows weekly or biweekly dosing, making it attractive when prolonged IV therapy is needed.

Current Evidence

- Not included in guideline-recommended first-line IE therapy.
- *Increasingly used off-label in*:
  - Patients unable to remain hospitalized or maintain long-term IV access.
  - Step-down therapy after initial stabilization.
  - Salvage therapy when standard regimens are not tolerated/feasible.
- Case series, observational cohorts, and small trials suggest efficacy in both native and prosthetic valve IE, particularly MRSA and enterococcal infections.
- *Reported outcomes*: High clinical success and fewer rehospitalizations, though data are limited and heterogeneous.
- No large randomized controlled trials in IE; hence, dalbavancin should be considered only as an alternative/adjunct, ideally within a multidisciplinary endocarditis team.

Fungal Endocarditis

- *Causative agents:* Most often *Candida* and *Aspergillus*; less frequently histoplasma or cryptococcus.
- *Risk factors:* Prosthetic heart valves, immunodeficiency, prior cardiac surgery, intravenous drug use, and long-term central venous catheters.
- *Clinical features:* Typically, culture-negative endocarditis with large vegetations and high embolic risk.
- *Diagnosis:* Blood cultures are usually positive for *Candida* but rarely for *Aspergillus*. Histopathology of surgical specimens and tissue/blood PCR aid diagnosis. Serum galactomannan supports the diagnosis of aspergillosis.
- *Treatment*
  - *Candida:* Liposomal amphotericin B 3–5 mg/kg/day ± flucytosine 25 mg/kg q24h; step-down to fluconazole if the strain is susceptible. High-dose echinocandins are an alternative if amphotericin is contraindicated.
  - *Aspergillus:* Voriconazole 6 mg/kg q12h for two doses, then 4 mg/kg q12h.
- *Surgical role:* Early valve surgery is indicated in most patients, followed by ≥6 weeks of antifungal therapy, then lifelong azole suppressive therapy to reduce relapse risk.

SURGICAL MANAGEMENT OF INFECTIVE ENDOCARDITIS

Surgery is integral to IE management when antimicrobial therapy alone cannot control infection or when structural complications occur. Radical debridement—removal of vegetations, abscesses, fistulae, and infected prosthetic material—is the cornerstone. Valve repair is prioritized, particularly for the mitral valve, to preserve native tissue and limit prosthetic-related complications **(Table 12)**.

Surgical Techniques

- *Aortic valve IE*: Valve replacement is standard; repair feasible only in select cases.
- *Mitral valve IE*: Repair preferred whenever technically possible.
- *Tricuspid valve IE*: Repair is first choice; if not feasible, replacement with a biological prosthesis is favored over mechanical.
- *Peri-annular complications*: Abscesses, pseudoaneurysms, or fistulae require

TABLE 12: Indications and timing of surgery in infective endocarditis.

When is surgery needed?	Urgency of surgery
Severe valvular lesions → refractory heart failure or cardiogenic shock (leaflet perforation or rupture leading to new severe valvular regurgitation, intracardiac fistulae, vegetation causing mal-coaptation, ischemia from coronary embolism)	Emergency (≤24 hours)
Persistent heart failure symptoms despite medical management	Urgent (3–5 days)
Severe valvular regurgitation without heart failure	Elective
Uncontrolled infection—persistent bacteremia, septic shock, abscess, persistent infection (persistent fever and positive blood cultures after 7 days of appropriate antibiotic therapy and ruling out septic embolic complications), increasing vegetation size, perivalvular extension leading to new AV block, resistant or virulent organisms such as MRSA, VRE, non-HACEK GNB (if not responding to therapy) and fungi	Urgent
• Embolic risk (vegetation ≥10 mm)—surgery must be performed if already embolic manifestations or another indication for surgery. Weaker indication for vegetations >10 mm but no embolism or another indication for surgery • Most commonly to the brain and spleen	Urgent
• Early PVE (<6 months of surgery)	Urgent/early
• CIED-related IE • Requires complete extraction	Immediate
Ischemic stroke	No delay
Hemorrhagic stroke	Delay suggested
Persistent AV block	Immediate pacemaker

aggressive debridement and reconstruction using patches, conduits, or homografts.

Choice of Prosthetic Material (Infective Endocarditis Surgery)

- *Biological valves:* Often preferred when long-term anticoagulation is undesirable (e.g., older patients, bleeding risk, and IVDU), with durability acceptable for life expectancy. Current evidence does not show lower reinfection versus mechanical; outcomes are broadly similar, so selection is individualized.
- *Mechanical valves:* Reasonable in younger patients with longer life expectancy when anticoagulation is acceptable/indicated.
- *Homografts/valved conduits:* Reserved for extensive destructive disease (e.g., annular/root abscess, invasive PVE) and aortic root involvement, where radical debridement and root replacement may be required **(Flowchart 1)**.

COMPLICATIONS

- *Neurological complications:* Commonly include ischemic or hemorrhagic stroke, transient ischemic attacks, silent emboli, cerebral abscesses, meningitis, encephalopathy, and seizures. In patients with embolic stroke, thrombolysis is contraindicated, while mechanical thrombectomy may be considered if appropriate. Mycotic aneurysms, though rare, can cause fatal intracerebral or subarachnoid hemorrhage. If suspected, CT is superior MR cerebral angiography is recommended; digital subtraction angiography (DSA) is indicated when suspicion

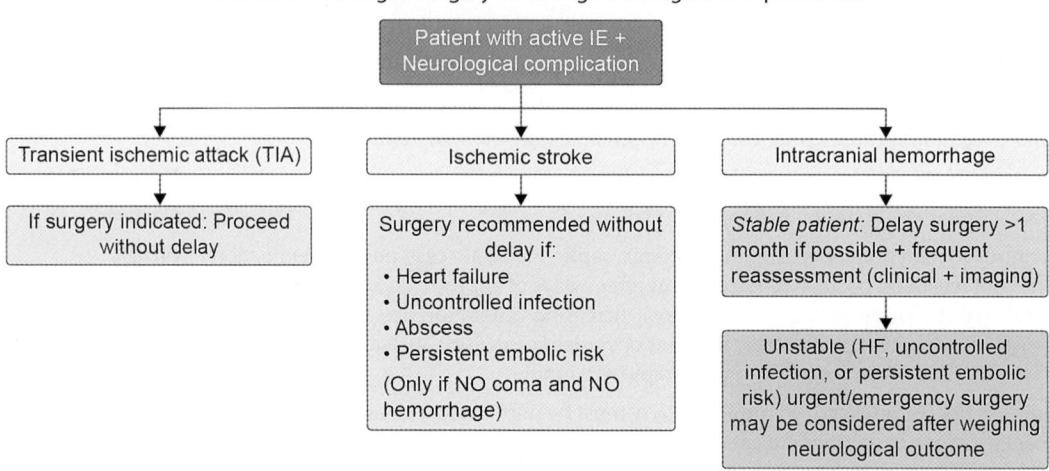

Flowchart 1: Timing of surgery following neurological complications.

persists despite negative imaging. Ruptured aneurysms, or large unruptured aneurysms that enlarge despite antibiotics, warrant surgical or percutaneous treatment. The safety of pre-existing anticoagulation remains uncertain; a retrospective analysis found that anticoagulation did not significantly affect the risk of stroke, intracranial hemorrhage, or short-term mortality in left-sided IE and may be continued when needed.[33]

- *Splenic complications:* Splenic infarction occurs in up to 40% of cases, usually asymptomatic, while splenic abscesses develop in ~5%. Splenectomy (ideally before cardiac surgery) is indicated for large or refractory abscesses, whereas percutaneous drainage is reserved for high-risk surgical candidates.
- *Myocarditis and pericarditis:* Purulent pericarditis may arise from rupture of a pseudoaneurysm or fistula and require urgent surgical drainage.
- *Conduction disturbances:* Typically result from perivalvular extension of infection. Risk factors include preexisting conduction abnormalities, *S. aureus* infection, tricuspid valve involvement, and aortic root abscesses.
- *Acute renal failure:* Multifactorial, related to immune complex glomerulonephritis, renal emboli, sepsis, hemodynamic compromise, cardiac surgery, and nephrotoxic medications.
- *Musculoskeletal manifestations:* They include arthralgia, myalgia, peripheral arthritis (~14%), and spondylodiscitis (3–15%).

INFECTIVE ENDOCARDITIS IN SPECIFIC SETTING

Prosthetic Valve Endocarditis

Prosthetic valve endocarditis (PVE) occurs in 1–6% of patients with prosthetic valves[34] and carries a high in-hospital mortality of 20–40%.[35] It is reported to be more frequent with bioprosthetic valves.[36] Early PVE is typically caused by *S. aureus, S. epidermidis*, gram-negative bacilli, or fungi, whereas late PVE resembles native valve endocarditis (NVE) in microbial profile. *Mycobacterium chimaera*, acquired from contaminated cardiopulmonary bypass heater–cooler units, is a rare cause that usually presents late.

Transesophageal echocardiography is essential for diagnosis due to its higher sensitivity for detecting vegetations and peri-annular complications. Cardiac CT angiography (CTA) is useful when echocardiography is inconclusive, particularly for identifying prosthetic dehiscence, abscesses, pseudoaneurysms, and fistulae. FDG-PET/CT and WBC-SPECT/CT significantly improve diagnostic accuracy in suspected PVE and are incorporated as major imaging criteria in the modified Duke–ESC criteria.

Management includes pathogen-directed antibiotic therapy (as detailed earlier). Surgery with complete debridement and prosthesis replacement is recommended urgently for early PVE. Selected cases of non-staphylococcal late PVE may be managed conservatively with close follow-up. Prognosis is worse compared with NVE, both in-hospital and long-term.

Endocarditis After Transcatheter Aortic Valve Implantation

Endocarditis following transcatheter aortic valve implantation (TAVI) occurs at a rate of 0.3–1.9 per 100 patient-years,[37] independent of valve type. Clinical presentation may be atypical, especially in elderly patients where fever is often absent. Diagnostic challenges arise due to frequent absence of vegetations, metallic artefacts from stent frames (especially self-expanding valves), vegetations located on the stent frame rather than valve leaflets, and occasionally involvement of structures remote from the prosthesis (e.g., mitral valve). CTA, FDG-PET, and intracardiac echocardiography may enhance diagnostic yield. Prognosis is poor due to advanced age and comorbidities, and surgical management is technically challenging given adhesions between the stent frame and surrounding tissue. Medical and surgical principles remain similar to PVE.

Cardiac Implantable Electronic Device Infections

Cardiac implantable electronic device infections range from superficial wound infections to isolated pocket infections and systemic infections with or without vegetations on leads or right-sided valves. S. aureus and CONS are the predominant pathogens. CONS commonly cause chronic pocket infections. Other organisms include *Enterococcus, Streptococcus spp., Cutibacterium*, gram-negative bacilli (e.g., *Pseudomonas, Serratia*), and fungi.[30]

Risk factors include renal failure, diabetes, repeat interventions, CRT systems, temporary pacing, prolonged procedures, hematoma formation, and surgical re-exploration.[38] Standard peri-procedural antibiotic prophylaxis targeting S. aureus is recommended (Class I). Prophylaxis for dental, genitourinary, gastrointestinal, or respiratory procedures is not recommended. Suggested regimens include *flucloxacillin (1–2 g iv), cefazolin (1–2 g iv), or vancomycin (1–2 g iv over 60–90 minutes)* when β-lactam allergy or MRSA prevalence is high.

Diagnosis requires three sets of blood cultures, TTE/TEE in all patients (repeatable after 7 days if suspicion persists), and adjunctive imaging such as FDG-PET or WBC-SPECT/CT. Intracardiac echocardiography may help assess right-sided leads when TEE is inconclusive. Sonication of removed hardware can increase pathogen detection when cultures are negative or discordant.[39]

Treatment is pathogen-directed IV therapy, with typical durations calculated from the first negative culture or definitive source control:
- *No vegetations and non-S. aureus*: ~2 weeks
- *Vegetations and/or S. aureus*: ~4 weeks
- *Septic emboli or associated prosthetic valve infection*: ~6 weeks

Complete device and lead extraction is strongly recommended, with earlier removal improving outcomes. In patients with large vegetations (>20 mm), percutaneous debulking or aspiration may be performed prior to extraction to reduce embolic risk. Extraction is also advised in patients with persistent or relapsing gram-positive bacteremia or fungemia, even without visible lead infection. Re-implantation must occur at a new site (contralateral or alternative) only after infection resolution and sustained negative blood cultures ≥72 hours (≥2 weeks if vegetations were present) (Class I). Leadless pacemakers may be considered to minimize recurrence risk.

Prevention strategies are guided by the PADIT risk score,[40] which stratifies patients undergoing CIED procedures. In high-risk patients, use of antibacterial envelopes (e.g., TYRX™) can reduce major device-related infections. A randomized trial of ~7,000 patients showed a ~40% relative reduction in major infections at 12 months (0.7% vs. 1.2%), with benefits extending to 3 years, particularly for pocket infections, without increasing complications[41] **(Table 13)**.

The AngioVac system provides a minimally invasive method for percutaneous removal of large right-sided vegetations in infective endocarditis, most often on the tricuspid valve or infected pacemaker/ICD leads (>20 mm). By using vacuum-assisted aspiration and extracorporeal filtration, it can significantly reduce vegetation size, bacterial burden, and the risk of septic pulmonary embolism, while facilitating safer device or lead extraction. It is particularly useful in patients who are poor surgical candidates or as a bridge to definitive surgery, with high procedural success rates and low complication rates. However, its role is adjunctive rather than curative, since it cannot replace prolonged antibiotic therapy or surgery when indicated, and its use is largely limited to right-sided IE in specialized centers.

Right sided IE: 5–10% of all patients with IE.[42] Predisposing factors include—iv drug abuse, immunodeficiency, central catheters, and congenital heart diseases. Tricuspid valve is involved much more commonly than the pulmonary valve with *Staphylococcus aureus* being the most common implicated bacteria. Interestingly,

TABLE 13: PADIT risk score.

Variable	Points
Age <60 years	1
Renal insufficiency (eGFR <30 mL/min/ 1.73 m² or dialysis)	1
Immunocompromised state (chronic steroids, chemotherapy, etc.)	1
Diabetes mellitus	1
Procedure type:	
• Generator replacement, upgrade, or revision	1
• Addition of new leads	2
• Cardiac resynchronization therapy (CRT) device	2
Hospitalization for procedure (vs. outpatient/short stay)	1

PADIT score	Risk of CIED infection (1 year)
0–4 (Low)	~0.5%
5–6 (Intermediate)	~1.4%
≥7 (High)	~3.4%

eustachian valve, if present, may also be involved. A randomized controlled trial[43] suggested that a 2-week antibiotic course with oxacillin or cloxacillin without an aminoglycoside may be adequate for immunocompetent patients without prosthetic heart valves with MSSA infections with vegetations <20 mm, and no pulmonary complications and who achieve clinical response within 96 hours for selected patients. Uncomplicated *S. aureus* right-sided IE in iv drug abusers, may be treated with oral ciprofloxacin (750 mg twice daily) plus rifampin (300 mg twice daily), provided the strain is susceptible and adherence is closely monitored.[44] For non-*S. aureus* organisms, management in PWID does not differ from that in other patient populations. *Surgical treatment* of right-sided IE on appropriate antibiotics is indicated for persistent bacteremia >1 week, severe tricuspid regurgitation causing

TABLE 14: Prevention of infective endocarditis.

Section	Details
1. Patients at risk	*High risk—prophylaxis recommended* • Previous IE • Prosthetic valves (surgical or transcatheter) or prosthetic repair material • *Congenital heart disease*: Unrepaired cyanotic lesions—repaired with prosthetic material/conduits/shunts (first 6 months, or lifelong if residual defect) • Ventricular assist devices (destination therapy) • Recently implanted closure devices, LAA occluders, vascular grafts, VA shunts (within 6 months) *Intermediate risk—no routine prophylaxis, preventive measures essential* • Rheumatic heart disease • Degenerative valve disease • Congenital valve abnormalities (including bicuspid aortic valve) • Hypertrophic cardiomyopathy • Cardiovascular implantable electronic devices (CIEDs)
2. Procedures and prophylaxis	*Dental (prophylaxis in high-risk patients only)* • Tooth extractions • Oral, periodontal, or implant surgery • Oral biopsies • Procedures involving gingiva or periapical tissues (e.g., scaling, root canal) *Non-dental* • No routine prophylaxis; consider only in selected high-risk cases (respiratory, GI, GU, skin, musculoskeletal interventions) • Strict asepsis for all invasive procedures *Cardiac and vascular interventions* • Always require perioperative prophylaxis when prosthetic valves/devices/grafts/occluders are implanted • Screen for nasal *Staphylococcus aureus* before elective cardiac surgery/TAVI; decolonize carriers with mupirocin/chlorhexidine • Eliminate dental sepsis ≥2 weeks before elective prosthetic implantation (when feasible)
3. Antibiotic prophylaxis regimens (dental procedures)	*Adults (no penicillin/ampicillin allergy)* • Amoxicillin 2 g orally, or • Ampicillin 2 g IV/IM *Adults (penicillin/ampicillin allergy)* • Cephalexin 2 g orally* • Cefazolin or ceftriaxone 1 g IV/IM* • Azithromycin or clarithromycin 500 mg orally • Doxycycline 100 mg orally *Avoid cephalosporins if immediate penicillin anaphylaxis/angioedema/urticaria*
4. General prevention measures (high and intermediate risk)	• Maintain twice-daily brushing and flossing • Professional dental cleaning—twice yearly (high risk), yearly (others) • Maintain skin hygiene; treat chronic dermatoses • Prompt wound disinfection; treat bacterial infections appropriately • Avoid tattoos and piercings • Minimize use of infusion catheters; adhere to infection-prevention bundles for lines • No self-prescription of antibiotics

*Should not be used in an individual with a history of anaphylaxis, angioedema, or urticarial with penicillin or ampicillin.

right ventricular dysfunction unresponsive to diuretics, respiratory failure after recurrent pulmonary emboli, involvement of left-sided structures, or large residual tricuspid vegetations >20 mm.

Infective endocarditis in solid organ transplant recipients: Left-sided involvement is more common, and they frequently have atrial or ventricular vegetations versus leaflet vegetations (mural IE).[45] *S. aureus* is most common followed by Enterococci and Streptococci. Post cardiac transplant, mitral valve is most frequently involved followed by mural IE and tricuspid valve in that order with causative agents being *S. aureus*>fungi>enterococcus.

Non-bacterial thrombotic endocarditis (NBTE): It is an uncommon disorder that occurs in individuals with predisposing conditions or hypercoagulable states, such as systemic lupus erythematosus (SLE), antiphospholipid syndrome (APS, also known as Libman–Sacks endocarditis), malignancies (marantic endocarditis), disseminated intravascular coagulation (DIC), or other chronic diseases such as tuberculosis and autoimmune disorders. A recent registry reported that 41% of NBTE patients had cancer, 33% had SLE, and 36% had APS, with 21% exhibiting both SLE and APS. Among cancer-associated cases, lung adenocarcinoma, breast cancer, and pancreatic cancer were most common.[46] Clinically, stroke was the predominant presentation (60%), followed by heart failure (21%) and acute coronary syndrome (7%). Mitral valve was more frequently affected (62%) than the aortic valve (24%). Libman–Sacks vegetations can vary in shape (sessile, tubular, and coalescent), echogenicity (homogeneous or heterogeneous), and size, and are typically located near the leaflet edges, sometimes extending toward mid or basal portions. *Anticoagulation is generally recommended for all patients, balancing against bleeding risk.* Options include low-molecular-weight heparin, unfractionated heparin, or vitamin K antagonists, whereas direct oral anticoagulants are not supported.

▪ PREVENTION

Prevention of infective endocarditis has been compiled in **Table 14**.

▪ CONCLUSION

Infective endocarditis is a serious infection requiring early diagnosis with multimodal imaging and prompt, pathogen-directed antibiotics. Surgery is indicated for uncontrolled infection or structural complications. Step-down or outpatient therapy may be used in stable patients. Special cases include prosthetic valves, TAVI, CIEDs, right-sided IE, fungal, and culture-negative infections. Prevention and multidisciplinary care are key to improving outcomes.

▪ REFERENCES

1. Slipczuk L, Codolosa JN, Davila CD, et al. Infective endocarditis epidemiology over five decades: a systematic review. PLoS One. 2013;8:e82665.
2. Chen H, Zhan Y, Zhang K, et al. The global, regional, and national burden and trends of infective endocarditis from 1990 to 2019: results from the Global Burden of Disease Study 2019. Front Med. 2022;9:774224.
3. Murdoch DR, Corey GR, Hoen B, et al. Clinical presentation, etiology, and outcome of infective endocarditis in the 21st century: the International Collaboration on Endocarditis–Prospective Cohort Study. N Engl J Med. 2009;360(5):491-502.
4. Habib G, Erba PA, Lung B, et al. Clinical presentation, aetiology and outcome of infective endocarditis: results of the ESC-EORP EURO-ENDO (European infective endocarditis) registry. Eur Heart J. 2019;40(39):3222-32.
5. Habib G, Lancellotti P, Lung B. 2023 ESC Guidelines for the management of endocarditis. Eur Heart J. 2023;44(39):3948-4043.
6. Bosshard PP, Abels S, Zbinden R, et al. Ribosomal DNA sequencing for identification of aerobic Gram-positive rods in the clinical laboratory. J Clin Microbiol. 2003;41(9):4134-40.

7. Fenollar F, Raoult D. Molecular diagnosis of bloodstream infections caused by non-cultivable bacteria. Int J Antimicrob Agents. 2007;30 Suppl 1:S7-15.
8. Sandoe JA, Wysome J, West AP, et al. Measurement of bacterial DNA in cardiac valve tissue from patients with infective endocarditis by quantitative PCR. J Clin Microbiol. 2003;41(7):3129-31.
9. Wilson MR, Sample HA, Zorn KC, et al. Clinical metagenomic sequencing for diagnosis of meningitis and encephalitis. N Engl J Med. 2019;380(24):2327-40.
10. Blauwkamp TA, Thair S, Rosen MJ, et al. Analytical and clinical validation of a microbial cell-free DNA sequencing test for infectious disease. Nat Microbiol. 2019;4(4):663-74.
11. Seng P, Drancourt M, Gouriet F, et al. Ongoing revolution in bacteriology: routine identification of bacteria by matrix-assisted laser desorption ionization time-of-flight mass spectrometry. Clin Infect Dis. 2009;49(4):543-51.
12. Fournier PE, Thuny F, Richet H, et al. Comprehensive diagnostic strategy for blood culture-negative endocarditis: a prospective study of 819 new cases. Clin Infect Dis. 2010;51(2):131-40.
13. Millar BC, Jugo J, Moore JE. Fungal endocarditis in the 21st century. Emerg Infect Dis. 2005;11(7):1112-8.
14. Li JS, Sexton DJ, Mick N, et al. Proposed modifications to the Duke criteria for the diagnosis of infective endocarditis. Clin Infect Dis. 2000;30:633-8.
15. Habib G, Derumeaux G, Avierinos JF, et al. Value and limitations of the Duke criteria for the diagnosis of infective endocarditis. J Am Coll Cardiol. 1999;33:2023-9.
16. Vieira ML, Grinberg M, Pomerantzeff PM, et al. Repeated echocardiographic examinations of patients with suspected infective endocarditis. Heart. 2004; 90:1020-24.
17. Hill EE, Herijgers P, Claus P, et al. Abscess in infective endocarditis: the value of transesophageal echocardiography and outcome: a 5-year study. Am Heart J. 2007;154:923-8.
18. Scholtens AM, Swart LE, Verberne HJ, et al. Confounders in FDG-PET/CT imaging of suspected prosthetic valve endocarditis. JACC Cardiovasc Imaging. 2016;9:1462-5.
19. Pizzi MN, Roque A, Cuellar-Calabria H, et al. (18)F-FDG-PET/CTA of prosthetic cardiac valves and valve- tube grafts: infective versus inflammatory patterns. JACC Cardiovasc Imaging. 2016;9:1224-7.
20. Roque A, Pizzi MN, Fernandez-Hidalgo N, et al. Morpho-metabolic post-surgical patterns of non-infected prosthetic heart valves by [18F]FDG PET/CTA: "normality" is a possible diagnosis. Eur Heart J Cardiovasc Imaging. 2020;21:24-33.
21. Dahl A, Fowler VG, Miro JM, et al. Sign of the times: updating infective endocarditis diagnostic criteria to recognize Enterococcus faecalis as a typical endocarditis bacterium. Clin Infect Dis. 2022;75:1097-1102.
22. Anis HK, Miller EM, George J, et al. Incidence and characteristics of osteoarticular infections in patients with infective endocarditis. Orthopedics. 2020;43:24-9.
23. Carbone A, Lieu A, Mouhat B, et al. Spondylodiscitis complicating infective endocarditis. Heart. 2020;106:1914-8.
24. Arvieux C, Common H. New diagnostic tools for prosthetic joint infection. Orthop Traumatol Surg Res. 2019;105:S23-S30.
25. Holland TL, Baddour LM, Bayer AS, et al. The Duke-ISCVID criteria for infective endocarditis: 2023 update. Clin Infect Dis. 2023;76(7):e118-4.
26. Le Bot A, Lecomte R, Gazeau P, et al. Is rifampin use associated with better outcome in staphylococcal prosthetic valve endocarditis? A multicenter retrospective study. Clin Infect Dis. 2021;72:e249-55.
27. Iversen K, Ihlemann N, Gill SU, et al. Partial oral versus intravenous antibiotic treatment of endocarditis. N Engl J Med. 2019;380:415-24.
28. Ramos-Martinez A, Munoz Serrano A, et al. Gentamicin may have no effect on mortality of staphylococcal prosthetic valve endocarditis. J Infect Chemother. 2018;24:555-62.
29. Pericas JM, Cervera C, del Rio A, et al. Changes in the treatment of Enterococcus faecalis infective endocarditis in Spain in the last 15 years: from ampicillin plus gentamicin to ampicillin plus ceftriaxone. Clin Microbiol Infect. 2014;20:O1075-83.

30. Delgado V, Ajmone Marsan N, de Waha S, et al. 2023 ESC Guidelines for the management of endocarditis. Eur Heart J. 2023;44(39):3948-4042.
31. Hidalgo-Tenorio C, Vinuesa D, Plata A, et al. DALBACEN cohort: dalbavancin as consolidation therapy in infective endocarditis. J Antimicrob Chemother. 2019;74(4):1104-9.
32. Durante-Mangoni E, Signoriello G, Andini R, et al. Dalbavancin for infective endocarditis: a multicenter experience. Int J Antimicrob Agents. 2020;56(3):106108.
33. Davis KA, Huang G, Petty SA, et al. The effect of preexisting anticoagulation on cerebrovascular events in left-sided infective endocarditis. Am J Med. 2020;133(3):360-9.
34. Vongpatanasin W, Hillis LD, Lange RA. Prosthetic heart valves. N Engl J Med. 1996;335:407-16.
35. Glaser N, Jackson V, Holzmann MJ, et al. Prosthetic valve endocarditis after surgical aortic valve replacement. Circulation. 2017;136:329-31.
36. Brennan JM, Edwards FH, Zhao Y, et al. Long-term safety and effectiveness of mechanical versus biologic aortic valve prostheses in older patients: results from the Society of Thoracic Surgeons adult cardiac surgery national database. Circulation. 2013;127:1647-55.
37. Stortecky S, Heg D, Tueller D, et al. Infective endocarditis after transcatheter aortic valve replacement. J Am Coll Cardiol. 2020;75: 3020-30.
38. Birnie DH, Wang J, Alings M, et al. Risk factors for infections involving cardiac implantable electronic devices. JAMA. 2017;318(10):967-76
39. Nagpal A, Patel R, Greenwood-Quaintance KE, et al. Sonication of CIEDs to enhance microbial detection. Am J Cardiol. 2015;115(7):912-7.
40. Krahn AD, Longtin Y, Philippon F, et al. Prevention of Arrhythmia Device Infection Trial: The PADIT Trial. J Am Coll Cardiol. 2018;72(24):3098-3109.
41. Tarakji KG, Mittal S, Kennergren C, et al; WRAP-IT Investigators. Antibacterial envelope to prevent cardiac implantable device infection. N Engl J Med. 2019;380(20):1895-905.
42. Lassen H, Nielsen SL, Gill SUA, et al. The epidemiology of infective endocarditis with focus on non-device related right-sided infective endocarditis: a retrospective register-based study in the region of southern Denmark. Int J Infect Dis. 2020;95:224-30.
43. Ribera E, Gomez-Jimenez J, Cortes E, et al. Effectiveness of cloxacillin with and without gentamicin in short-term therapy for right-sided Staphylococcus aureus endocarditis. A randomized, controlled trial. Ann Intern Med. 1996;125:969-74.
44. Al-Omari A, Cameron DW, Lee C, et al. Oral antibiotic therapy for the treatment of infective endocarditis: a systematic review. BMC Infect Dis. 2014;14:140.
45. Martinez-Selles M, Valerio-Minero M, Farinas MC, et al. Infective endocarditis in patients with solid organ transplantation. A nationwide descriptive study. Eur J Intern Med. 2021;87:59-65.
46. Zmaili MA, Alzubi JM, Kocyigit D, et al. A contemporary 20-year Cleveland clinic experience of nonbacterial thrombotic endocarditis: etiology, echocardiographic imaging, management, and outcomes. Am J Med. 2021;134:361-9.

CHAPTER 13

Advances in Atrial Fibrillation Ablation: Technology and Technique

Sebastian E Beyer, Salil K Midha, Leon M Ptaszek

■ INTRODUCTION

The prevalence of atrial fibrillation (AF) is steadily increasing, driven largely by the aging of the global population.[1] A growing body of evidence indicates that utilization of an early, aggressive rhythm control strategy for AF is associated with improved patient outcomes.[2] Although clinicians can use either antiarrhythmic drug therapy or catheter ablation as part of a rhythm control strategy for managing AF, catheter ablation has consistently demonstrated superiority over medical therapy across a variety of patient populations.[3-5]

The combination of rising AF prevalence and the expanded indications for ablation therapy has led to a marked increase in the number of AF ablation procedures performed worldwide. In many regions, electrophysiology (EP) laboratories have needed to adjust procedural workflow to meet the growing demand for ablation procedures. Recent advances in ablation technology, most notably the development of pulsed field ablation (PFA), have improved both the safety profile and efficiency of the procedure. These innovations have allowed EP laboratories to perform more ablation procedures without compromising procedural safety or effectiveness.

■ EXPANDING INDICATIONS FOR RHYTHM CONTROL MANAGEMENT OF ATRIAL FIBRILLATION

The *EAST-AFNET 4* trial[2] established that an early, aggressive rhythm control strategy improves outcomes in patients with AF. In this study, patients were randomized to receive an early aggressive rhythm control strategy or a rate control strategy. The 2,789 patients treated according to a rhythm control strategy in this study (antiarrhythmic drugs and catheter ablation) within 1 year of the initial diagnosis of AF exhibited a lower likelihood of meeting the composite study endpoint of cardiovascular death, stroke, or hospitalization for acute decompensated heart failure or acute coronary syndrome.

Catheter ablation has become the cornerstone of AF management as it has been shown to be more effective in reducing the burden of AF than antiarrhythmic drug therapy.[3-5] Contemporary guideline statements reflect expanded indications for the use of ablation therapy.[6] Multiple randomized controlled trials (RCTs) have demonstrated the superiority of catheter ablation over antiarrhythmic therapy, particularly with respect to freedom from AF recurrence and improvement in AF-related symptoms. The *STOP-AF*,[3] *EARLY-AF*,[4] and *THERMOCOOL*[5] trials reported significantly higher rates of freedom from AF compared with medical therapy. While most RCTs have enrolled patients with paroxysmal AF, the *SARA* trial demonstrated similar benefits in those with persistent AF.[7]

The *CABANA* trial,[8] the largest RCT comparing catheter ablation with medical therapy, did not meet its primary composite endpoint; however, ablation was associated with substantially lower rates of AF recurrence in the study population. Further evidence of the benefits of ablation therapy was provided by the *SHAM-PVI* trial,[9] which confirmed a direct causal effect of ablation on symptom improvement, and demonstrated significant improvement in quality-of-life outcomes among patients randomized to ablation versus a sham procedure.

The impact of catheter ablation is particularly striking in patients with AF and concomitant heart failure. In the *CASTLE-AF* trial,[10] which enrolled patients with left ventricular ejection fraction <35% and NYHA class II–IV symptoms, ablation reduced both all-cause mortality [hazard ratio (HR) 0.53; 95% confidence interval (CI) 0.32–0.86; $p = 0.01$] and hospitalizations for worsening heart failure (HR 0.56; 95% CI 0.37–0.83; $p = 0.004$). These results support an especially central role for catheter ablation in this high-risk population.

Taken together, the findings from these RCTs support the hypothesis that catheter ablation is the most effective strategy for reducing AF burden. Updated versions of AF treatment guidelines now include ablation as part of the first line of treatment for AF. The resultant increases in demand for AF ablation procedures have tested the capacity limits of many EP laboratories.

NEW ABLATION THERAPIES AND TECHNIQUES

The three most widely used techniques for catheter-based AF ablation are PFA, radiofrequency ablation (RFA) ablation, and cryoablation (CA). The key characteristics of these techniques are summarized in **Table 1**. The ablation catheters available for use with PFA, RFA, and CA are described in **Table 2**. Open-chest ablation strategies are not included in this document.

RFA and CA are thermal modalities that achieve tissue necrosis and electrical inactivation through tissue heating (RFA) or freezing (CA). In contrast, PFA generates a strong electrical field that produces cellular death through electroporation, which is generally not associated with thermal injury.[11,12] PFA lesions tend to not affect tissues outside of the heart,[13] thereby reducing the risk of collateral injury to adjacent structures (e.g., esophagus and phrenic nerve) as compared with RFA and CA.

The first PFA catheter ablation system to treat cardiac arrhythmias was approved by the US Food and Drug Administration in 2023. This is much more recent than the approval of the cryoballoon (2010) and the open-irrigated RFA catheter (2008). Despite its recent arrival, PFA is already the most commonly utilized ablation system in many hospitals worldwide. The rapid adoption of PFA has been attributed to its favorable safety profile and reduction in ablation procedure time as compared with RFA and CA. Utilization of PFA technology has helped many EP laboratories keep up with the ever-increasing clinical demand for AF ablation.

RADIOFREQUENCY ABLATION

RFA is the most extensively studied technique for AF ablation, with well-established safety characteristics and postablation outcomes.[5,14] While effective, RFA carries notable limitations, including the risk of collateral injury to surrounding structures due to tissue heating. In addition, many available RFA ablation catheters deliver ablation lesions at single points of the tissue. Effective isolation of pulmonary veins (or other atrial structures) requires delivery of multiple adjacent point lesions, which is relatively time-consuming.[14] In addition, gaps between ablation lesions can lead to pulmonary vein reconnection and AF recurrence.

Recent innovations have shortened RFA procedure time. High-power, short-duration (HPSD) ablation delivers higher energy (up to 90 W) over shorter intervals (4–10 seconds), compared with conventional settings (20–35 W for 20–40 seconds). Shorter lesion delivery times translate to shorter procedure times. The HPSD

TABLE 1: Attributes of the most commonly utilized ablation techniques.

	Pulsed field	Radiofrequency	Cryoablation	References
Mechanism	Irreversible electroporation	Thermal injury: Heating	Thermal injury: Freezing	12,24
Myocardial tissue selectivity	High	Low with higher risk of damage to adjacent structures	Low with higher risk of damage to adjacent structures	13
Procedure time	Fastest	Slowest	Intermediate	25,26
Acute procedural success	98–99.9%	95–99%	98–99%	25,27
Major complication rate	~1%	~1%	~1%	11,14
Risk of esophageal fistula	Not reported	Possible, <0.1%	Possible, <0.1%	11,28,29
Risk of phrenic nerve injury	Low, reported cases have been transient	Possible, <0.5%	Possible, 1–2%	11,14,30
Risk of pulmonary vein stenosis	Not reported	<1%	<1%	31,32
Risk of coronary artery spasm	High if ablation is performed adjacent to coronary artery	Not reported	Not reported	21,33
Ablation of extra-pulmonary vein lesions	Concern for limited durability	Possible	Limited	23
Ablation catheter types available	Both multipoint and single-point catheters available (multipoint most common)	Both multipoint and single-point catheters available (single-point most common)	Both multipoint and single-point catheters available (balloon catheter more common for AF)	
Cost	Highest	Intermediate	Lowest	25

RFA approach also produces more superficial lesions, thus reducing the risk of collateral damage to adjoining structures. Trials such as *POWER-AF*[15] and *FAST AND FURIOUS*[16] have demonstrated the efficiency benefits of the HPSD RFA strategy.

Additional advances involve integration of RFA with artificial intelligence (AI)-guided mapping. For example, the Volta Medical system analyzes spatiotemporal electrogram dispersion to identify ablation targets. In the *TAILORED-AF* trial,[17] pulmonary vein isolation (PVI) plus AI-guided ablation was compared with PVI alone. The AI-guided strategy was associated with significantly lower AF recurrence at 1 year; however, no difference was observed in freedom from any atrial arrhythmias.

Multi-electrode RFA catheters that can ablate multiple points in space simultaneously have been described **(Table 2)**. Utilization of such catheters can increase the speed of RFA procedures by increasing the amount of tissue that is ablated per unit of time. These multi-electrodes are not as commonly used as single-point RFA catheters.

During RFA lesion delivery, sudden increase in tissue temperature are possible. These temperature spikes can produce "steam pops" which are a major safety concern as they can cause considerable damage to cardiac tissue as well as cardiac tamponade. Steam pops are not observed for CA or PFA.

TABLE 2: Description of novel ablation catheters that can be utilized with each type of ablation technique.

	Pulsed field	Radiofrequency	Cryo
Single point	Sphere-9 Catheter with Affera mapping system (Medtronic)[34]	• QDOT MICRO RF catheter (Johnson and Johnson)[16] • DiamondTemp RF catheter (Medtronic)[35] • TactiFlex catheter (Abbott)[36]	Not used for atrial fibrillation ablation
Multispline array	• Farawave catheter (Boston Scientific)[20] • Varipulse catheter (Johnson and Johnson)[37] • PulseSelect catheter (Medtronic)[38] • Volt system (Abbott)[39] • Omnypulse (Johnson and Johnson)[40] • Globe (Kardium)[41]	N/A	N/A
Balloon	N/A	• Luminize RF balloon catheter (Boston Scientific)[42] • Heliostar (Johnson and Johnson)[43]	• PolarX (Boston Scientific)[44] • Arctic Front (Medtronic)[45]

■ CRYOABLATION

Cryoablation of AF is typically performed using balloon-tipped catheters, which are positioned at the pulmonary vein ostia. Temperature of the balloon is decreased leading to freezing of all cardiac tissue in contact with the surface of the balloon. CA balloon catheters are intended to contact the tissue through the entirety of the circumference of a pulmonary vein ostium, thus facilitating "single-shot" pulmonary vein isolation. The randomized *FIRE AND ICE* trial[18] demonstrated noninferiority of CA compared with RFA for the composite endpoint of AF or atrial tachycardia (AT) recurrence during a mean follow-up period of 1.5 years. Safety outcomes were similar for RFA and CA, but procedure times were shorter for CA.

Recent advances in cryoballoon design have resulted in lower nadir temperatures and improvements in procedural efficacy, with acute pulmonary vein isolation success rates of approximately 99%.[19] Despite this improvement, cryoballoon ablation can lead to incomplete pulmonary vein isolation due to incomplete contact between spherical balloons and sometimes irregularly-shaped pulmonary vein ostia. Other drawbacks associated with cryoballoon use include the inability to address arrhythmia substrates outside of the pulmonary veins. Although single-point CA catheters are available, they are not frequently used for AF ablation because of the relatively long time required to deliver a CA lesion. Another key limitation of CA is the risk of phrenic nerve palsy, which is reported in up to 2.5% of patients in recent meta-analyses.[19]

CA is potentially better-suited for use in resource-constrained areas than RFA and PFA. CA does not require use of an electroanatomic mapping system and is potentially more straightforward to maintain. In addition, CA systems tend to be less expensive than RFA and PFA systems.

Advances in Atrial Fibrillation Ablation: Technology and Technique

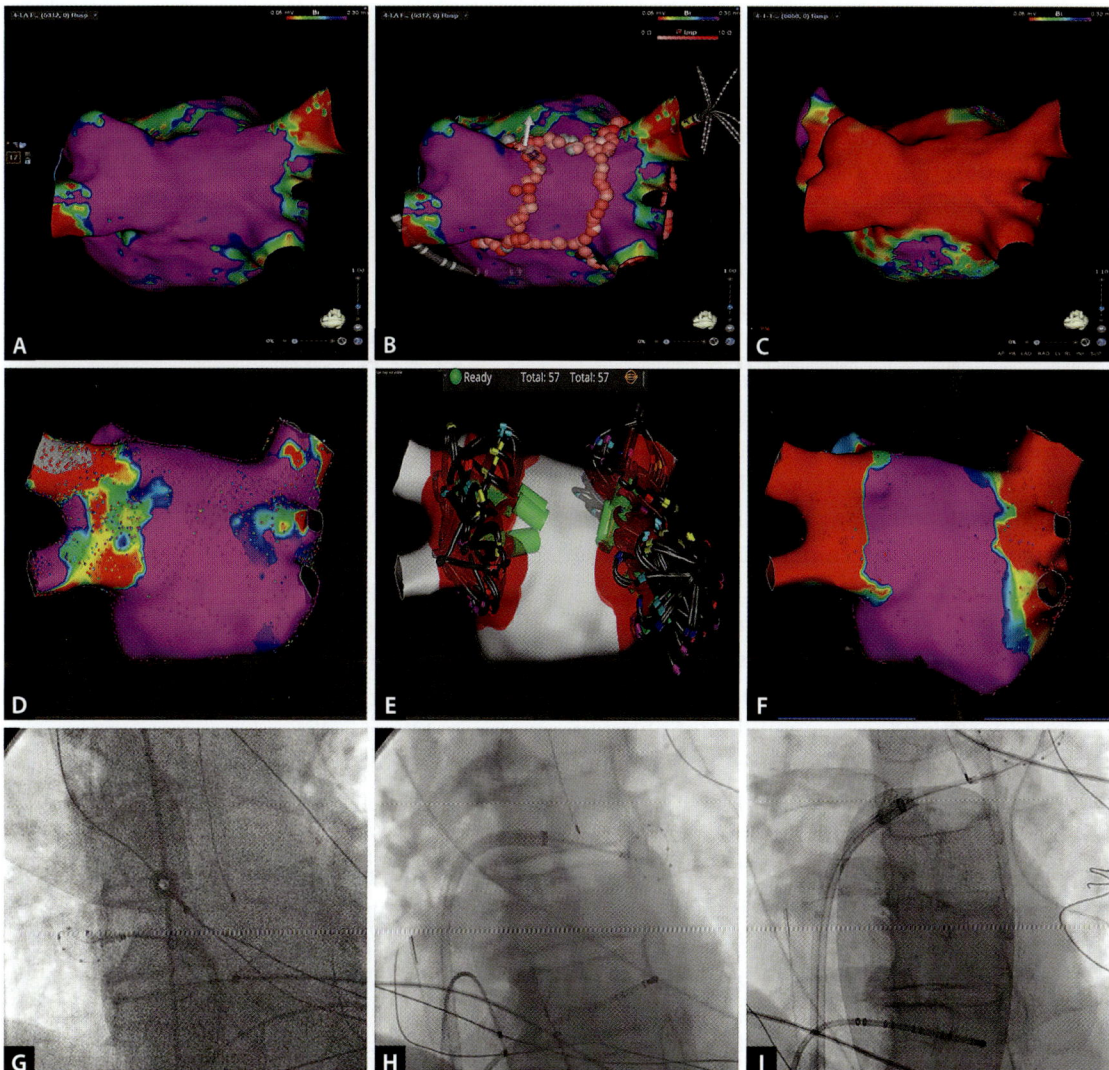

Figs. 1A to I: Electroanatomic maps and fluoroscopy images of pulmonary vein isolation achieved with point-by-point RFA, "single-shot" PFA, and cryoballoon ablation. (A) The electroanatomic posterior-anterior voltage maps of the left atrium prior to ablation with radiofrequency (RF); (B) The point-by-point ablation lesions performed using an RF catheter; (C) The voltage map following ablation. Mapping was performed using the multi-spline catheter and electroanatomic mapping software. Purple areas indicate normal voltage, while red areas indicate low voltage; (D) The posterior-anterior voltage maps of the left atrium prior to ablation with pulsed-field ablation (PFA); (E) The sets of ablation lesions produced by a "single-shot" PFA catheter; (F) The voltage map following ablation; (G) The fluoroscopic images obtained during cryoablation of the right inferior; (H) Left inferior; (I) Left superior pulmonary veins.

PULSED FIELD ABLATION

The electroporation produced by PFA has been shown to be less likely to damage structures adjacent to the heart than RFA and CA.[12,13] The randomized *ADVENT* trial[20] compared PFA with RFA and CA in patients with drug-refractory, paroxysmal AF. In this study, PFA demonstrated noninferiority to RFA and CA with respect to procedural success and serious adverse events. Limitations of this study included relatively small sample size which could limit detection of rare complications such as phrenic nerve injury or atrial-esophageal fistula formation. The larger *MANIFEST 17k* registry[11] reported no esophageal complications, pulmonary vein stenosis, or persistent phrenic nerve palsy among >17,000 PFA procedures.

Several PFA systems are currently available. Some of the most widely used systems are listed in **Table 1**. Many PFA platforms employ catheters designed for simultaneous multipoint ablation **(Figs. 1A to I; Table 2)**. These "single-shot" catheters enable pulmonary vein isolation with fewer ablation applications. The lower number of ablation applications is associated with markedly reduced time required to achieve pulmonary vein isolation as compared with point-by-point RFA.

Despite its favorable safety profile, several PFA-specific complications have been described. These include coronary vasospasm when energy is delivered near coronary arteries. PFA-mediated coronary vasospasm can typically be mitigated with nitroglycerin but can prolong total procedure times.[21] PFA also produces intravascular hemolysis, which can lead to hemoglobinuria and acute kidney injury, especially when large numbers of PFA applications are delivered.[22] In addition, concerns also remain regarding PFA lesion durability in certain anatomical locations such as the coronary sinus and mitral isthmus.[23]

Perhaps the most significant limitation of PFA is cost. As PFA is the newest ablation modality, PFA-based ablation systems and their associated single-use components (notably ablation catheters) are significantly more expensive than RFA or CA platforms. Consequently, hospitals considering the adoption of PFA must weigh the high initial investment and per-procedure costs against the potential gains in procedural efficiency.

CONCLUSION

Catheter ablation is the most effective strategy for maintaining sinus rhythm in patients with AF. The number of ablation procedures continues to rise each year, driven by both the increasing prevalence of AF and the expanded indications for ablation in recently released treatment guidelines. The most commonly used catheter ablation techniques are RFA, CA, and PFA. Each of these techniques is associated with distinct advantages and limitations that may influence their suitability for different practice settings.

PFA is associated with shorter procedure times and lower complication rates than RFA and CA. However, the higher costs associated with PFA systems and their associated single-use catheters present a significant economic barrier to adoption. For many hospitals, the resources required to establish and maintain a PFA program may be prohibitive. Even hospitals that can afford the initial cost of establishing a PFA system may not have sufficient AF ablation volumes to make it feasible to maintain a PFA program long-term. These factors underscore the need to balance safety and efficiency gains against economic feasibility when considering use of PFA against lower-cost options such as RFA and CA.

REFERENCES

1. Kornej J, Börschel CS, Benjamin EJ, et al. Epidemiology of atrial fibrillation in the 21st Century: Novel methods and new insights. Circ Res. 2020;127(1):4-20.

2. Kirchhof P, Camm AJ, Goette A, et al. Early rhythm-control therapy in patients with atrial fibrillation. N Engl J Med. 2020;383(14):1305-16.
3. Wazni OM, Dandamudi G, Sood N, et al. Cryoballoon ablation as initial therapy for atrial fibrillation. N Engl J Med. 2021;384(4):316-24.
4. Andrade JG, Wells GA, Deyell MW, et al. Cryoablation or drug therapy for initial treatment of atrial fibrillation. N Engl J Med. 2021;384(4):305-15.
5. Wilber DJ, Pappone C, Neuzil P, et al. Comparison of antiarrhythmic drug therapy and radiofrequency catheter ablation in patients with paroxysmal atrial fibrillation: a randomized controlled trial. JAMA. 2010;303(4):333-40.
6. Joglar JA, Chung MK, Armbruster AL, et al. 2023 ACC/AHA/ACCP/HRS guideline for the diagnosis and management of atrial fibrillation: A report of the American College of Cardiology/American Heart Association Joint Committee on Clinical Practice Guidelines. Circulation. 2024;149(1):e1-156.
7. Mont L, Bisbal F, Hernández-Madrid A, et al. Catheter ablation vs. antiarrhythmic drug treatment of persistent atrial fibrillation: a multicentre, randomized, controlled trial (SARA study). Eur Heart J. 2014;35(8):501-7.
8. Packer DL, Piccini JP, Monahan KH, et al. Ablation versus drug therapy for atrial fibrillation in heart failure: Results from the CABANA trial. Circulation. 2021;143(14):1377-90.
9. Dulai R, Sulke N, Freemantle N, et al. Pulmonary vein isolation vs sham intervention in symptomatic atrial fibrillation: The SHAM-PVI randomized clinical trial. JAMA. 2024;332(14):1165-73.
10. Marrouche NF, Brachmann J, Andresen D, et al. Catheter ablation for atrial fibrillation with heart failure. N Engl J Med. 2018;378(5):417-27.
11. Ekanem E, Neuzil P, Reichlin T, et al. Safety of pulsed field ablation in more than 17,000 patients with atrial fibrillation in the MANIFEST-17K study. Nat Med. 2024;30(7):2020-9.
12. Kotnik T, Rems L, Tarek M, et al. Membrane electroporation and electropermeabilization: Mechanisms and models. Annu Rev Biophys. 2019;48:63-91.
13. Cochet H, Nakatani Y, Sridi-Cheniti S, et al. Pulsed field ablation selectively spares the oesophagus during pulmonary vein isolation for atrial fibrillation. Europace. 2021;23(9):1391-9.
14. Hsu JC, Darden D, Du C, et al. Initial Findings From the national cardiovascular data registry of atrial fibrillation ablation procedures. J Am Coll Cardiol. 2023;81(9):867-78.
15. Wielandts JY, Kyriakopoulou M, Almorad A, et al. Prospective randomized evaluation of high power during CLOSE-guided pulmonary vein isolation: The POWER-AF Study. Circ Arrhythm Electrophysiol. 2021;14(1):e009112.
16. Richard Tilz R, Sano M, Vogler J, et al. Very high-power short-duration temperature-controlled ablation versus conventional power-controlled ablation for pulmonary vein isolation: The fast and furious - AF study. Int J Cardiol Heart Vasc. 2021;35:100847.
17. Deisenhofer I, Albenque JP, Busch S, et al. Artificial intelligence for individualized treatment of persistent atrial fibrillation: a randomized controlled trial. Nat Med. 2025;31(4):1286-93.
18. Kuck KH, Brugada J, Fürnkranz A, et al. Cryoballoon or radiofrequency ablation for paroxysmal atrial fibrillation. N Engl J Med. 2016;374(23):2235-45.
19. du Fay de Lavallaz J, Knecht S, Reichlin T, et al. Novel vs established cryoballoon ablation system for atrial fibrillation: A systematic review and meta-analysis. Heart Rhythm O2. 2025;6(1):21-31.
20. Reddy VY, Gerstenfeld EP, Natale A, et al. Pulsed field or conventional thermal ablation for paroxysmal atrial fibrillation. N Engl J Med. 2023;389(18):1660-71.
21. Reddy VY, Petru J, Funasako M, et al. Coronary arterial spasm during pulsed field ablation to treat atrial fibrillation. Circulation. 2022;146(24):1808-19.
22. Popa MA, Venier S, Menè R, et al. Characterization and clinical significance of hemolysis after pulsed field ablation for atrial fibrillation: Results of a multicenter analysis. Circ Arrhythm Electrophysiol. 2024;17(10):e012732.
23. La Fazia VM, Mohanty S, Gianni C, et al. Feasibility and safety of pulsed field ablation for coronary sinus and left atrial appendage isolation and mitral isthmus ablation: Acute and chronic findings. Circ Arrhythm Electrophysiol. 2025;18(9):e014026.
24. Brasca FM, Curti E, Perego GB. Thermal and non-thermal energies for atrial fibrillation ablation. J Clin Med. 2025;14(6):2071.
25. Calvert P, Mills MT, Xydis P, et al. Cost, efficiency, and outcomes of pulsed field ablation vs thermal

ablation for atrial fibrillation: A real-world study. Heart Rhythm. 2024;21(9):1537-44.
26. Nakasone K, Della Rocca DG, Magnocavallo M, et al. Pulsed field ablation in the elderly by a pentaspline multielectrode catheter: Safety, efficacy, and comparison with cryoballoon and radiofrequency devices. Heart Rhythm. 2025;22(7):e30-9.
27. Vetta G, Della Rocca DG, Parlavecchio A, et al. Multielectrode catheter-based pulsed electric field vs. cryoballoon for atrial fibrillation ablation: a systematic review and meta-analysis. Europace. 2024;26(12):euae293.
28. John RM, Kapur S, Ellenbogen KA, et al. Atrioesophageal fistula formation with cryoballoon ablation is most commonly related to the left inferior pulmonary vein. Heart Rhythm. 2017;14(2):184-9.
29. Pappone C, Vicedomini G, Santinelli V. Atrio-esophageal fistula after AF ablation: pathophysiology, prevention, & treatment. J Atr Fibrillation. 2013;6(3):860.
30. Tachibana S, Miyazaki S, Nitta J, et al. Incidence of phrenic nerve injury during pulmonary vein isolation using different cryoballoons: data from a large prospective ablation registry. Europace. 2024;26(4):euae092.
31. Teunissen C, Velthuis BK, Hassink RJ, et al. Incidence of pulmonary vein stenosis after radiofrequency catheter ablation of atrial fibrillation. JACC Clin Electrophysiol. 2017;3(6):589-98.
32. Tokutake K, Tokuda M, Yamashita S, et al. Anatomical and procedural factors of severe pulmonary vein stenosis after cryoballoon pulmonary vein ablation. JACC Clin Electrophysiol. 2019;5(11):1303-15.
33. Zhang C, Neuzil P, Petru J, et al. Coronary artery spasm during pulsed field vs radiofrequency catheter ablation of the mitral isthmus. JAMA Cardiol. 2024;9(1):72-7.
34. Anter E, Mansour M, Nair DG, et al. Dual-energy lattice-tip ablation system for persistent atrial fibrillation: a randomized trial. Nat Med. 2024;30(8):2303-10.
35. Kautzner J, Albenque JP, Natale A, et al. A novel temperature-controlled radiofrequency catheter ablation system used to treat patients with paroxysmal atrial fibrillation. JACC Clin Electrophysiol. 2021;7(3):352-63.
36. Abbott. Ablation Catheters. [Online] Available from https://www.cardiovascular.abbott/us/en/hcp/products/electrophysiology/ablation-technology.html [Last accessed November, 2025].
37. Duytschaever M, De Potter T, Grimaldi M, et al. Paroxysmal atrial fibrillation ablation using a novel variable-loop biphasic pulsed field ablation catheter integrated with a 3-dimensional mapping system: 1-year outcomes of the multicenter inspIRE study. Circ Arrhythm Electrophysiol. 2023;16(3):e011780.
38. Verma A, Haines DE, Boersma LV, et al. Pulsed field ablation for the treatment of atrial fibrillation: PULSED AF pivotal trial. Circulation. 2023;147(19):1422-32.
39. Abbott. Volt Pulse Field Ablation (PFA) Clinical Evidence. [Online] Available from https://www.cardiovascular.abbott/us/en/ep-clinical-evidence/volt-clinical-evidence.html [Last accessed November, 2025].
40. Duytschaever M, Grimaldi M, De Potter T, et al. PVI with CF-sensing large-tip focal PFA catheter with 3D mapping for paroxysmal AF: Omny-IRE 3-month results. JACC Clin Electrophysiol. 2025;11(8):1769-82.
41. Kardium. Globe Pulsed Field System. [Online] Available from https://kardium.com/globe-system/ [Last accessed November, 2025].
42. Reddy VY, Al-Ahmad A, Aidietis A, et al. A Novel visually guided radiofrequency balloon ablation catheter for pulmonary vein isolation: One-year outcomes of the multicenter AF-FICIENT I trial. Circ Arrhythm Electrophysiol. 2021;14(10):e009308.
43. Bordignon S, My I, Tohoku S, et al. Efficacy and safety in patients treated with a novel radiofrequency balloon: a two centres experience from the AURORA collaboration. Europace. 2023;25(5):euad106.
44. Knecht S, Sticherling C, Roten L, et al. Efficacy and safety of a novel cryoballoon ablation system: multicentre comparison of 1-year outcome. Europace. 2022;24(12):1926-32.
45. Boveda S, Metzner A, Nguyen DQ, et al. Single-procedure outcomes and quality-of-life improvement 12 months post-cryoballoon ablation in persistent atrial fibrillation: Results from the multicenter CRYO4PERSISTENT AF trial. JACC Clin Electrophysiol. 2018;4(11):1440-7.

Microvascular Angina: How to Diagnose and Manage It

CHAPTER 14

Viveka Kumar, Anil Yadav, Sangeeta Dhir, Mitendra Singh Yadav, Anupam Goel

INTRODUCTION

Ischemia with no obstructive coronary artery disease (INOCA) is increasingly recognized in contemporary cardiovascular practice, affecting a substantial proportion of patients undergoing diagnostic angiography for suspected CAD.[1] Microvascular angina (MVA)—a clinical manifestation of coronary microvascular dysfunction (CMD)—is a major contributor to INOCA. Data from the Women's Ischemia Syndrome Evaluation (WISE) program estimate that 3-4 million individuals in the United States alone have vasomotor dysfunction without obstructive CAD, with similar prevalence patterns reported in other regions.[2] Contrary to earlier perceptions of a benign syndrome, robust longitudinal data demonstrate that MVA is associated with:

- *Increased major adverse cardiovascular events (MACE):* Myocardial infarction (MI), stroke, HFpEF, and cardiovascular death[2-7]
- Reduced quality of life and functional capacity[2,4]
- Increased healthcare utilization—recurrent hospitalizations and repeat investigations.[2]

CMD is demonstrable in a large proportion of patients with suspected MVA or vasospastic angina.[1] Women, particularly postmenopausal, are disproportionately affected, though the condition is increasingly recognized in men[1,2]

PATHOPHYSIOLOGY

Anatomy of the Coronary Microcirculation

- *Epicardial vessels:* ≥500 µm—conductance vessels.
- *Microvasculature:* <500 µm—prearterioles, arterioles, and capillaries—the principal site of resistance regulation.
- Microvascular resistance accounts for >50% of total coronary resistance.[8]

Endotypes of Coronary Microvascular Dysfunction

- *Structural CMD:*
  - Arteriolar wall thickening, reduced lumen diameter, and perivascular fibrosis.
  - Increased microvascular resistance and impaired vasodilatory capacity.
- *Functional CMD:*
  - Abnormal vasomotor tone regulation.
  - Impaired endothelial-dependent and/or nonendothelial-dependent vasodilation.
  - Microvascular spasm.

Mechanistic Pathways

- Endothelial dysfunction →↓ nitric oxide bioavailability; ↑ endothelin-1 → vasoconstriction, platelet aggregation.
- Smooth muscle hyperreactivity → exaggerated constriction to vasoconstrictor stimuli.

- Microvascular rarefaction → capillary density loss → subendocardial hypoperfusion.
- Autonomic imbalance → increased sympathetic tone.
- Inflammatory injury → microvascular remodeling and fibrosis.[8,9]

Sex-specific Differences
- Women have greater microvascular reactivity and autonomic sensitivity.
- Estrogen deficiency postmenopause exacerbates endothelial dysfunction.
- Hormonal modulation may partly explain symptom variability.[1,2]

EPIDEMIOLOGY AND RISK FACTORS (TABLE 1)

Special associations: Autoimmune disorders (SLE, RA), infiltrative cardiomyopathies, hypertrophic cardiomyopathy, prior myocarditis.[1,8]

PROGNOSTIC SIGNIFICANCE

Historically labeled "benign angina" or "cardiac syndrome X," MVA is now firmly established as a condition with significant long-term risk.

TABLE 1: Epidemiology and risk factors.

Risk factor	Mechanism in CMD
Hypertension	Arteriolar remodeling; ↑ wall: lumen ratio
Diabetes mellitus	Advanced glycation end-products, oxidative stress, ↓ nitric oxide
Dyslipidemia	Endothelial injury; micro-atheroma
Smoking	Impaired endothelial vasodilation; oxidative stress
Ageing	Arterial stiffening; rarefaction; ↓ vasodilator reserve
Systemic inflammation	Immune-mediated microvascular injury

Key Prognostic Insights
- *WISE:* CFR <2.32 predicted a 5-year MACE rate of 27% versus 9.3% with CFR >2.32 ($p = 0.01$)[2]
- *iPOWER:* Coronary flow velocity reserve (CFVR) <2.33 independently predicted MI and heart failure hospitalization over 4.5 years (HR 1.07 per 0.1-unit decrease; $p < 0.001$)[3]
- *Zhou et al.:* Stress-CMR-derived myocardial perfusion reserve index (MPRI) <1.47 predicted 5-year MACE (HR 3.14)[6]
- *Murthy et al.:* PET-derived CFR <2.0 linked to higher risk of cardiac death and MI over 3 years.[5]
- *Meta-analysis (Gdowski et al.):* CMD associated with >5-fold increased odds of MACE (OR 5.16; 95% CI 2.81–9.47).[7]

Practical implication: Prognostic stratification is critical. Functional assessment [e.g., CFR, index of microvascular resistance (IMR)] should not be considered optional—it guides therapy and helps predict outcomes.[1,10,11]

INVESTIGATIONS

Initial Evaluation
- *History:* Symptom onset, triggers, duration, nitrate response, and atypical sites (jaw, back, epigastrium).
- *Risk factor assessment:* Hypertension, diabetes, dyslipidemia, smoking, and menopausal status.
- *Physical examination:* Often normal between episodes; assess for hypertension, murmurs, systemic disease features.
- *Resting ECG:* May be normal; baseline Q waves, LVH, or repolarization changes possible.

Stepwise Diagnostic Framework

The diagnostic process aims to:
- Confirm symptoms are ischemic in origin.
- Exclude obstructive CAD.

- Demonstrate objective evidence of ischemia.
- Confirm CMD and classify mechanism[1,10] **(Flowchart 1)**

Noninvasive Investigations (Table 2)

Stress Electrocardiogram

- Resting ECG may be normal.
- Exercise ECG sensitivity for MVA is modest (≈30–50%) due to diffuse subendocardial ischemia.
- ST-segment depression during exercise or recovery is suggestive.[1,10]

Myocardial Perfusion Imaging ((Single Photon Emission Computed Tomography/Positron Emission Tomography)

- *SPECT:* Perfusion defects possible; limited spatial resolution for microvascular disease.
- *PET:* Gold standard for noninvasive quantification of CFR; tracers include ^{13}N, ^{82}Rb, ^{18}F. PET-CFR <2.0 is associated with adverse outcomes.[5]

Stress Cardiac Magnetic Resonance

- Measures MPRI; MPRI ≤1.84 suggests CMD.
- *Advantages:* No radiation, high spatial resolution, tissue characterization.[1,6]

Transthoracic Doppler Echocardiography

- Measures CFVR in the left anterior descending (LAD) artery.
- CFVR ≤2.0–2.3 is abnormal; predicts prognosis (iPOWER)[3]
- *Limitations:* Operator-dependent.

Computed Tomography Myocardial Perfusion

- Combines anatomic CTA with perfusion imaging.
- Limited validation in MVA; radiation and contrast-load considerations.[1,10]

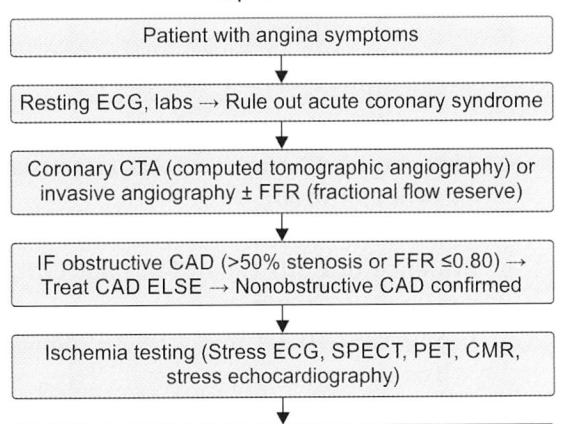

Flowchart 1: Overall diagnostic algorithm for suspected MVA.

TABLE 2: Noninvasive diagnostic modalities in MVA.

Modality	Advantages	Limitations	Diagnostic cut-off	ESC 2019 Class/LOE
PET	Quantitative CFR; prognostic data	Cost; availability	CFR <2.0	IIb/B
CMR	No radiation; high resolution	Limited availability	MPRI ≤1.84	IIb/B
TTDE	Inexpensive; portable	Operator-dependent	CFVR ≤2.3	IIb/B
CT perfusion	Anatomy + perfusion	Radiation; contrast	Not standardized	

Invasive Coronary Function Testing

Principles

- Gold standard for mechanism-based diagnosis.
- Evaluates:
  - *Structural CMD:* Reduced CFR; elevated IMR.
  - *Microvascular spasm:* Reproduction of symptoms with ischemic ECG changes during acetylcholine infusion without epicardial spasm.
  - *Macrovascular spasm:* >90% epicardial constrictio.[1,4,12]

Preparation

- Withhold vasoactive drugs (nitrates, calcium-channel blockers) per protocol.
- Anticoagulation with unfractionated heparin (70–100 U/kg).

Measurement Steps

- Position Doppler or thermodilution wire in proximal LAD.
- Record baseline average peak velocity (APV) or resting transit time.
- Adenosine infusion → measure hyperemia → calculate CFR.
- Acetylcholine infusion (graded doses) → assess vasomotor response.
- Nitroglycerin bolus → assess endothelium-independent epicardial dilation.[4,12]

Diagnostic Thresholds

- CFR ≤2.0 = abnormal (structural CMD).
- IMR ≥25 = abnormal microvascular resistance.
- *Coronary spasm:* Angina + ischemic ECG changes ± epicardial constriction per COVADIS[4,12] **(Flowchart 2)**.

Integrated Diagnostic Criteria–COVADIS

- *Definitive MVA:*
  - Symptoms of ischemia;

Flowchart 2: Invasive CFT protocol.

Baseline measurement:
- Place Doppler or thermodilution wire in proximal LAD
- Record resting coronary flow

↓

Adenosine infusion:
- Measure coronary flow reserve (CFR)
- Calculate index of microvascular resistance (IMR)

↓

If CFR low and IMR high → *Diagnosis:* Structural CMD

↓

Acetylcholine infusion (graded from low to high dose):
- Monitor symptoms and ECG changes
- Perform angiography after each dose

↓

- If symptoms + ECG changes and no epicardial spasm → *Diagnosis:* Microvascular spasm
- If >90% epicardial constriction with symptoms/ECG changes → *Diagnosis:* Macrovascular spasm

- Absence of obstructive CAD (stenosis <50% or FFR >0.80);
- Objective evidence of ischemia; and
- Evidence of CMD (low CFR, high IMR, and/or microvascular spasm).
  - *Suspected MVA:* Criteria 1 + 2 + (either 3 or 4).[12]

■ MANAGEMENT

Management of MVA should be tailored to the underlying mechanism identified via invasive or noninvasive testing. Both the ESC 2019 Chronic Coronary Syndrome guideline and the ACC/AHA 2023 Chronic Coronary Disease guideline emphasize mechanism-based therapy.[1,4,10,11]

Goals of Therapy

- Relieve anginal symptoms
- Improve quality of life
- Reduce ischemia burden
- Address long-term cardiovascular risk.

Mechanism-based Algorithm

See **Flowchart 3**.

Pharmacologic Therapy

See **Table 3**.

Nonpharmacologic Therapy

- *Lifestyle modification:* Smoking cessation, Mediterranean diet, weight management.
- *Exercise training:* Improves endothelial function and symptoms.
- *Enhanced external counterpulsation (EECP):* Symptom relief; ↑ exercise tolerance.
- *Stress-reduction strategies:* Yoga, meditation, cognitive-behavioral therapy.[1,10]

Special Populations

- *Women:* Higher prevalence of microvascular spasm; CCBs often effective[1,2]
- *Diabetes mellitus:* SGLT2 inhibitors may improve vascular function; strict glycemic control.
- *Elderly:* Careful dose titration due to polypharmacy.

Ongoing Clinical Trials

See **Table 4**.

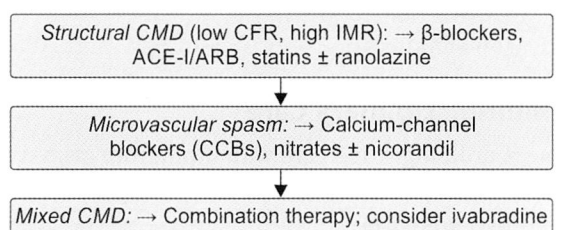

Flowchart 3: Treatment strategy for MVA.

TABLE 3: Pharmacologic options in MVA.

Class	Example	Dose range	Evidence	ESC COR/LOE
Statins	Atorvastatin	20–80 mg/day	Improves endothelial function; risk reduction in chronic coronary disease	I/B
ACE-I/ARB	Quinapril, Enalapril	Quinapril 80 mg/day; Enalapril 5 mg bid	Improves CFR; symptom reduction in selected studies	I/B
β-blockers	Nebivolol, Carvedilol	Nebivolol 5–10 mg/day	↓ heart rate; ↑ diastolic perfusion time	IIa/B
CCBs	Amlodipine, Verapamil	Amlodipine 5–10 mg/day	Effective for vasospasm	IIa/B
Nitrates	ISMN, GTN	ISMN 20–60 mg bid	Symptom relief (spasm-predominant)	IIb/C
Ranolazine	—	500–1,000 mg bid	Benefit in low CFR; mixed trial data	IIb/B
Ivabradine	—	5–7.5 mg bid	Heart-rate reduction; symptom improvement	IIb/B1-4,10,11

TABLE 4: Ongoing clinical trials.

Trial	Population	Intervention	Outcome
WARRIOR	Women with INOCA	Intensive medical therapy (statin + ACE-I/ARB + aspirin)	Cardiovascular events[13]
PRIZE	CMD	Zibotentan (endothelin-A antagonist)	CFR improvement[14]
MINOCA-BAT	MINOCA/INOCA	β-blocker + ACE-I/ARB	MACE reduction (ongoing)

FOLLOW-UP AND SECONDARY PREVENTION

Effective follow-up ensures sustained symptom control, optimized risk-factor management, and early detection of complications.

Follow-up Schedule

- *Initial postdiagnosis review:* 4–6 weeks after initiating therapy
- *Stable patients:* Every 6–12 months
- *High-risk or refractory symptoms:* Every 3–6 months[10,11]

Clinical Assessment at Each Visit

- Angina frequency and severity (e.g., Seattle Angina Questionnaire).
- Functional capacity (exercise tolerance, 6-minute walk).
- Adherence to medications and lifestyle changes.
- Side-effect monitoring (e.g., hypotension, bradycardia, and dizziness).

Repeat Investigations

- Noninvasive ischemia testing if symptoms change significantly.
- Consider repeat CFR/IMR measurement in research or refractory cases.
- *Risk-factor reassessment:* Blood pressure, lipids, HbA1c, renal function[10,11]

Secondary Prevention Strategies

See **Table 5.**

Patient Education and Engagement

- Educate on the nature of disease and prognosis.
- Emphasize importance of lifestyle measures.
- Encourage a symptom diary for angina tracking.

Multidisciplinary Care

- Cardiologist-led care with input from primary care, nutritionists, physiotherapists, and psychologists.
- Psychological support for anxiety/depression related to chronic symptoms[1,10]

FUTURE RESEARCH PRIORITIES

- *Outcome-focused trials:* While CorMicA has shown symptomatic benefit from tailored therapy, large-scale trials (e.g., WARRIOR, PRIZE) will clarify the impact on hard endpoints[4,13,14]
- *Novel therapeutics:* Endothelin-receptor antagonists, Rho-kinase inhibitors, and regenerative therapies hold promise for CMD treatment[1,14]
- *Sex-specific strategies:* Given the high prevalence in women, hormone-related

TABLE 5: Secondary prevention measures in MVA.

Measure	Target	Evidence/guidelines
Blood pressure control	<130/80 mm Hg	ESC CCS 2019; ACC/AHA 2023[10,11]
LDL-cholesterol	<55 mg/dL (very high risk)	ESC/EAS dyslipidemia guideline[15]
Glycemic control	HbA1c <7%	Major diabetes guidelines
Smoking cessation	Complete abstinence	I/A[10,11]
Physical activity	≥150 min/week moderate-intensity	WHO recommendations[16]
Weight management	BMI 20–25 kg/m²	I/B[10,11]

pathophysiological differences warrant further study[1,2]

- *Imaging biomarkers:* Quantitative CMR, PET, and CT perfusion may provide noninvasive surrogates for invasive measures[1,5,6]

KEY TAKE-HOME MESSAGES

- MVA is common, prognostically important, and mechanistically heterogeneous.[2-7]
- A comprehensive, guideline-aligned diagnostic algorithm improves accuracy and guides therapy.[1,10,11]
- Mechanism-based treatment can improve symptoms and functional outcomes.[4,10,11]
- Aggressive secondary prevention is essential to reduce cardiovascular risk.[10,11,15,16]

Ongoing trials will refine the therapeutic landscape and clarify long-term benefits.[13,14]

CONCLUSION AND FUTURE DIRECTIONS

Microvascular angina is firmly established as a clinically significant condition within the spectrum of INOCA, with a burden comparable to that of obstructive CAD. It is associated with increased risks of MACE, recurrent hospitalization, and impaired quality of life.[2-7] Mechanism-based diagnosis and treatment, aligned with contemporary ESC and ACC/AHA guidelines, can lead to substantial improvements in symptom control and functional capacity.[1,4,10,11]

A structured diagnostic approach integrating noninvasive ischemia testing and, where feasible, invasive coronary function testing enables precise phenotyping into structural CMD, microvascular spasm, or mixed forms. This precision facilitates tailored therapy—from β-blockers and ACE inhibitors for structural CMD to calcium-channel blockers and nitrates for vasospastic forms—complemented by aggressive risk-factor modification and patient education.[1,4,10,11]

REFERENCES

1. Kunadian V, Chieffo A, Camici PG, et al. An EAPCI Expert Consensus Document on Ischaemia with Non-Obstructive Coronary Arteries in collaboration with ESC Working Group on Coronary Pathophysiology & Microcirculation; endorsed by COVADIS. EuroIntervention. 2021;16(14):1049-69.
2. Bairey Merz CN, Pepine CJ, Walsh MN, et al. Ischemia and no obstructive coronary artery disease (INOCA): Developing evidence-based therapies and research agenda for the next decade. Circulation. 2017;135(11):1075-92.
3. Prescott E, Abildstrøm SZ, Aziz A, et al. Improving diagnosis of stable angina in women with suspected ischaemic heart disease: The iPOWER study. Eur Heart J. 2016;37(11):849-56.
4. Ford TJ, Stanley B, Good R, et al. Stratified medical therapy using invasive coronary function testing in angina: The CorMicA trial. J Am Coll Cardiol. 2018;72(23 Pt A):2841-55.
5. Murthy VL, Naya M, Taqueti VR, et al. Effects of sex on coronary microvascular dysfunction and cardiac outcomes. Circulation. 2014;129(24):2518-27.
6. Zhou W, Lee J, Feng Y, et al. Coronary microvascular dysfunction and prognosis in patients with chest pain, normal coronary arteries, and abnormal stress cardiac magnetic resonance tests. JACC Cardiovasc Imaging. 2020;13(9):1945-56.
7. Gdowski MA, Murthy VL, Doering M, et al. Coronary microvascular dysfunction is associated with poor outcomes: A systematic review and meta-analysis. J Am Coll Cardiol. 2020; 75(21):2414-22.
8. Camici PG, Crea F. Coronary microvascular dysfunction. N Engl J Med. 2007;356(8):830-40.
9. Taqueti VR, Di Carli MF. Coronary microvascular disease: Pathogenic mechanisms and therapeutic options. J Am Coll Cardiol. 2018;72(21):2625-41.
10. Knuuti J, Wijns W, Saraste A, et al. 2019 ESC Guidelines for the diagnosis and management of chronic coronary syndromes. Eur Heart J. 2020;41(3):407-77.
11. Gulati M, Levy PD, Mukherjee D, et al. 2023 ACC/AHA guideline for the management of patients

with chronic coronary disease. J Am Coll Cardiol. 2023;81(15):1443-574.
12. Ong P, Camici PG, Beltrame JF, et al. International standardization of diagnostic criteria for microvascular angina. Int J Cardiol. 2018;250:16-20.
13. Handberg EM, Bairey Merz CN, Cooper-DeHoff R, et al. Rationale and design of the Women's Ischemia Trial to Reduce Events in Non-Obstructive CAD (WARRIOR) trial. Am Heart J. 2021;237:90-103.
14. Ford TJ, Rocchiccioli P, McEntegart M, et al. The PRIZE trial: Evaluation of zibotentan for the treatment of coronary microvascular angina. Eur Heart J. 2023;44(Suppl 1):ehad103.3613.
15. Mach F, Baigent C, Catapano AL, et al. 2019 ESC/EAS Guidelines for the management of dyslipidaemias: Lipid modification to reduce cardiovascular risk. Eur Heart J. 2020;41(1):111-88.
16. WHO. Guidelines on physical activity and sedentary behaviour. Geneva: World Health Organization; 2020.

CHAPTER 15

Myocardial Bridging: Current Perspectives

Suman Bhandari, Atul Kaushik

INTRODUCTION

Myocardial bridging (MB) is a congenital coronary anomaly in which a segment of an epicardial coronary artery—normally situated on the surface of the heart—takes an intramyocardial (within the heart muscle) course. This tunneled segment is overlain by myocardial fibers, forming a "bridge" that compresses the artery during the cardiac cycle, especially in systole. While often considered benign, MB can become clinically significant, particularly in certain anatomical variants or comorbid settings.[1-5]

It has been observed that MB are common in left anterior descending (LAD) chronic total occlusion (CTO) (40.4% MB) as compared to LAD non-CTOs (25.8%). Moreover, the LAD CTOs had stent extended into an MB after which the target lesion failure was significantly higher.[6] MB also predisposes the patients with INOCA to coronary spasm.[7] These finding re-emphasize the need for look for MB in coronary arteries.

PREVALENCE

The incidence of MB varies significantly depending on the imaging modality:

- *Coronary angiography:* MB is detected in approximately 2–6% of patients undergoing conventional invasive coronary angiography.[1-3] This modality may underestimate prevalence due to its inability to detect subtle anatomical abnormalities or functional compression unless under stress.
- *Coronary computed tomography angiography (CCTA):* Offers a more sensitive assessment of coronary anatomy, detecting MB in 19–22% of patients.[2,4]
- *Autopsy studies:* Considered the most definitive method, autopsy reveals MB in 33–44% of cases, suggesting that most instances are subclinical and likely asymptomatic.[1,3]

LOCATION OF MYOCARDIAL BRIDGING

The LAD artery is the most involved coronary artery, especially its mid-segment. Studies report that 67–98% of MBs affect the LAD.[5,6] Sites other than LAD have been observed like, diagonal branches are involved in approximately 18%, Obtuse marginal branches in 40%, and right coronary artery (RCA) involvement is rare, reported in isolated case series.[8]

PATHOPHYSIOLOGY

MB alters normal coronary hemodynamics through a phenomenon known as the "milking effect," characterized by systolic compression of the bridged artery. While this effect is benign in most patients, it can compromise coronary perfusion, especially when:

- The bridge is deep (>2 mm) or long
- There is increased heart rate or myocardial contractility, reducing diastolic filling time
- It coexists with hypertrophic cardiomyopathy or microvascular dysfunction.[9]

Normally, coronary perfusion occurs predominantly during diastole (~85%). However, in MB, especially in symptomatic cases, compression may extend into early diastole, reducing perfusion by up to 30%, which may lead to myocardial ischemia.[10] Ischemia in MB may result from multiple mechanisms: Dynamic systolic and early diastolic compression of the artery, vasospasm triggered by endothelial dysfunction, increased intramural pressure leading to coronary flow reserve (CFR) reduction, disturbed shear stress, and proinflammatory endothelial activation.[11,12]

Proximal to the bridged segment, increased wall shear stress and turbulent flow result in plaque formation. The tunneled segment is generally protected from atherosclerosis due to consistent systolic compression and smooth muscle orientation, which is not conducive to plaque deposition.[11,12] This dynamic explains why CTOs in the LAD are frequently found just proximal to a bridged segment, especially in postmortem or IVUS studies.[6,13]

PRESENTATION

Although MB is often asymptomatic and found incidentally, symptomatic cases may present with exertional angina or chest pain, myocardial infarction (in absence of obstructive coronary disease), arrhythmias (due to ischemia-related electrical instability), syncope or presyncope, or sudden cardiac death, particularly in young athletes or in conjunction with structural heart disease.[5,9]

DIAGNOSIS

- *CT-CAG:* Provides high-resolution 3D imaging of the coronary arteries and surrounding myocardium, allowing precise assessment of bridge length, depth, and associated myocardial mass.[2,6]
- *IVUS:* Demonstrates the half-moon sign—a crescent-shaped echolucency between the bridged artery and overlying muscle.[10]
- *OCT:* Offers finer spatial resolution and characterizes the plaque morphology and arterial wall details, particularly useful in assessing the prebridged segment.[14]
- *Fractional flow reserve (FFR):* FFR assesses the physiological impact of MB. However, mean FFR may be misleading due to systolic compression not affecting perfusion.
  - Diastolic FFR offers more accurate ischemia detection.
  - Dobutamine challenge, rather than adenosine, is preferred to mimic physiological stress.[15,16]
- *Provocative pharmacological testing:* Nitroglycerin can worsen compression by relaxing the adjacent vessel and exaggerating the difference in wall tension—potentially increasing systolic narrowing from ~24 to ~65%.[9] It is therefore contraindicated in MB patients.[10,17]

CLASSIFICATION

Schwarz et al. proposed a clinically relevant classification to guide management:[18]

- *Type A:* Symptomatic without ischemia,
- *Type B:* Symptomatic with positive stress test (noninvasive ischemia),
- *Type C:* Symptomatic with hemodynamic changes seen on intracoronary techniques (QCA, CFR, Doppler).

MANAGEMENT

Medical management remains the first-line strategy for symptomatic MB:

- β-blockers reduce heart rate and contractility, enhancing diastolic perfusion, and reducing the milking effect.[19]
- Calcium channel blockers are effective in MB with associated vasospasm.[4]
- Nitrates are avoided due to their potential to exacerbate compression and worsen symptoms.[17]

Percutaneous Coronary Intervention

While technically feasible, PCI is reserved for rare refractory cases not amenable to medical or surgical therapy. PCI in MB has significant limitations like Stent fracture due to repetitive motion, in-stent restenosis, stent thrombosis, and coronary perforation in deep tunnels.[17,19,20]

Surgical Management

Surgical intervention is considered in patients with severe symptoms refractory to medical therapy or in cases with deep/long MB.

- Coronary artery bypass grafting (CABG) is preferred for long (>25 mm) or deep (>5 mm) MBs, bypassing the bridged segment entirely.[17,20]
- Surgical myotomy involves resecting the overlying myocardium, most effective in short, superficial bridges.[17]

CONCLUSION

The prognosis of MB is generally favorable in asymptomatic individuals. However, symptomatic MB, especially with demonstrable ischemia or structural anomalies, warrants careful evaluation, and tailored therapy. In athletes and patients with hypertrophic cardiomyopathy, MB carries a higher risk of sudden cardiac events, and exercise restriction or surgical evaluation may be indicated. Long-term follow-up with stress testing, imaging, and symptom monitoring is crucial to ensure patient safety and prevent progression of complications.

REFERENCES

1. Polacek P, Zechmeister A. The occurrence and significance of myocardial bridges and loops on coronary arteries. In: Krutna V (Ed). Monograph 36, Opuscola Cardiologica. Acta Facultatis Medicae Universitatis Brunenses. Brno: University J.E. Purkinje; 1968. pp. 1-99.
2. Roberts W, Charles SM, Ang C, et al. Myocardial bridges: a meta-analysis. Clin Anat. 2021;34(5):685-709.
3. Houstic S, Negoi I, Rusu MC, et al. Myocardial bridging: meta-analysis of prevalence. J Forensic Sci. 2018;63:1176-85.
4. Teragawa H, Fukuda Y, Matsuda K, et al. Myocardial bridging increases the risk of coronary spasm. Clin Cardiol. 2003;26:377-83.
5. Alegria JR, Herrmann J, Holmes DR Jr, et al. Myocardial bridging. Eur Heart J. 2005;26:1159-68.
6. Yamamoto K, Sugizaki Y, Karmpaliotis D, et al. Presence and relevance of myocardial bridge in LAD-PCI of CTO and Non-CTO lesions. JACC Cardiovasc Interv. 2024;17(4):491-501.
7. Teragawa H, Oshita C, Uchimura Y. The impact of myocardial bridging on the coronary functional test in patients with ischaemia with non-obstructive coronary artery disease. Life (Basel). 2022;12(10):1560.
8. Ge J, Erbel R, Gorge G, et al. High wall shear stress proximal to myocardial bridging and atherosclerosis: intracoronary ultrasound and pressure measurements. Br Heart J. 1995;73:462-5.
9. Corban MT, Hung OY, Eshtehardi P, et al. Myocardial bridging: contemporary understanding of pathophysiology with implications for diagnostic and therapeutic strategies. J Am Coll Cardiol. 2014;63:2346-55.
10. Sternheim D, Power DA, Samtani R, et al. Myocardial bridging: diagnosis, functional assessment, and management. JACC State-of-the-Art-Review. 2021;78(22):2196-212.
11. Möhlenkamp S, Hort W, Ge J, et al. Update on myocardial bridging. Circulation. 2002;106(20):2616-22.
12. Rajendran R, Hegde M. The prevalence of myocardial bridging on multidetector computed tomography and its relation to coronary plaques. Pol J Radiol. 2019;84:e478-83.
13. Escaned J, Cortés J, Flores A, et al. Importance of diastolic fractional flow reserve and dobutamine challenge in physiologic assessment of myocardial bridging. J Am Coll Cardiol. 2003;42:226-33.
14. Hakeem A, Cilingiroglu M, Leesar MA. Hemodynamic and intravascular ultrasound assessment of myocardial bridging: fractional flow reserve paradox with dobutamine versus adenosine. Catheter Cardiovasc Interv. 2010;75:229-36.
15. Hongo Y, Tada H, Ito K, et al. Augmentation of vessel squeezing at coronary-myocardial bridge by nitroglycerin: study by quantitative coronary

angiography and intravascular ultrasound. Am Heart J. 1999;138:345-50.
16. Ye Z, Lai Y, Yao Y, et al. Optical coherence tomography and intravascular ultrasound assessment of the anatomic size and wall thickness of a muscle bridge segment. Catheter Cardiovasc Interv. 2019;93:772-8.
17. Lee MS, Chen C-H. Myocardial bridging: an up-to-date review. J Invasive Cardiol. 2015;27:521-8.
18. Schwarz ER, Klues HG, vom Dahl J, et al. Functional, angiographic and intracoronary Doppler flow characteristics in symptomatic patients with myocardial bridging: effect of short-term intravenous beta-blocker medication. J Am Coll Cardiol. 1996;27:1637-45.
19. Schwarz ER, Gupta R, Haager PK, et al. Myocardial bridging in absence of coronary artery disease: proposal of a new classification based on clinical-angiographic data and long-term follow-up. Cardiology. 2009;112:13-21.
20. Doenst T, Haverich A, Serruys P, et al. PCI and CABG for treating stable coronary artery disease: JACC review topic of the week. J Am Coll Cardiol. 2019;73:964-76.

CHAPTER 16

Imaging as Class I Indication: Current Value of ICI and Strategies for Achieving Better Penetration in India

Palanivel Rajan, Karthikeyan B, Vijayakumar S

INTRODUCTION

Coronary angiography (CAG) provides the roadmap for percutaneous coronary intervention (PCI). However, it is limited by its lower resolution, angle dependency, vessel overlap, and fore shortening. In addition, it only provides a two-dimensional shadow of a three-dimensional structure (lumenogram) and does not provide complete information of the plaque characteristics.[1]

Intravascular imaging (IVI) provides cross-sectional images of the coronary arteries and helps the interventionist understand plaque morphology, vessel landing zone, results of stenting, and mechanism of stent failure (SF) enabling rational decision-making during PCI. It is an essential tool in every coronary catheterization laboratory as it adds objectivity to intraprocedural decision-making.[2] Current IVI modalities are either ultrasound based [intravascular ultrasound (IVUS)] or light based [optical coherence tomography (OCT)]. Following discussion summarizes the role of IVI in contemporary PCI optimization.

TECHNICAL FEATURES OF INTRAVASCULAR IMAGING SYSTEMS

The IVI system consists of three components: (1) A console, (2) an automatic pullback device, and (3) an imaging catheter. The miniature transducer or optical lens at the tip of the imaging catheter emits ultrasound waves or light photons respectively, that get reflected from the tissue interfaces back to the transducer. The transducer revolves around the circumference and acquires information. The signals received are decoded and reconstructed by the console into a cross-sectional image. The pullback device moves the catheter along the length of the vessel at a constant speed that creates the longitudinal image.

The currently available IVUS systems of different manufacturers use high frequency ultrasound probes between 20 and 60 MHz with variable bandwidth and either rotatory or solid-state models for image acquisition. The axial resolution varies between 60 and 150 μ. In contrast, the very high frequency provides the OCT, a resolution in the range of 15 μ. Compared to IVUS, OCT requires clearing of blood for image acquisition and is limited by its penetration.[3]

NORMAL VESSEL WALL CHARACTERS AND IMAGE INTERPRETATION

A typical IVUS/OCT image has four components: (1) *The catheter:* A circular structure inside the lumen. (2) *The guidewire:* It appears as a bright spot with a wedge-shaped shadow. (3) *The lumen:* In an optimally acquired OCT image, the lumen appears uniformly dark as the blood is cleared with contrast. In the IVUS image, blood speckles are visualized in the lumen. (4) *The vessel wall:* In both IVUS and OCT, the collagen and elastin rich intimal and adventitial layers appear bright, and the smooth muscle cell rich media appears dark.

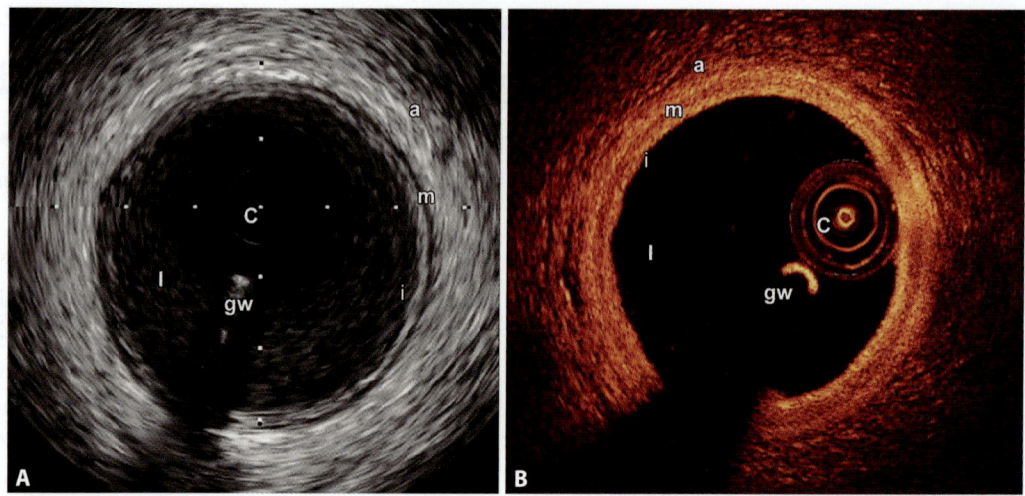

Figs. 1A and B: Normal coronary artery on IVUS (A)/OCT (B) has four components: (1) Imaging catheter (c); (2) Guidewire (gw); (3) Lumen (l, contains blood speckles in IVUS and echolucent in OCT); and (4) Three-layered vessel wall in bright–dark–bright pattern (i—intima, m—media, a—adventitia).

This gives the vessel wall a three-layered "bright–dark bright" pattern **(Figs. 1A and B)**.[3]

Atherosclerosis is a disease of intima, and the plaque morphology depends on the relative composition of fibrotic, calcific, lipid, and matrix tissue. Plaque characterization by gray scale IVUS is based on the echogenicity of the plaque with reference to the echogenicity of the adventitia: (1) Calcified plaque (hyperechoic to adventitia with acoustic shadowing or reverberations), (2) fibrous plaque (isoechoic to adventitia), (3) soft plaque (hypoechoic to adventitia), (4) mixed plaque (no single acoustic type constituting >80% of the plaque), (5) attenuated plaque (signal loss in the absence of superficial calcium), and (6) echolucent plaque (plaque with intraplaque echolucency) **(Figs. 2A to F)**.[2,4,5]

The plaque characterization by OCT is based on backscatter, attenuation, composition, and border features of the tissue: (1) Fibrous plaque (homogenous, high backscatter, and low attenuation), (2) lipidic plaque (homogenous, low backscatter, high attenuation, and diffuse borders), (3) fibrocalcific plaque (heterogenous, low backscatter, low attenuation, sharp borders), (4) red thrombus (intraluminal mass with high backscatter and high attenuation), (5) white thrombus (intraluminal mass with high backscatter and low attenuation), (6) recanalized thrombus (intraluminal mass with channels and intact media), (7) spontaneous coronary artery dissection (medial disruption with accumulation of blood), (8) thin cap fibroatheroma [lipid-rich plaque (LRP) with fibrous thickness <65 µ], (9) LRP—lipid occupying 180° of the cross-sectional image, (10) microchannels (intraplaque signal voids 50–300 µ in diameter), (11) macrophages (linear signal rich spots with signal attenuation), (12) spotty calcium (calcium with an arc <90°), (13) cholesterol crystals (linear, signal-rich structures with no signal attenuation), (14) healed plaque (layers with different optical properties), (15) plaque rupture (PR) (fibrous cap disruption with underlying LRP), (16) plaque erosion (PE) (intact fibrous cap with attached thrombus), (17) noneruptive calcified nodule (CN) (nodular calcium with intact fibrous cap),

Imaging as Class I Indication: Current Value of ICI and Strategies for Achieving Better Penetration in India

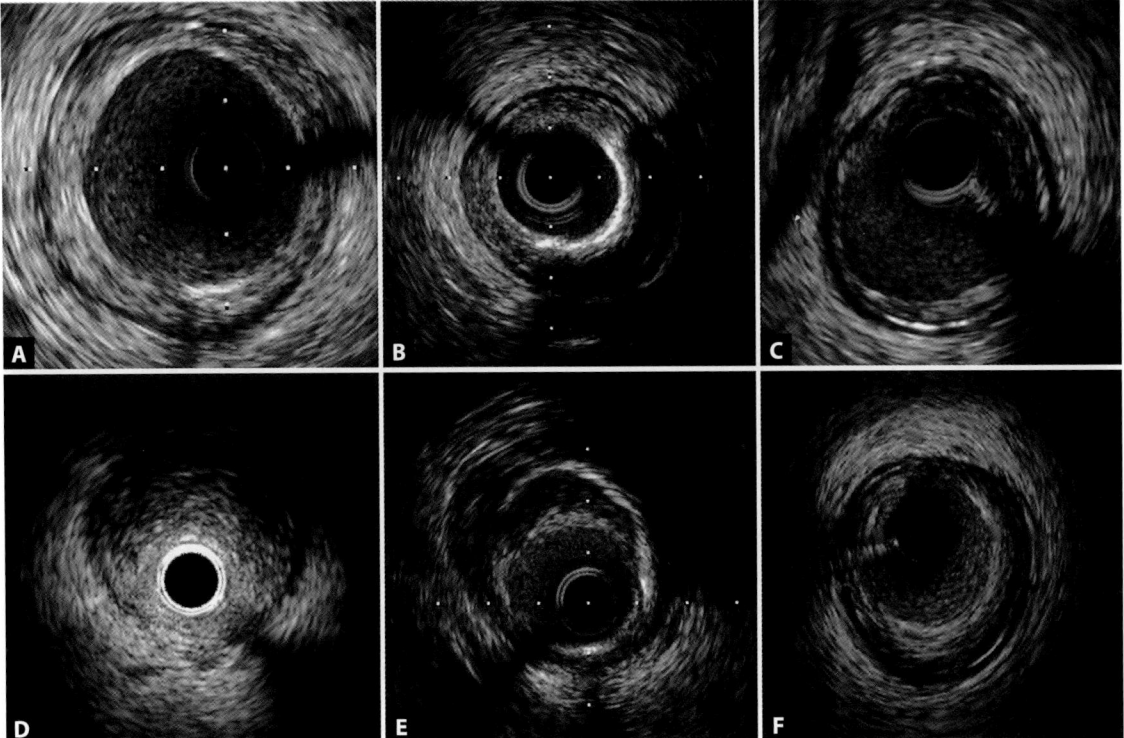

Figs. 2A to F: IVUS plaque characterization. (A) Fibrous plaque; (B) Calcific plaque; (C) Soft plaque; (D) Attenuated plaque; (E) Mixed plaque; and (F) Echolucent plaque.

(18) (protruding calcium with irregular surface and attached thrombus) **(Figs. 3A to R)**.[6]

INTRAVASCULAR IMAGING ARTIFACTS

Artifacts are commonly encountered in both IVUS and OCT imaging. They can degrade image quality, hinder accurate identification of true tissue structures, and at times be misinterpreted as pathological findings, potentially leading to unnecessary interventions. Since both modalities rely on similar imaging principles, and because mechanical IVUS and OCT systems utilize a drive cable and protective sheath, they share several types of artifacts.[3] **Table 1** summarizes the common artifacts with IVUS and OCT imaging **(Figs. 4A to R)**.

INTRAVASCULAR IMAGING MEASUREMENTS

Intravascular imaging modalities enable precise cross-sectional and longitudinal measurements. Both IVUS and OCT systems offer automatic measurement capabilities. In native vessels, three interfaces are identified: (1) Lumen–intima, (2) media–adventitia, and (3) external elastic lamina (EEL). In stented vessels, the interfaces are (a) lumen–neointima, (b) stent, and (c) EEL. All measurements are taken from leading edge to leading edge through the center of the lumen.[3] Common measurements are listed in **Table 2**.

ASSESSMENT OF LESION SEVERITY

Intravascular imaging is currently not recommended for the assessment of lesion severity in

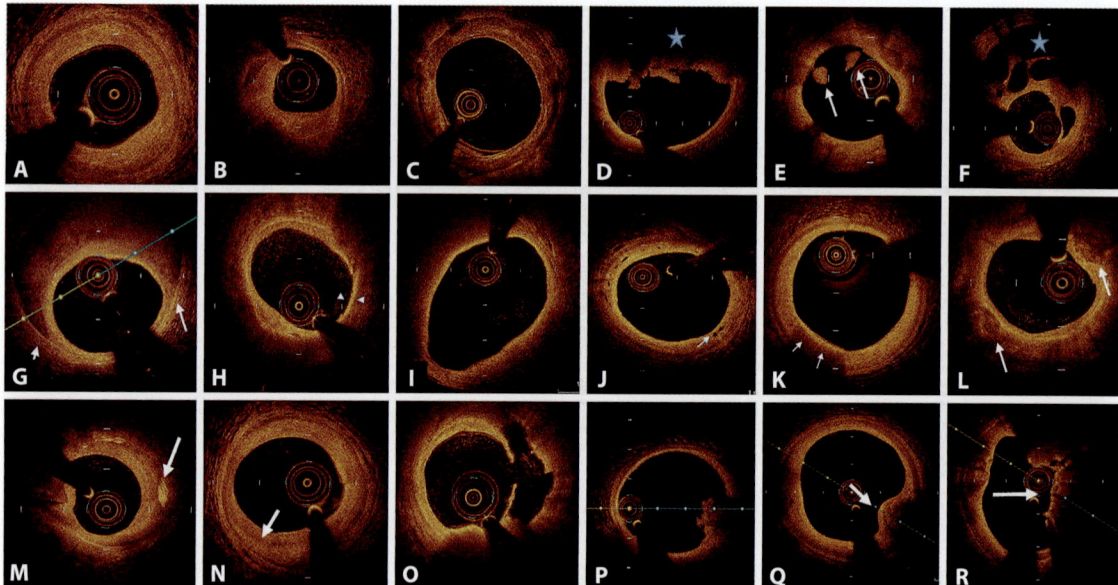

Figs. 3A to R: OCT plaque characterization. (A) Fibrous plaque; (B) Lipidic plaque; (C) Fibrocalcific plaque; (D) Red thrombus (star); (E) White thrombus; (F) Recanalized thrombus; (G) Spontaneous coronary artery dissection (arrows indicating medial split); (H) Thin cap fibroatheroma (arrowheads indicating fibrous cap); (I) Lipid-rich plaque; (J) Microchannels (arrow); (K) Macrophages (arrows); (L) Spotty calcium (arrows); (M) Cholesterol crystals (arrow); (N) Healed plaque; (O) Plaque rupture; (P) Plaque erosion; (Q) Noneruptive calcified nodule (arrow); and (R) Eruptive calcified nodule (arrow).

Artifact	Cause	Appearance on IVUS/OCT	Clinical impact/pitfall
TABLE 1: Common IVUS and OCT artifacts.			
Artifacts common to IVUS and OCT			
Nonuniform rotational distortion (NURD)	Uneven drag/friction on drive cable; tortuous vessel, stenosis, tight hemostatic valve, and defective catheter	Smearing/geometric distortion in part of the circumference	Conceals structures in that part of the vessel; inaccurate cross-sectional measurement
Motion/sew-up (seamline)	Rapid movement of artery or catheter during acquisition	Malalignment along circumference	Misrepresentation of vessel wall
Obliquity	Catheter noncoaxial in large/curved vessels	Elliptical cross section	Inaccurate diameter/area measurements
Shadow artifact	Strong reflectors (guidewire, stent struts, thrombus, and RBCs) block signal	Signal dropout behind reflector	Hides underlying lumen and vessel wall details
Multiple reflections/reverberations	Sound/light bouncing between specular surfaces (catheter facets and stent struts)	Ghost circular lines or extra strut layers	May be mistaken for additional interfaces

Contd...

Contd...

Artifact	Cause	Appearance on IVUS/OCT	Clinical impact/pitfall
Artifacts specific to IVUS			
Ring-down artifact	High frequency oscillations close to the surface of the catheter	Luminous halos of different thickness around the surface of the catheter	Hinders evaluation of the area in the proximity of the catheter
Air bubble artifact	Small air bubbles trapped in the protective sheath	Poor image quality, reverberations, ring-down artifact	Difficult to interpret images
Blood speckles	Slow moving blood/obstruction/high frequency ultrasound transducer	Spontaneous echo contrast in the lumen	Obscure the lumen—intima interface
Side lobe	Reflection of side beams from highly reflective structures	Bright linear or arc like ghost echoes along the circumference	Appearance of malapposition or dissection
Artifacts specific to OCT			
Residual blood artifact	Incomplete flushing of blood in the vessel	Swirls in varying forms	Misinterpreted as thrombus; obscures vessel wall details
Fold-over	Vessel diameter > field of view (~10 mm) → Aliasing in Fourier transformation	Far field vessel wall folded into lumen	False vessel duplication; common at side branches
Saturation	Excessive backscatter (stent struts, guidewire) overwhelms detector	Very bright A-lines	Loss of detail; obscures strut edges
Blooming	Intense stent reflections of the stent struts	Glare-axial thickening of struts	Hinders stent edge identification; errors in strut apposition analysis
Proximity artifact	Eccentric catheter position	Artificially bright adjacent tissues	May exaggerate wall brightness
Tangential signal dropout	Catheter in contact with wall; light parallel to wall	Superficial bright layer with deeper signal loss	Mimics thin-cap fibroatheroma (TCFA)
Merry-go-round effect	Reduced lateral resolution; incomplete flushing	Apparent lateral elongation of stent struts	May falsely suggest stent deformation
Sunflower effect	Eccentric catheter in stented vessel; reflection from strut edge	Struts oriented toward the catheter	Mimics stent malapposition; overestimates strut–wall distance

(IVUS: intravascular ultrasound; OCT: optical coherence tomography)

non-LMCA territory in view of poor correlation between IVI minimum lumen area and fractional flow reserve. Two recent trials reported noninferior outcomes with IVI-based assessment compared to the FFR.[7,8] In the FORZA (FFR or OCT Guidance to RevasculariZe Intermediate Coronary Stenosis Using Angioplasty) trial, 350 patients with angiographically intermediate (30–80% diameter stenosis) lesions were randomly allocated to either an FFR-based (≤0.80) or to an

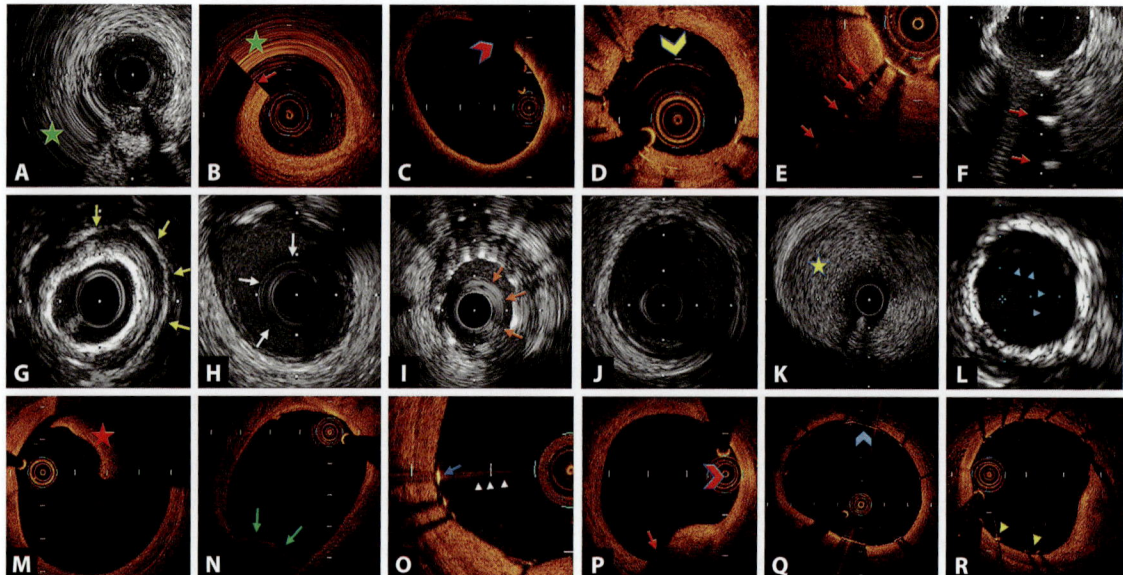

Figs. 4A to R: Artifacts observed in intravascular imaging. (A to F) Artifacts common to intravascular ultrasound (IVUS) and optical coherence tomography (OCT): (A and B) Nonuniform rotational deformity (green stars) and sew-up artifact (red arrow); (C) Obliquity artifact, with shadowing from the guidewire indicated by the red arrowhead; (D) Multiple reflection artifact (yellow arrowhead); (E and F) Stent reverberations (red arrows); (G to L) IVUS-specific artifacts; (G) Calcium reverberation (yellow arrows); (H) Ring-down artifact (white arrows); (I) Air bubble with associated ring-down artifact (orange arrows); (J) Air bubble artifact with degraded image quality; (K) Blood speckle artifact (yellow star); (L) Side-lobe artifact (blue arrowheads); (M to R) OCT-specific artifacts: (M) Residual blood artifact (red star); (N) Fold-over artifact (green arrows); (O) Saturation artifact (white arrowheads) and blooming artifact (blue arrow); (P) Proximity artifact (red arrowhead) and tangential signal dropout (red arrow); (Q) Merry-go-round artifact (blue arrowhead); and (R) Sunflower artifact (yellow arrowheads).

OCT-based revascularization decision-making (>75% area stenosis, or 50–75% area stenosis with minimal luminal area <2.5 mm^2, or presence of PR). The composite of MACE or significant angina was significantly lower in the OCT group at 13 months (8% vs. 14.8%, p <0.001).[7] In the FLAVOUR (Fractional Flow Reserve and IVUS for Clinical Outcomes in Patients With Intermediate Stenosis) study, 1,682 patients with intermediate stenosis (40–70% stenosis), were randomized either to FFR (≤0.80) or IVUS guidance (lumen areas <3 mm^2 or 3–4 mm^2 with plaque burden >70%) revascularization. The MACE (composite of death, MI, or revascularization) at 24 months the IVUS-guided strategy was noninferior to the FFR-guided strategy (8.5% vs. 8.1%, p <0.01 for noninferiority).[8]

■ PRESTENT ASSESSMENT

Systematic prestenting IVI assessment remains the cornerstone of optimal post-PCI outcomes. The major roles of pre-PCI IVI are: (1) Decision regarding lesion preparation, (2) selecting appropriate landing zones, (3) stent sizing, and (4) poststent optimization balloon sizing. Presence of significant calcification at the lesion site suggests the need for appropriate calcium modification. Ideal landing zones are the ones with no plaque. However, atherosclerosis is typically diffuse and often angiographically silent. In vessels with

TABLE 2: Intravascular imaging (IVI) measurements.

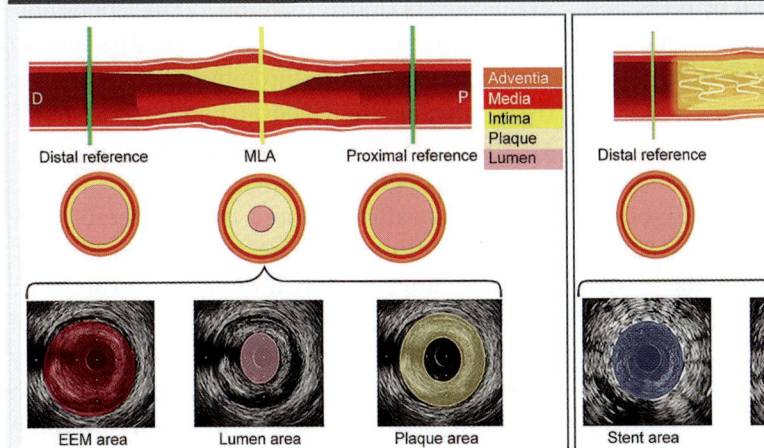
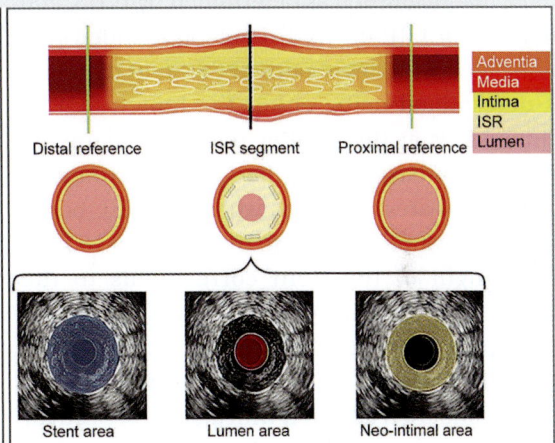

Vessel/external elastic lamina (EEL) area: Area bounded by the media-adventitia interface	*Stent CSA:* Area circumscribed by the stent border
Lumen cross-sectional area (CSA): Area circumscribed by the lumen border	*Proximal and distal reference:* The sites with largest lumen areas on either side of the stent and within 5 mm of the edges
Minimal lumen area (MLA): Smallest CSA in the lesion segment	*Maximum (max) and minimum (min) stent diameters (SD):* The longest and shortest diameters measured through the center of the stent
Maximum and minimum EEL diameters: The longest and shortest EEL distances measured through the center of the lumen	*Minimal stent CSA* = Smallest stent CSA
Maximum and minimum lumen diameters: The longest and shortest lumen distances measured through the center of the lumen	*Stent expansion:* Minimal stent CSA in correlation with reference lumen CSA (proximal, distal, or average)
Proximal and distal reference: The sites with largest lumen areas on either side of the lesion within 10 mm and in the same segment	*Stent symmetry* = Max SD – Min SD/Max SD
Plaque + Media area = EEL area – Lumen CSA	*Neointimal area* = Stent CSA – Lumen CSA
Plaque burden = EEL CSA – Lumen CSA/EEL CSA × 100	*In-stent lumen area stenosis* = The reference lumen CSA – minimal in-stent CSA/reference lumen CSA × 100
Lumen area stenosis: The reference lumen CSA – minimal lumen CSA/reference lumen CSA × 100	*Maximum and minimum neointimal thickness:* The longest and shortest dimensions between the lumen border of the neointima to the adluminal stent border along the line passing through the center of the lumen
Remodeling: Change in vessel size at the site of the lesion. *Positive remodeling:* Lesion EEL/average reference EEL >1.05. *Negative remodeling:* Lesion EEL/average reference EEL <0.95	*% neo intimal area* = Neointimal CSA/stent CSA

diffuse disease, selecting a landing zone with <50% plaque burden as determined by IVUS, and absence of LRP on OCT, is recommended and associated with lower rates of SF. Stent diameter is determined using either the lumen or EEL dimensions at the smaller reference diameter. With lumen-based sizing, the stent size is rounded up to the nearest 0.25 mm, while with EEL-based sizing it is rounded down to the nearest 0.25 mm. The length of the stent corresponds to the distance between the reference zones. If there is a discrepancy between the reference zones, a stent capable of expanding to the larger reference is chosen and then adjusted with a balloon sized for the larger reference **(Figs. 5A to F)**.[9]

POSTSTENT ASSESSMENT

After stent implantation and optimization according to prestenting IVI measurements, and once angiographic success has been confirmed, IVI is performed again to determine if further optimization is necessary. The following parameters of suboptimal stent implantation are evaluated: (1) Underexpansion, (2) malapposition, (3) geographic miss, (4) edge dissection/hematoma, (5) tissue/thrombus protrusion, and (6) unintended stent deformation **(Figs. 6A to K)**.

- *Underexpansion:* Stent expansion refers to the degree to which the lumen area is restored after PCI and is considered a key factor affecting long-term outcomes.[10,11] There are currently no universal criteria for optimal expansion, as studies utilize different measures. Stent expansion can be assessed by absolute lumen area or by comparing it with the reference lumen area. Absolute lumen area thresholds range from 5.0–5.5 mm² for IVUS and 4.5 mm² for OCT outside LMCA regions.[9] In small vessels, the optimal OCT area is 3.5 mm². Relative expansion may use distal reference, combined reference, or both, with cutoffs ranging from 70% to 100%.[12] The prevailing guidelines suggest an absolute area of 5 mm² for IVUS and 4.5 mm² for OCT, or

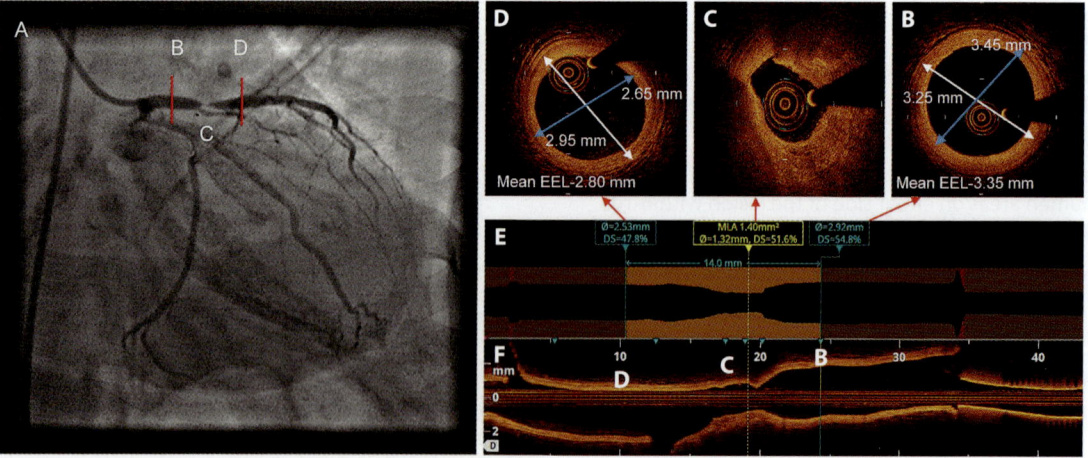

Figs. 5A to F: Stent sizing with OCT. Coronary angiogram showing a tight stenosis in the proximal left anterior descending coronary artery (A). OCT imaging was acquired following predilatation with a 2 mm balloon. In the first step, the lesion (C) is located on the lumen profile (E) and then the cursor is moved both proximally and distally to identify the disease-free reference segments (B and D). The average of maximum and the minimum lumen and external elastic membrane (EEL) diameters at each reference segments are measured. As the reference segments are free of disease, the stent is sized to the distal mean EEL diameter (2.80 mm). The distance between these reference segments is the length of the stent (14 mm). Hence, a 2.75 × 18 mm stent was chosen; and (F) Longitudinal view.

Imaging as Class I Indication: Current Value of ICI and Strategies for Achieving Better Penetration in India

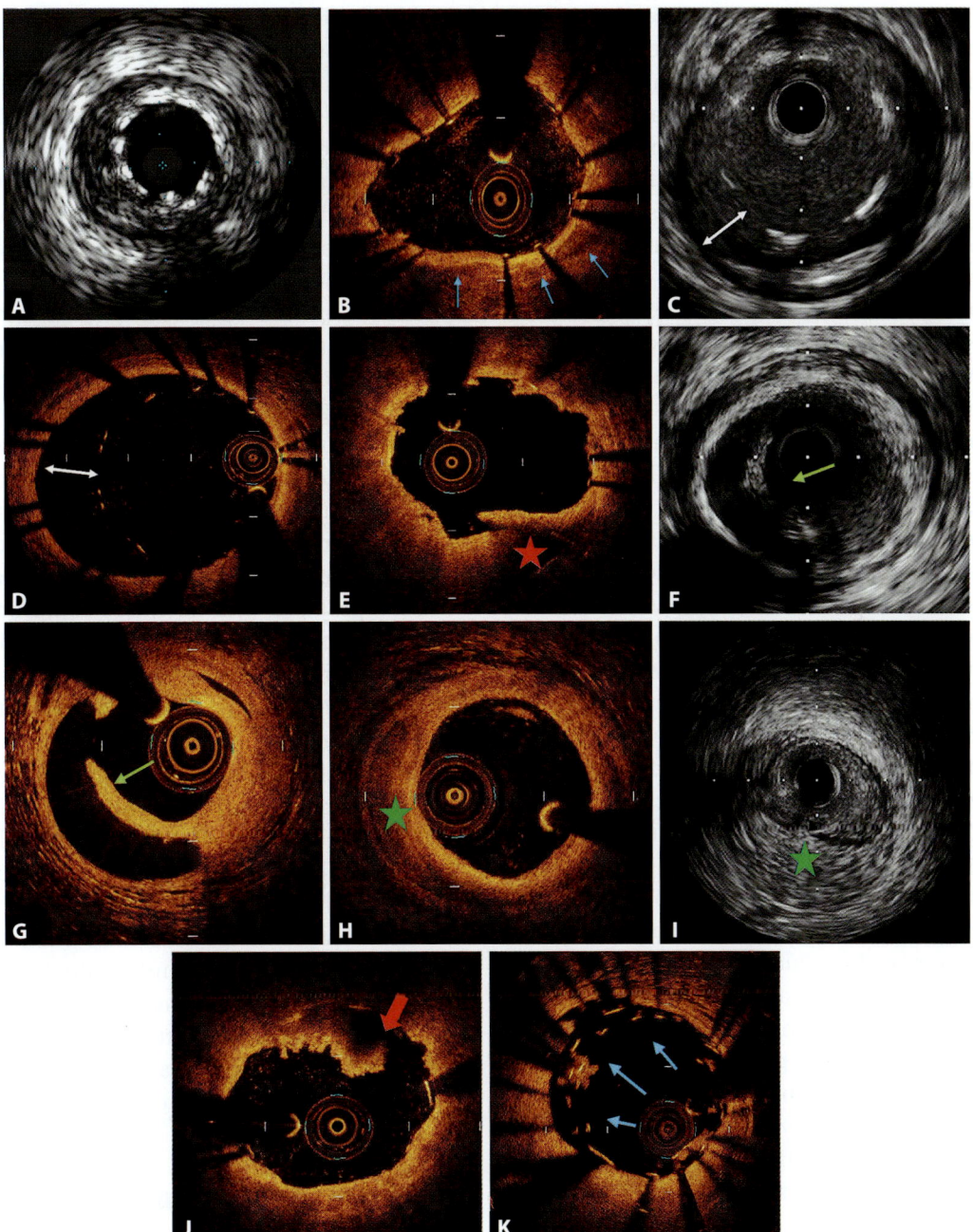

Figs. 6A to K: Postpercutaneous coronary intervention complications. (A and B) Underexpansion. (A) Underexpansion related to under deployed stent; (B) Underexpansion related to underlying calcium (blue arrows); (C and D) Malapposition (double headed white arrows); (E) Geographic miss—stent landed in the lipid plaque (red star); (F and G) Major edge dissections. Green arrows indicate dissection flap; (H and I) Intramural hematoma (green stars); (J) Irregular tissue protrusion (red arrow); and (K) Unintended stent deformation induced by guide catheter (blue arrows showing two stent layers).

<80% of the combined reference. If significant underexpansion is identified, additional high-pressure postdilatation with an appropriately sized noncompliant balloon is advised.[9]
- *Malapposition:* Malapposition refers to the lack of contact between the stent strut and the vessel wall not overlying a side branch. It occurs either acutely during the procedure or identified during the follow-up IVI. Acute malapposition is related to undersizing, underexpansion, or underlying calcified plaque. Acute malapposition in a well-expanded stent has not been shown to be associated with adverse outcomes. Most of the malappositions resolve by neointimal growth.[13] Malapposition during follow-up occurs due to persistence of acute malapposition, resolution of thrombus behind the stent struts or acquired from toxicity related to drug or polymer.[13,14] Vessel wall toxicity related malapposition has been shown to be associated with increased incidence of very late stent thrombosis.[15] The current consensus recommends correction of malappositions >400 µ and longitudinal extension >1 mm.[9]
- *Geographic miss:* Coronary atherosclerosis is frequently diffuse and often not evident angiographically. Landing zone disease is a major predictor of edge-related SF. In the presence of residual disease within 5 mm of stent edges with a plaque burden of >50% on IVUS or lumen areas <4.5 mm^2 on OCT additional stenting should be considered if anatomically feasible.[16]
- *Edge dissection/hematoma:* IVI identifies more edge dissections than coronary angiogram, while OCT detects more than IVUS due to higher resolution. Most dissections seen by IVI are minor and clinically insignificant. Cross-sectional imaging from IVI reveals the circumferential and axial extent of dissections. Treatment is generally needed when circumferential spread exceeds 60°, axial extension reaches the media, or length is over 2 mm.[9] Distal edge dissections pose greater risks than proximal ones. Edge hematomas pose more risk when left untreated and about one-third are angiographically silent. When a lumen compromising hematoma is detected by IVI, additional stenting with adequate length extending well beyond the distal extent of the hematoma needs to be done.[17]
- *Tissue/thrombus prolapse:* Protrusion of intrastent thrombus or plaque occurs often during PCI for ACS. OCT detects more plaque prolapse than IVUS. The exact clinical consequences of IVI-detected tissue prolapse are not well studied. An OCT study showed that irregular tissue prolapse was associated with adverse outcomes compared to smooth or disrupted fibrous tissue prolapse.[18] A large tissue prolapse with flow area compromise may require prolonged low-pressure balloon dilatation or additional stenting.
- *Unintended stent deformation:* Stent deformation during PCI is not uncommon and is associated with a very high incidence of SF. It is recognized with IVI by the presence more than one layer of the stent struts where only one stent is implanted or malapposed struts with loss of stent tubularity without obvious cause. It occurs more often during LMCA/bifurcation PCI and results from the interaction of guide/balloon/imaging catheter with the stent, and unintentional abluminal wiring. Identification and correction of deformation during procedure reduces adverse events.[19]

INTRAVASCULAR IMAGING IN SPECIAL SUBSETS

Vulnerable Plaque Assessment

Vulnerable plaque is a plaque, which is prone to produce clinical events either from rapid progression or from thrombosis. It is characterized by large lipid content/necrotic core, thin fibrous cap, expansive remodeling, inflammation, spotty calcification, intraplaque hemorrhage, and neoangiogenesis.[20] The current IVI modalities differ in their ability to detect the features of plaque vulnerability to a varying extent. In the PROSPECT (Providing Regional Observations to Study Predictors of Events in the Coronary Tree) study, the presence of grayscale IVUS plaque burden ≥70%, a luminal area ≤4 mm^2, and virtual histology thin cap fibroatheroma in nonculprit lesions were associated with a 3-year MACE rate of 18.2% compared to 1.9% in lesions without these features (HR: 11.05, CI: 4.39–27.82, p <0.001).[21] The NIRS IUVS identifies the presence of lipid in the plaque with high accuracy compared to other IVI modalities. In the LRP study, a NIRS IVUS maximum 4 mm Lipid Core Burden Index (maxLCBI 4 mm) of >400 predicted higher risk of MACE in nonculprit lesions in patients undergoing PCI at 2 years follow-up (HR: 3.39, CI: 1.85–6.20, p < 0.0001).[22] OCT by virtue of its high resolution enables accurate assessment of fibrous cap thickness (FCT), and detection of macrophages, cholesterol crystals, and spotty calcification. In the CLIMA (Coronary pLaque morphology of the left Anterior descending artery and twelve Months clinicAl outcome) study, an MLA <3.5 mm^2, FCT <75 µm, lipid arc >180°, and presence of macrophages in proximal LAD lesions significantly increased the risk of MACE at 12 months (HR: 7.54, 95% CI: 3.1–18.6).[23] The PREVENT (Preventive percutaneous coronary intervention versus optimal medical therapy alone for the treatment of vulnerable atherosclerotic coronary plaques) trial showed PCI of IVI-detected nonflow limiting vulnerable lesions (IVUS/OCT MLA ≤4.0 mm^2, IVUS plaque burden >70%, NIRS maxLCBI 4 mm >315 and OCT/VH TCFA) reduced clinical events compared to optimal medical therapy alone at 2 years (0.4% vs. 3.4%, p = 0.0003).[24] However, the natural history of vulnerable plaque is too complex, with most of the TCFA stabilize and few thick cap fibroatheromas transform into TCFA. Thus, the treatment of vulnerability remains at the patient level rather than at the plaque level.[25]

Acute Coronary Syndrome

Intravascular imaging plays a pivotal role in the management of patients with ACS. OCT with its high resolution is better suited for this purpose than IVUS. The various roles include (1) Identification of the culprit lesion by when there is more than one significant stenosis (presence of thrombus); (2) categorization of the underlying pathology that enables appropriate treatment strategy; (3) estimation of thrombus burden and the need for thrombus aspiration; (4) prediction of the risk of no-reflow; (5) accurate estimation vessel dimensions and extent of disease for stent sizing; and (6) stent optimization.[3,26]

Coronary thrombosis in ACS commonly results from three basic mechanisms. *PR* results from the disruption of thin fibrous cap overlying a large necrotic core in a TCFA. The exposure of highly thrombogenic necrotic material to the circulating blood promotes thrombosis. It accounts for 65% of all cases of ACS.[27] *PE* constitutes about 25–30% of cases of ACS and results from damage to the endothelial layer of the plaque. In contrast to PR, in PE, the fibrous cap is intact and is associated with lesser plaque burden and a larger residual lumen area. Hence, many of these patients may be treated conservatively without stenting.[27,28] *CN* accounts for about 2–8% of the ACS cases. Here, thrombosis is caused by disruption of the fibrous cap by protruding fragmented nodular calcification. Compared to PR and PE, CN has been associated with a very high rate of repeat revascularization.[29] In addition, OCT also enables the diagnosis of nonatherosclerotic causes of ACS like spontaneous coronary artery dissection and coronary spasm.[26]

Chronic Total Occlusion

Intravascular ultrasound imaging plays a pivotal role in improving procedure success during CTO revascularization.[30-33] Recent introduction of a CTO-specific IVUS catheter (AnteOwl, Terumo, Japan) further advanced the utility of IVUS for this purpose.[34,35] During antegrade CTO PCI, IVUS helps in wire crossing when the angiographic information is inadequate. In case of proximal cap ambiguity, side branch IVUS helps in identifying the exact location of the proximal cap and in addition, provides information about the plaque morphology. Once the cap is entered, it confirms wire position in the center of the plaque which facilitates intraplaque advancement. If the wire inadvertently enters the subintimal space, real-time subintimal IVUS-guided 3D wiring using tip detection technique helps in distal true lumen entry either by intimal plaque tracking or antegrade dissection re-entry.[34,35] During retrograde CTO PCI, IVUS helps in resolving wire position in two situations. When the CTO is in the ostioproximal right coronary artery or proximal left main branches, IVUS confirms intraplaque location of the retrograde guidewire and thus prevents inadvertent aortic dissection and branch occlusion, respectively.[33] In case of difficult reverse controlled antegrade-retrograde tracking, IVUS identifies relative position of the antegrade and retrograde guidewires and facilitates wire crossing into the true lumen.[30-32] After successful wire crossing, IVI helps in stent sizing by identifying the appropriate landing zones and differentiating between diffuse disease and negative remodeling.[36]

LEFT MAIN CORONARY ARTERY DISEASE

Assessment of unprotected LMCA (ULMCA) by angiography is largely inaccurate with an interobserver variability as high as 50%.[37] Importantly, angiography-guided LMCA interventions were associated with high rates of MACE and stent thrombosis.[38] Hence, IVI is essential to guide revascularization in LMCA disease. IVUS with its large field of view, higher tissue penetration and ability to visualize the ostium, is the modality of choice for guiding LMCA revascularization. The various roles of IVUS during PCI are: (1) Resolving angiographic ambiguity such as haziness (thrombus, CN, or ruptured plaque), (2) Assessing angiographically intermediate lesions: revascularization can be deferred if the IVUS MLA is >6 mm^2,[39] (3) *Stenting strategy:* A side branch MLA of <3.7 mm^2 and a plaque burden of >56% predicts side branch compromise following crossover stenting and favors an upfront two-stent strategy,[40] (4) *Lesion preparation:* Presence and severity of calcification helps in selecting appropriate debulking strategy, (5) stent sizing and identification of appropriate landing zones, (6) confirming adequacy of crushing, appropriate side branch cell crossing and identification of abluminal wire position, (7) stent optimization: stent expansion in various segment of the bifurcation (MLA in each segment >90% of the reference or absolute areas of 5 mm^2, 6 mm^2, 7 mm^2, and 8 mm^2 at LCX ostium, LAD ostium, polygon of confluence, and distal LMCA, respectively), malapposition, residual disease/dissection at the stent edges, and unintended stent deformation.[41,42]

Bifurcation Lesions

Coronary bifurcation lesions constitute 15–20% of all PCIs and are characterized by lower procedural success rate and a higher rate of SF compared to nonbifurcation PCIs.[43] IVI, specifically OCT with its higher resolution and 3D capabilities, provides valuable insights during various stages of the procedure, that improve procedure outcomes. Preprocedure IVI provides information on the side branch lumen area, plaque distribution/composition, and disease extent. It helps in identifying the exact cause of side branch compromise by differentiating true ostial side branch disease from the main vessel disease mimicking SB disease.[44] A side branch lumen area of <2.4 mm^2 and a plaque burden of >50%, predicts postprocedure positive FFR and the need for two-stent strategy.[45] Presence of eyebrow sign or spiky carina, carina tip angle of <50° and branch point to bifurcation tip angle of <1.7 mm, and plaque distribution opposite to the SB increase the risk of carina shift and side branch compromise.[46] Post main vessel stenting, 3D OCT reveals the strut morphology across the side branch ostium and confirms appropriate cell crossing. It also identifies incomplete crushing of the side branch stent struts and inadvertent abluminal wire crossing.[47] Final imaging identifies stent underexpansion, particularly at the side branch ostium, incomplete opposition, residual disease at the stent edges, and unintended stent deformation. In the recent OCTOBER trial, systematic usage of OCT during bifurcation PCI resulted in significant reduction of 2 years MACE.[42]

Calcified Lesions

Severe coronary artery calcification (CAC) is a strong predictor of failure of device delivery, stent underexpansion, procedural complications, and poor long-term outcomes.[48] IVI is more sensitive than CAG to detect coronary calcification and in addition, it identifies morphological characteristics that predict stent underexpansion. Both IVUS and OCT clearly delineate the location, circumferential, and longitudinal extent of calcification. With the ability of light to penetrate calcium, OCT provides additional information regarding plaque calcium thickness.[49] IVUS and OCT-based calcium scoring systems developed from retrospective studies help in identifying lesions at risk of underexpansion and thus the need for calcium modification.[50-52] The IVUS imaging characteristics include 360° arc of superficial calcification, calcium angle of >270° for a length of >5 mm, vessel diameter <3.5 mm, and presence of CN.[50] The OCT imaging features include 360° arc of superficial calcification, calcium angle of >270° for a length of >3 mm, and calcium thickness of >0.5 mm.[52] Presence of two or more features increases the risk of underexpansion and consideration for aggressive calcium modification.[50,52] In addition, it aids in the selection of an appropriate calcium modification strategy based on these morphological features. Further, IVI also helps in the assessment of response to lesion modification in the form of calcium fractures and dissections. Finally, it helps in stent optimization by identifying gross underexpansion.[49]

Stent Failure

Intravascular imaging plays a major role in the evaluation of underlying cause of SF and in addition, helps in planning appropriate management strategy. OCT, with its better tissue characterization capabilities, is well suited for this purpose. SF can result from mechanical, biological, or combined causes. The common mechanical causes include underexpansion, malapposition, stent edge issues (geographic miss, dissection, or hematoma), tissue prolapse, and stent structural problems such as fracture, gap, or longitudinal deformation. Biological factors comprise neointimal hyperplasia (NIH), neoatherosclerosis, and uncovered stent struts. Predominant underexpansion with minimal NIH can be addressed using high-pressure balloon dilatation alone. Edge stenosis, stent fracture, longitudinal deformation, and stent gap are treated with additional stenting. NIH is classified into heterogenous, layered, and homogenous patterns. Homogenous and layered pattern ISRs are treated with either DES or DCB after appropriate lesion preparation assessed by OCT.

Heterogenous NIH is considered to result from abnormal response to the polymer or drug and hence treated with plain balloon dilatation alone, if the lumen gain is adequate. Neoatherosclerosis is either lipid-rich or calcified. Calcified neoatherosclerosis requires preparation with appropriate calcium modification tools. In case of stent thrombosis with predominant uncovered stent struts, indefinite dual antiplatelet therapy should be considered.[26,53]

CURRENT EVIDENCE BASE AND GUIDELINE RECOMMENDATIONS

Multiple randomized studies and meta-analysis **(Tables 2 and 3)** are now available which have demonstrated the incremental value of IVI-guided PCI in terms of angiographic results and long-term outcomes.[42,54-60] Based on the recent studies showing incremental benefits with imaging-guided PCI compared to conventional angiographic guidance, the current guidelines on acute and chronic coronary syndromes have recommended a class I indication for intracoronary imaging in complex angioplasty subsets such as left main, true bifurcation, long diffuse disease, and SF.[61,62]

IMPROVING IVI ADOPTION AND UTILIZATION IN INDIA

Intravascular imaging has emerged as a transformative tool in cardiovascular care, yet its adoption remains uneven. To unlock its full potential, a concerted effort is needed across individual, institutional, industry, and insurance domains.

At the individual level, addressing knowledge gaps with structured training, including online modules, onsite proctoring, and remote troubleshooting to support clinicians during initial learning will help to improve adoption of the technology. Standardizing best practices and offering clear learning pathways will improve confidence and consistent IVI use.

Hospitals can explore methods to safely and effectively reuse imaging accessories, potentially reducing technology costs for patients. Institutions may also consider implementing policies that integrate IVI into complex PCI procedures without significantly increasing overall procedural costs, as such integration has been associated with improved safety and long-term outcomes, which may influence the number of patients undergoing complex procedures **(Table 3)**.

TABLE 3: Landmark clinical trials and meta-analyses comparing intravascular imaging and coronary angiography-guided PCI.

Study	Modality	Population	Follow-up	Outcomes
IVUS-XPL[54]	IVUS	IVUS-guided PCI (n = 700) vs. angiography-guided PCI (n = 700)	5 years	• *MACE:* HR: 0.50 (0.34–0.75) • *Cardiac death:* HR: 0.43 (0.17–1.12) • *TL-MI:* HR: 0.67 (0.19–2.36) • *ID-TLR:* HR: 0.54 (0.33–0.89) • *ST:* HR: 1.00 (0.14–7.10)
ULTIMATE[55]	IVUS	IVUS (n = 724) vs. CAG (n = 724)	3 years	• *TVF:* HR: 0.60 (0.42–0.87) • *Cardiac death:* HR: 0.68 (0.34–1.37) • *TV-MI:* HR: 0.46 (0.19–1.14) • *CD-TLR:* HR: 0.64 (0.41–1.00)
RENOVATE-COMPLEX PCI[56]	IVUS (73.3%) OCT (25.5%)	Complex coronary artery lesions, IVI (1092, IVUS—800 and OCT—278) vs. CAG (547)	25 months	• *TVF:* HR: 0.64 (0.45–0.89) • *Cardiac death:* HR: 0.47 (0.24–0.93) • *TV-MI:* HR: 0.74 (0.45–1.22) • *TLR:* HR: 0.69 (0.40–1.18)

Contd...

Contd...

Study	Modality	Population	Follow-up	Outcomes
ILUMIEN IV[57]	OCT	Diabetes mellitus, complex coronary artery lesions, OCT (n = 1,233) vs. CAG (n = 1,254)	2 years	• *TVF:* HR: 0.90 (0.67–1.19) • *Cardiac death:* HR: 0.57 (0.25–1.29) • *TV-MI:* HR: 0.77 (0.48–1.22) • *ID-TVR:* HR: 0.99 (0.71–1.40)
OCTOBER[42]	OCT	Complex true bifurcation lesions OCT (n = 600) or CAG (n = 601)	2 years	• *MACE:* HR: 0.70 (0.50–0.98) • *Cardiac death:* HR: 0.53 (0.22–1.25) • *TL-MI:* HR: 0.90 (0.60–1.34) • *ID-TLR:* HR: 0.61 (0.32–1.13)
OCCUPI[58]	OCT	Complex coronary artery lesions OCT (n = 803) or CAG (n = 801)	1 year	• *MACE:* HR: 0.62 (0.41–0.93) • *Cardiac death:* HR: 0.20 (0.03–1.71) • *TV-MI:* HR: 0.72 (0.45–1.16) • *ID-TLR:* HR: 0.36 (0.18–0.69)
Stone et al.[59]	IVI	22 studies, 15,694 patients	–	• *Mortality:* OR: 0.75 (0.6–0.93) • *CV mortality:* OR: 0.55 (0.41–0.75) • *MI:* OR: 0.83 (0.71–0.99) • *ST:* OR: 0.52 (0.34–0.81) • *TVR:* OR: 0.64 (0.38–1.07) • *TLR:* OR: 0.72 (0.60–0.86)
Sreenivasan et al.[60]	IVI	16 studies, 7,814 patients	–	• *MACE:* OR: 0.67 (0.55–0.82) • *Mortality:* OR: 0.75 (0.55–1.02) • *CV mortality:* OR: 0.49 (0.34–0.71) • *ST:* OR: 0.63 (0.40–0.99) • *TVR:* OR: 0.60 (0.45–0.80) • *TLR:* OR: 0.67 (0.49–0.91)

(CD-TLR: clinically driven TLR; CV: cardiovascular; ID-TLR: ischemia-driven TLR; ILUMIEN IV: Optical Coherence Tomography (OCT)-guided coronary stent implantation compared with angiography; IVI: intravascular imaging; IVUS: intravascular ultrasound; IVUS-XPL: impact of intravascular ultrasound guidance on outcomes of xience prime stents in long lesions; MACE: major adverse cardiovascular events; MI: myocardial infarction; OCCUPI: Optical Coherence Tomography-guided Versus Angiography-guided Percutaneous Coronary Intervention for Patients With Complex Lesion; OCT: optical coherence tomography; OCTOBER: European Trial on Optical Coherence Tomography Optimized Bifurcation Event Reduction; RENOVATE-COMPLEX-PCI: randomized controlled trial of intravascular imaging guidance versus angiography-guidance on clinical outcomes after complex percutaneous coronary intervention; ST: stent thrombosis; TL-MI: target lesion–related MI; TLR: target lesion revascularization; TVR: target vessel revascularization; ULTIMATE: intravascular ultrasound-guided Drug-eluting stents implantation In "All-Comers" Coronary Lesions)

Insurance providers should acknowledge the long-term benefits of IVI in enhancing patient outcomes and minimizing repeat procedures. Promoting coverage approval, along with informing patients about the advantages of imaging-guided interventions, may contribute to increased demand and broader acceptance.

Finally, government policies promoting indigenous IVI solutions, lowering hardware costs, and procuring imaging systems to government hospitals help to expand access to this technology for the public. Making IVI as part of the cardiology training may enhance the early adoption of the technology.

CONCLUSION

Intravascular imaging is an invaluable addition in every catheterization laboratory which enables enhanced decision-making and improve long-term outcomes of PCI. Hybrid systems incorporating multiple modalities of imaging in a single catheter have now become a reality, leveraging the strengths of each technology. The seamless integration of IVI and coregistration with angiogram during PCI will further improve safety, efficacy, and long-term benefits of PCI. Artificial intelligence enabled plaque characterization, vessel size measurements, and landing zone selection will further simplify PCI workflow and enhance wider adoption of IVI.

REFERENCES

1. DeRouen TA, Murray JA, Owen W. Variability in the analysis of coronary arteriograms. Circulation. 1977;55:324-8.
2. Mintz GS, Nissen SE, Anderson WD, et al. American college of cardiology clinical expert consensus document on standards for acquisition, measurement and reporting of intravascular ultrasound studies (IVUS). A report of the American College of Cardiology Task Force on clinical expert consensus documents. J Am Coll Cardiol. 2001;37:1478-92.
3. Subban V, Raffel OC, Vasu N, et al. Intravascular ultrasound and optical coherence tomography for the assessment of coronary artery disease and percutaneous coronary intervention optimization: The basics. Indian Heart J Interv. 2018;1:71-94.
4. Saito Y, Kobayashi Y, Fujii K, et al. CVIT 2025 clinical expert consensus document on intravascular ultrasound. Cardiovasc Interv Ther. 2025;40:211-25.
5. Pu J, Mintz GS, Biro S, et al. Insights into echo-attenuated plaques, echolucent plaques, and plaques with spotty calcification: Novel findings from comparisons among intravascular ultrasound, near-infrared spectroscopy, and pathological histology in 2,294 human coronary artery segments. J Am Coll Cardiol. 2014;63:2220-33.
6. Ong DS, Jang IK. Fundamentals of Optical Coherence Tomography: Image Acquisition and Interpretation. Interv Cardiol Clin. 2015;4:225-37.
7. Koo BK, Hu X, Kang J, et al. Fractional flow reserve or intravascular ultrasonography to guide PCI. N Engl J Med. 2022;387:779-89.
8. Burzotta F, Leone AM, Aurigemma C, et al. Fractional flow reserve or optical coherence tomography to guide management of angiographically intermediate coronary stenosis. JACC Cardiovasc Interv. 2020;13:49-58.
9. Raber L, Mintz GS, Koskinas KC, et al. Clinical use of intracoronary imaging. Part 1: Guidance and optimization of coronary interventions. An expert consensus document of the European Association of Percutaneous Cardiovascular Interventions. Eur Heart J. 2018;39:3281-300.
10. Castagna MT, Mintz GS, Leiboff BO, et al. The contribution of "mechanical" problems to in-stent restenosis: An intravascular ultrasonographic analysis of 1090 consecutive in-stent restenosis lesions. Am Heart J. 2001;142:970-4.
11. Cheneau E, Leborgne L, Mintz GS, et al. Predictors of subacute stent thrombosis: Results of a systematic intravascular ultrasound study. Circulation. 2003;108:43-7.
12. Matsuo Y, Kubo T, Aoki H, et al. Optimal threshold of postintervention minimum stent area to predict in-stent restenosis in small coronary arteries: An optical coherence tomography analysis. Catheter Cardiovasc Interv. 2016;87:E9-E14.
13. Attizzani GF, Capodanno D, Ohno Y, et al. Mechanisms, pathophysiology, and clinical aspects of incomplete stent apposition. J Am Coll Cardiol. 2014;63:1355-67.
14. Karalis I, Ahmed TA, Jukema JW. Late acquired stent malapposition: why, when and how to handle? Heart. 2012;98:1529-36.
15. Lee SY, Ahn JM, Mintz GS, et al. Ten-Year Clinical Outcomes of Late-Acquired Stent Malapposition After Coronary Stent Implantation. Arterioscler Thromb Vasc Biol. 2020;40:288-95.
16. Ali Z, Landmesser U, Karimi Galougahi K, et al. Optical coherence tomography-guided coronary stent implantation compared to angiography: a multicentre randomised trial in PCI - design

17. Maehara A, Mintz GS, Bui AB, et al. Incidence, morphology, angiographic findings, and outcomes of intramural hematomas after percutaneous coronary interventions: An intravascular ultrasound study. Circulation. 2002;105:2037-42.
18. Soeda T, Uemura S, Park SJ, et al. Incidence and Clinical Significance of Poststent Optical Coherence Tomography Findings: One-Year Follow-Up Study From a Multicenter Registry. Circulation. 2015;132:1020-9.
19. Andreasen LN, Neghabat O, Laanmets P, et al. Unintended Deformation of Stents During Bifurcation PCI: An OCTOBER Trial Substudy. JACC Cardiovasc Interv. 2024;17:1106-15.
20. Sinclair H, Bourantas C, Bagnall A, et al. OCT for the identification of vulnerable plaque in acute coronary syndrome. JACC Cardiovasc Imaging. 2015;8:198-209.
21. Stone GW, Maehara A, Lansky AJ, et al. A prospective natural-history study of coronary atherosclerosis. N Engl J Med. 2011;364:226-35.
22. Waksman R, Mario C, Torguson R, et al. Identification of patients and plaques vulnerable to future coronary events with near-infrared spectroscopy intravascular ultrasound imaging: a prospective, cohort study. Lancet. 2019; 394: 1629-37.
23. Prati F, Romagnoli E, Gatto L, et al. Relationship between coronary plaque morphology of the left anterior descending artery and 12 months clinical outcome: the CLIMA study. Eur Heart J. 2020; 41:383-91.
24. Park SJ, Ahn JM, Kang DY, et al. Preventive percutaneous coronary intervention versus optimal medical therapy alone for the treatment of vulnerable atherosclerotic coronary plaques (PREVENT): a multicentre, open-label, randomised controlled trial. Lancet. 2024;403:1765.
25. Narula J, Kovacic JC. Putting TCFA in clinical perspective. J Am Coll Cardiol. 2014;64:681-3.
26. Subban V, Raffel OC, Vasu N, et al. Intravascular ultrasound and optical coherence tomography for the assessment of coronary artery disease and percutaneous coronary intervention optimization: Specific lesion subsets. Indian Heart J Interv. 2018;1:95-123.
27. Yahagi K, Kolodgie FD, Otsuka F, et al. Pathophysiology of native coronary, vein graft, and in-stent atherosclerosis. Nat Rev Cardiol. 2016;13:79-98.
28. Hu S, Zhu Y, Zhang Y, et al. Management and outcome of patients with acute coronary syndrome caused by plaque rupture versus plaque erosion: An intravascular optical coherence tomography study. J Am Heart Assoc. 2017;6:e004730.
29. Lee T, Mintz GS, Matsumura M, et al. Prevalence, predictors, and clinical presentation of a calcified nodule as assessed by optical coherence tomography. JACC Cardiovasc Imaging. 2017; 10:883-91.
30. Kimura M, Asakura Y. IVUS-guided CTO-PCI. In: Waksman R, Saito S (Eds). Chronic total occlusions: A guide to recanalization, 2nd edition. New Jersey: Wiley; 2013. pp. 67-77.
31. Tsuchikane E. IVUS-guided recanalization of CTO. In: Waksman R, Saito S (Eds). Chronic total occlusion: A guide to recanalization, 2nd edition. New Jersey: Wiley; 2013. pp. 105-8.
32. Sumitsuji S. Intravascular ultrasound applications for chronic total occlusion percutaneous intervention. In: Thompson CA, (Ed). Textbook of Cardiovascular Intervention, 1st edition. London: Springer-Verlag; 2014. pp. 311-16.
33. Huang WC, Teng HI, Hsueh CH, et al. Intravascular ultrasound guided wiring re-entry technique for complex chronic total occlusions. J Interv Cardiol. 2018;31:572-9.
34. Okamura A, Iwakura K, Iwamoto M, et al. Tip Detection Method Using the New IVUS Facilitates the 3-Dimensional Wiring Technique for CTO Intervention. JACC Cardiovasc Interv. 2020;13:74-82.
35. Tanaka K, Okamura A, Yoshikawa R, et al. Tip Detection-Antegrade Dissection and Re-Entry With New Puncture Wire in CTO Intervention: Revolution Through 3D-Wiring. JACC Asia. 2024;4:359-72.
36. Neishi Y, Okura H, Kume T, et al. Prediction of chronic vessel enlargement by a novel intra-vascular ultrasound finding. Circ J. 2015;79:607-12.
37. Lindstaedt M, Spiecker M, Perings C, et al. How good are experienced interventional cardiologists

at predicting the functional significance of intermediate or equivocal left main coronary artery stenoses? Int J Cardiol. 2007;120:254-61.
38. Morice MC, Serruys PW, Kappetein AP, et al. Five-year outcomes in patients with left main disease treated with either percutaneous coronary intervention or coronary artery bypass grafting in the Synergy Between Percutaneous Coronary Intervention with Taxus and Cardiac Surgery trial. Circulation. 2014;129:2388-94.
39. de la Torre Hernandez JM, Hernandez Hernandez F, Alfonso F, et al. Prospective application of pre-defined intravascular ultrasound criteria for assessment of intermediate left main coronary artery lesions results from the multicenter LITRO study. J Am Coll Cardiol. 2011;58:351-8.
40. Kang SJ, Ahn JM, Kim WJ, et al. Functional and morphological assessment of side branch after left main coronary artery bifurcation stenting with cross-over technique. Catheter Cardiovasc Interv. 2014;83:545-52.
41. Kang SJ, Ahn JM, Song H, et al. Comprehensive intravascular ultrasound assessment of stent area and its impact on restenosis and adverse cardiac events in 403 patients with unprotected left main disease. Circ Cardiovasc Interv. 2011;4:562-9.
42. Holm NR, Andreasen LN, Neghabat O, et al. OCT or Angiography Guidance for PCI in Complex Bifurcation Lesions. N Engl J Med. 2023; 389:1477-87.
43. Iakovou I, Ge L, Colombo A. Contemporary stent treatment of coronary bifurcations. J Am Coll Cardio. 2005;46:1446-55.
44. Furukawa E, Hibi K, Kosugi M, et al. Intravascular ultrasound predictors of side branch occlusion in bifurcation lesions after percutaneous coronary intervention. Circ J. 2005;69:325-30.
45. Kang SJ, Mintz GS, Kim WJ, et al. Preintervention angiographic and intravascular ultrasound predictors for side branch compromise after a single-stent crossover technique. Am J Cardiol. 2011;107:1787-93.
46. Watanabe M, Uemura S, Sugawara Y, et al. Side branch complication after a single-stent crossover technique: Prediction with frequency domain optical coherence tomography. Coron Artery Dis. 2014;25:321-9.
47. Okamura T, Nagoshi R, Fujimura T, et al. Impact of guidewire recrossing point into stent jailed side branch for optimal kissing balloon dilatation: Corelab 3D optical coherence tomography analysis. Eurointervention. 2018;13:e1785-93.
48. Madhavan MV, Tarigopula M, Mintz GS, et al. Coronary artery calcification: Pathogenesis and prognostic implications. J Am Coll Cardiol. 2014;63:1703-14.
49. Mehanna E, Abbott JD, Bezerra HG. Optimizing percutaneous coronary intervention in calcified lesions: Insights from optical coherence tomography of atherectomy. Circ Cardiovasc Interv. 2018;11:e006813.
50. Zhang M, Matsumura M, Usui E, et al. Intravascular Ultrasound-Derived Calcium Score to Predict Stent Expansion in Severely Calcified Lesions. Circ Cardiovasc Interv. 2021;14:e010296.
51. Fujino A, Mintz GS, Matsumura M, et al. A new optical coherence tomography-based calcium scoring system to predict stent underexpansion. EuroIntervention. 2018;13:e2182-e2189.
52. Sato T, Matsumura M, Yamamoto K, et al. A Revised Optical Coherence Tomography-Derived Calcium Score to Predict Stent Underexpansion in Severely Calcified Lesions. JACC Cardiovasc Interv. 2025;18:622-33.
53. Subban V, Raffel OC. Optical coherence tomography: fundamentals and clinical utility. Cardiovasc Diagn Ther. 2020;10:1389-414.
54. Hong SJ, Mintz GS, Ahn CM, et al. Effect of intravascular ultra-sound-guided drug-eluting stent implantation: 5-year follow-up of the IVUS-XPL randomized trial. JACC Cardiovasc Interv. 2020;13:62-71.
55. Gao XF, Ge Z, Kong XQ, et al. 3-year outcomes of the ULTIMATE trial comparing intravascular ultrasound versus angiography-guided drug-eluting stent implantation. JACC Cardiovasc Interv. 2021;14:247-57.
56. Lee JM, Choi KH, Song YB, et al. Intravascular imaging-guided or angiography-guided complex PCI. N Engl J Med. 2023;388:1668-79.
57. Ali ZA, Landmesser U, Maehara A, et al. Optical coherence tomography-guided versus angiography-guided PCI. N Engl J Med. 2023; 389:1466-76.

58. Hong SJ, Lee SJ, Lee SH, et al. Optical coherence tomography-guided versus angiography-guided percutaneous coronary intervention for patients with complex lesions (OCCUPI): an investigator-initiated, multicentre, randomised, open-label, superiority trial in South Korea. Lancet. 2024; 404:1029-39.
59. Stone GW, Christiansen EH, Ali ZA, et al. Intravascular imaging-guided coronary drug-eluting stent implantation: an updated network meta-analysis. Lancet. 2024;403(10429):824-37.
60. Sreenivasan J, Reddy RK, Jamil Y, et al. Intravascular Imaging-Guided Versus Angiography-Guided Percutaneous Coronary Intervention: A Systematic Review and Meta-Analysis of Randomized Trials. J Am Heart Assoc. 2024;13: e031111.
61. Vrints C, Andreotti F, Koskinas KC, et al. 2024 ESC guidelines for the management of chronic coronary syndromes. Eur Heart J. 2024;45:3415-537.
62. Rao SV, O'Donoghue ML, Ruel M, et al. 2025 ACC/AHA/ACEP/NAEMSP/SCAI guideline for the Management of Patients with Acute Coronary Syndromes: A report of the American College of Cardiology/American Heart Association joint committee on clinical practice guidelines. Circulation. 2025;151:e771-862.

CHAPTER 17

Cardiogenic Shock: Diagnosis and Early Management—Status 2025

Siddarth Varshney, Deepti Yadav, Sonali Bansal, Praveen Chandra

INTRODUCTION

Cardiogenic shock (CS) is a complex, heterogeneous, and multifactorial clinical syndrome characterized by inadequate tissue perfusion resulting from primary cardiac dysfunction. This inadequate cardiac output leads to systemic hypoperfusion and progressive end-organ failure. CS remains a leading cause of admissions to contemporary cardiac intensive care units (CICUs) and is associated with persistently high morbidity and mortality despite advances in care. The short-term mortality rate for CS ranges between 30% and 40%, while 1-year mortality may approach or even exceed 50%.[1]

Historically, the majority of clinical trials and therapeutic strategies have focused on CS secondary to acute myocardial infarction (AMI-CS), which is the most extensively studied subtype of cardiogenic shock. However, over the past decade, the incidence of non-AMI causes of CS—particularly heart failure-related cardiogenic shock (HF-CS)—has been steadily increasing, especially in developing countries such as India. These patients often present with distinct baseline characteristics, comorbidities, patterns of resource utilization, and clinical outcomes when compared to AMI-CS cohorts.

Despite substantial improvements in revascularization strategies and the widespread adoption of temporary mechanical circulatory support (tMCS) devices over the last two decades, randomized controlled trials (RCTs) have generally failed to demonstrate significant reductions in mortality, except in the context of early revascularization for AMI-CS.[2] A notable exception is the Danish–German Cardiogenic Shock (DanGer Shock) trial, which was the first to report a mortality benefit from mechanical circulatory support (MCS). In this trial, the early use of a percutaneous microaxial flow pump (Impella CP) in carefully selected patients with ST-segment elevation myocardial infarction (STEMI)-related shock significantly improved 180-day survival compared to standard therapy.

Modern management emphasizes not just revascularization, but early hemodynamic stabilization and organ perfusion restoration. Two emerging metrics have become critical:

- *Door-to-support time:* The time from hospital arrival to initiation of pharmacologic or mechanical support
- *Door-to-lactate-free time:* The time it takes to normalize lactate levels, indicating reversal of systemic hypoperfusion

These time-sensitive goals reflect that shock is both a structural and metabolic emergency. Persistent hyperlactatemia (>2 mmol/L) is a marker of ongoing tissue ischemia and correlates strongly with poor outcomes. Reducing lactate levels through timely PCI, inotropes, and MCS correlates with survival, making "lactate clearance" a new bedside target.

PATHOPHYSIOLOGY OF CARDIOGENIC SHOCK (INTERVENTIONAL PERSPECTIVE)

Cardiogenic shock is a serious condition where the heart fails to pump enough blood to meet the body's requirement. As a result, vital organs such as the brain, kidneys, and liver do not receive adequate oxygen, leading to rapid deterioration if not promptly treated. For interventional cardiologists, especially in acute care settings such as the catheterization laboratory, understanding the evolving physiology behind CS is essential for choosing the right mechanical and pharmacological strategies.

What Triggers Cardiogenic Shock?

The most common cause remains AMI, especially large anterior myocardial infarctions (MIs). However, CS can also be triggered by:
- Mechanical complications (e.g., VSD and papillary muscle rupture)
- Severe valvular disease
- Fulminant myocarditis
- Arrhythmias (e.g., sustained VT/VF).

In all these cases, there is a sudden drop in cardiac output, which leads to low blood pressure, reduced perfusion, and end-organ damage.

Vicious Cycle

Once the heart's pumping ability drops:
- Blood pressure falls, reducing coronary perfusion—further weakening the heart
- The lungs fill with fluid due to backward pressure from the failing LV → pulmonary congestion
- *Compensatory mechanisms start:*
  - Heart rate increases to maintain output
  - Blood vessels constrict, raising afterload
  - Kidneys retain fluid, increasing preload.

These responses initially help but soon become harmful—raising myocardial oxygen demand and worsening the cycle of ischemia → dysfunction → hypoperfusion.

Why Just Increasing Blood Pressure is not Enough?

Even if we manage to raise the blood pressure with fluids or inotropes, the tiny blood vessels (microcirculation) might still be unable to deliver oxygen effectively. In this "cryptic shock" state:
- The patient looks better hemodynamically, *but*
- Lactate remains high, *and*
- Organs continue to deteriorate.

Thus, our goal must shift from just fixing BP to restoring oxygen delivery at the cellular level. Hence, "door-to-lactate-free time" is now becoming a key quality indicator, like door-to-balloon in STEMI.[3]

EARLY IDENTIFICATION AND RISK STRATIFICATION

Early diagnosis of CS is often the difference between organ preservation and irreversible multiorgan failure. In busy emergency rooms and catheterization laboratories, especially in Indian settings where time and resources may be limited, clinicians must rely on a mix of bedside assessment, rapid biomarkers, and smart use of imaging to make timely decisions.

Clinical Diagnosis First

Cardiogenic shock remains a clinical diagnosis, built on:
- Hypotension (SBP <90 mm Hg or MAP <65 mm Hg for >30 minutes)
- *Signs of hypoperfusion:* Cold extremities, low urine output, and altered sensorium
- *Evidence of cardiac dysfunction:* Elevated JVP, pulmonary congestion, and gallop rhythm.

In India, where invasive monitors may not be immediately available, bedside clinical clues still hold major value.

Role of Point-of-Care Tools

Role of point-of-care tools is as follows:
- *ECG:* Often the first clue—identify STEMI, LBBB, or arrhythmias.
- *POCUS (point-of-care ultrasound):*
  - Assess LV function and RV size.
  - Rule out tamponade and massive PE.

- *Bedside ECHO (or catheterization laboratory ECHO):*
  - Global/regional wall motion abnormalities
  - Mechanical complications
- *Chest X-ray:* It is useful for pulmonary edema and device positioning.

Laboratory and Hemodynamic Monitoring

Laboratory and hemodynamic monitoring include:
- *Serum lactate:* Rising trend—worsening shock
- *NT-proBNP/Troponin:* Cardiac stress and injury
- *ABG:* Acidosis is a red flag.
- *Creatinine/LFTs:* Assess end-organ damage.

In advanced centers, pulmonary artery catheters or noninvasive cardiac output monitors can offer additional insights—but most decisions in CS are clinical and should not be delayed waiting for numbers.

Risk Stratification Models

Several scoring systems have emerged, but their bedside use remains limited. However, they offer perspective on prognosis:
- *Intra-aortic balloon pump (IABP)-SHOCK II risk score*
- *CardShock risk score*
- *SCAI shock staging (now commonly used):*[4] SCAI staging is now widely adopted and particularly helpful for Indian catheterization laboratories to communicate team decisions and plan stepwise escalation. It is summarized in **Table 1**.

EARLY MANAGEMENT AND REVASCULARIZATION

Once cardiogenic shock is identified, time-sensitive management becomes critical. The goal is not only to restore perfusion but to preserve organ function, stabilize the myocardium, and prevent irreversible injury. For interventional cardiologists, the first hour after diagnosis is a golden window where coordinated procedural, pharmacological, and mechanical strategies must be rapidly initiated.

Initial Stabilization

Initial stabilization requires:
- Hemodynamic goals
  - Systolic BP >90 mm Hg or MAP >65 mm Hg
  - Lactate clearance as a marker of improving perfusion
  - Urine output >0.5 mL/kg/hour
  - Normalize mental status and acid–base profile.

  These are signs that perfusion is being restored—not just pressure.
- Oxygen and ventilation
  - Supplemental oxygen to maintain SpO_2 >94%
  - Early noninvasive or invasive ventilation may be needed in pulmonary edema or respiratory failure
- Vascular access
  - Secure two large-bore IV lines or a central line.
  - Consider arterial line for continuous BP monitoring if available.

Pharmacotherapy in Cardiogenic Shock

While procedural intervention is key, medical management remains foundational, especially in the precatheterization and periprocedural phases. Various pharmacological agents are summarized in **Table 2**.

Vasopressors and Inotropes

- Norepinephrine is the first-line vasopressor to maintain MAP ≥65 mm Hg.
- Dobutamine is preferred for inotropic support in low-output states without marked hypotension.

TABLE 1: SCAI shock classification.

Stage	Label	Clinical features	Hemodynamics	Biochemical/organ perfusion markers	Typical support
A	At risk	• Patient at risk for shock (e.g., ACS, decompensated HF, myocarditis, valvular disease) • No hypotension or hypoperfusion	• SBP ≥100 mm Hg, MAP ≥65 mm Hg • CI >2.2 L/min/m² • PCWP may be elevated	• Lactate normal • Normal creatinine • Urine output preserved	No inotropes/pressors, observation, and medical therapy
B	Beginning (pre-shock)	• Relative hypotension or narrow pulse pressure • Tachycardia • Mild symptoms (dyspnea, diaphoresis, and anxiety) without overt hypoperfusion	• SBP <100 mm Hg or MAP <65 mm Hg but responsive to fluids • CI often preserved (>2.2 L/min/m²) • PCWP often elevated	• Lactate normal • Mild rise in creatinine possible	May need low-dose inotrope/pressor and close monitoring
C	Classic Shock	• Hypotension with clear hypoperfusion • Altered mentation, oliguria, and cool extremities • Pulmonary congestion possible	• SBP <90 mm Hg or MAP <65 mm Hg despite fluids • CI <2.2 L/min/m² • PCWP >15 mm Hg	• Elevated lactate >2 mmol/L • Rising creatinine, LFTs	Requires vasopressors/inotropes ± IABP, Impella, ECMO (depending on cause)
D	Deteriorating	• Worsening shock despite therapy • Escalating vasopressor/inotrope doses • Progressing multi-organ dysfunction	• Persistent MAP <65 mm Hg despite support • CI <2.0 L/min/m² • Worsening filling pressures	• Rising lactate, metabolic acidosis • Worsening renal/hepatic indices	• MCS escalation (Impella CP/5.5, TandemHeart, VA-ECMO) • Multimodal organ support
E	Extremis	• Refractory shock with circulatory collapse • Ongoing cardiac arrest/need for CPR • Agonal or pulseless state	• No meaningful perfusion • CI unmeasurable • MAP unmaintainable	• Severe metabolic acidosis • Lactate very high (>5–10 mmol/L) • Multiorgan failure	• ACLS + maximal MCS • ECMO in ECPR setting

- Epinephrine reserved for refractory cases increases myocardial oxygen demand.
- Avoid dopamine due to arrhythmic potential.

Vasodilators and Diuretics

- Use vasodilators cautiously in hypertensive CS or afterload-sensitive LV failure.
- Use loop diuretics for pulmonary congestion but avoid in preload-dependent states.

Anti-ischemic and Adjunctive Therapy

- Aspirin, statins, and dual antiplatelet therapy (DAPT) as per ACS protocols
- Early heparin unless contraindicated

TABLE 2: Latest advances in cardiogenic shock.

Domain	Key updates	Indian context
SCAI shock classification	Dynamic staging better predicts outcome; electronic medical record/application-based classification tools are emerging	Being adopted in tertiary centers; potential for mobile-based use in tier-2 cities
Door-to-lactate-free protocols	Lactate normalization <6 hours is a predictor of survival; used for early escalation decisions	Piloted in select Indian cardiac centers
Early MCS strategy	Shift toward early MCS ("Impella-first"); hybrid MCS (e.g. ECMO + IABP) for refractory shock	Impella use increasing in metros; ECMO + IABP used in few high-volume centers
Culprit-only PCI	Reinforced by trials (e.g. CULPRIT-SHOCK); nonculprit lesions treated later unless unstable	Supported by experience in resource-limited PCI settings
Biomarkers and precision triage	ST2, adrenomedullin, hs-Troponin + NT-proBNP combinations under research	Limited access currently; AI-based tools under development
Shock team standardization	ESC/AHA endorse shock teams; tiered team-based response and tele-triage showing benefit	Shock teams piloted in metro CICUs; telemedicine support in district hospitals
Novel therapies	Selatogrel (SC P2Y12), Levosimendan analogs, sGC modulators are under trial	Access in India limited to research/compassionate use
India-specific trends	INDECMO registry launched; AI-based deterioration alerts; ECMO under PM-JAY in select states	National data being compiled; alerts integrated at AIIMS and few private hospitals

- Intravenous fluids should be guided by dynamic assessment—avoid overload.

Role of Glucose, Temperature, and pH Management

- Maintain glucose <180 mg/dL
- Prevent hypothermia and correct metabolic acidosis.
- Address hypomagnesemia, hypokalemia—common postrevascularization.

REVASCULARIZATION: HEART OF THE MATTER

In AMI-related CS, emergent revascularization remains the single most important intervention that improves survival. Data from the SHOCK trial[5] and subsequent registries have reinforced the need for timely PCI in patients with infarct-related CS.

Culprit-only versus Multivessel Percutaneous Coronary Intervention

Recent evidence favors culprit-lesion only PCI during the index procedure in patients with multivessel disease.[6] Multivessel PCI during the same sitting can lead to longer procedure times, more contrast load, and potential hemodynamic worsening.

Culprit-only PCI is strongly recommended unless:
- The patient has ongoing ischemia in non-culprit territories.
- Cardiogenic shock is refractory despite revascularization.

Multivessel PCI/Coronary artery bypass grafting can be planned as a staged procedure once the patient stabilizes.

Timing is Crucial

Early revascularization, ideally within 90 minutes of first medical contact, is associated with better outcomes. However, real-world data from Indian centers often show delays due to late referrals, nonavailability of catheterization laboratories in peripheral hospitals, and patient financial constraints.

This necessitates:
- Streamlined referral networks
- Prehospital triage systems
- Shock team activation alongside STEMI code.

Access Considerations

Following are the access considerations:
- Radial access is preferred for its lower bleeding risk, but in profound shock, femoral access allows easier use of large-bore catheters and rapid MCS deployment if needed.
- Operators must be prepared for rapid hemodynamic collapse during balloon inflation—have inotropes and IABP/Impella ready.

Indian Practical Points

- Door-to-balloon + Door-to-lactate-free targets should be integrated into every PCI protocol.
- Simultaneous stabilization and revascularization—a dual track approach—is key.
- In selected patients, PCI + IABP upfront in the same suite improves outcomes.
- There is a strong need for national protocols on AMI-CS revascularization and interhospital transfer agreements.

Revascularization remains the most powerful intervention in patients with AMI-related CS. Based on the CULPRIT-SHOCK trial and recent 2023–24 registry data:[7]

- *Culprit-lesion only PCI* is preferred in the acute setting
- Nonculprit lesions can be staged later once the patient stabilizes.

Door-to-reperfusion Targets

- *Door-to-reperfusion targets include:* Aim for door-to-wire crossing within 90 minutes.
- If possible, minimize delays by pre-alerting catheterization laboratory and starting pharmacologic support in ER.

MECHANICAL CIRCULATORY SUPPORT IN 2025

In the last decade, MCS has transformed from a salvage measure to a proactive component of CS management. In appropriate patients, early MCS can unload the ventricle, stabilize perfusion, and provide a bridge to recovery or decision. However, access, cost, and expertise limit its widespread use—especially in low- and middle-income countries like India.

Why Mechanical Circulatory Support? Understanding Physiology

In CS, the failing heart struggles against systemic vascular resistance, worsening myocardial oxygen demand and ischemia. Inotropes help but increase metabolic demand and arrhythmogenic risk.

Mechanical circulatory support devices offload the heart, support forward flow, reduce LV wall stress, and improve perfusion—buying time for revascularization and myocardial recovery.

Types of MCS devices: With limited randomized, head-to-head evidence among tMCS modalities, clinicians must weigh expected benefit against the risks of bleeding, vascular and neurologic complications, infection, and other device-related harms **(Fig. 1)**.[1] The most commonly used devices in India include:

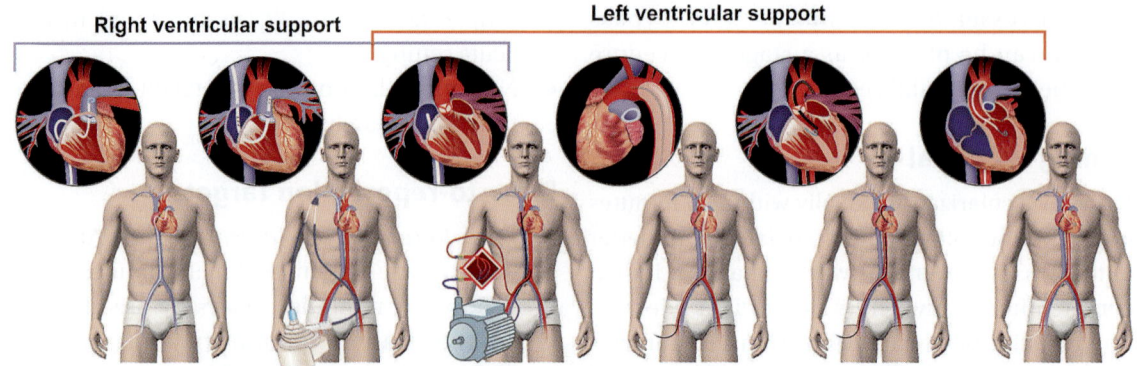

	Impella RP Flex	RA-PA pVAD	VA-ECMO	IABP	Impella CP	Impella 5.5
Max flow	3.0–4.0 L/min	4.0–5.0 L/min	5.0–7.0 L/min	0.5–1.0 L/min	3.0–4.3 L/min	5.0–6.0 L/min
Max pump speed	33,000 rpm	7,500 rpm	6,000 rpm	NA	46,000 rpm	33,000 rpm
Mechanism	Axial flow continuous pump (RA-to-PA)	Centrifugal flow continuous pump (RA-to-PA)	Centrifugal flow continuous pump (RA-to-AO)	Balloon inflation-deflation (AO)	Axial flow continuous pump (LV-to-AO)	Axial flow continuous pump (LV-to-AO)
Sheath size	23 F venous peel-away	29 or 31 F venous (inflow)	15–24 F arterial 19–25 F venous	7–8 F arterial	14 F arterial peel-away	23 F arterial peel-away
Typical insertion/ placement	Internal jugular vein	Internal jugular vein	Femoral vein (drain) Femoral artery (return)	Femoral artery or Axillary artery	Femoral artery or Axillary artery	Axillary artery
Direct LV unloading	–	–	–	–	+++	+++
Direct RV unloading	+	+	+	–	–	–
Afterload	–	–	↑↑↑	↓↓	↓	↓
Coronary perfusion	–	–	↑↑	↑↑	↑↑	↑↑

Fig 1: Types of MCS devices.

- *Intra-aortic balloon pump (IABP):* It provides diastolic support and is widely available. Although the survival benefit is modest, it remains useful if applied early.
- *Impella:* It offers active LV unloading and is particularly useful in AMI with high LVEDP. Requires expertise and has higher costs, hence limited to select centers.
- *VA-ECMO:* It provides full biventricular and oxygenation support, indicated in refractory or biventricular failure. Its use is increasing in tertiary centers with ECMO programs.
- *Tandem heart:* It creates left atrial to femoral bypass support. Its use is limited in India due to availability and expertise constraints.

Early MCS (within 2 hours of shock onset) has a survival advantage. Shock teams and hub-spoke models can optimize deployment.

Current Recommendations (2025 Updates)

Current recommendations include:

- Routine MCS in all CS patients is not supported.
- *Selective early use in:*
  - Persistent hypotension despite inotropes
  - Rising lactate >4 mmol/L
  - Large anterior MI with low EF (<25%)
  - Shock + mechanical complications
  - Pre-PCI stabilization in very high-risk cases

The CULPRIT-SHOCK sub-analyses and recent global registries (e.g., DanGer Shock) suggest that earlier MCS may reduce mortality if deployed pre-PCI in selected patients.

Decision-making Framework: "Stepwise MCS Ladder"

- Inotropes + vasopressors
- IABP (early in post-MI shock or as bridge to PCI)
- Impella or VA-ECMO for nonresponders or severe biventricular failure
- Hybrid support (ECMO + Impella/IABP) in extreme cases
- Bridge to recovery or durable VAD/transplant.

LATEST ADVANCES IN CARDIOGENIC SHOCK

Latest advances in cardiogenic shock are given in **Table 2**.

CONCLUSION

Cardiogenic shock remains a time-critical, high-mortality syndrome that demands rapid recognition, structured triage, and coordinated multidisciplinary action. Advances over the past decade—particularly the refinement of SCAI shock staging, adoption of door-to-support and door-to-lactate-free metrics, and selective early use of mechanical circulatory support—have shifted management from reactive to proactive, physiology-guided care. Early culprit-only revascularization continues to be the cornerstone in AMI-related shock, while rising rates of HF-related shock underscore the need for broader diagnostic precision and individualized strategies. In resource-variable settings such as India, integration of shock teams, tele-triage, and standardized referral pathways is essential to improve outcomes. As evidence continues to evolve, a structured, timely, and patient-specific approach remains central to breaking the cycle of hypoperfusion and improving survival in cardiogenic shock.

REFERENCES

1. Naidu SS, Baran DA, Jentzer JC, et al. SCAI SHOCK stage classification expert consensus update: a review and incorporation of validation studies. J Am Coll Cardiol. 2022;79(9):933-46.
2. Moller JE, Engstrom T, Jensen LO, et al. Microaxial flow pump or standard care in infarct related cardiogenic shock. N Engl J Med. 2024;390: 1382-93.
3. Naidu SS. Cardiac Intervention Today. (2025). A Cardiogenic Shock Challenge: Achieving 24-Hour Door-to-Lactate Clearance. Cardiac Intervention Today. [online] Available from https://citoday.com/articles/2025-digital-exclusive-3/a-cardiogenic-shock-challenge-achieving-24-hour-door-to-lactate-clearance [Last accessed November, 2025].
4. Kapur NK, Kanwar M, Sinha SS, et al. Criteria for defining stages of cardiogenic shock severity. J Am Coll Cardiol. 2022;80:185-98.
5. Hochman JS, Sleeper LA, Webb JG, et al. Early revascularization in acute myocardial infarction complicated by cardiogenic shock. N Engl J Med. 1999;341:625-34.
6. Thiele H, Akin I, Sandri M, et al. PCI strategies in patients with acute myocardial infarction and cardiogenic shock. N Engl J Med. 2017;377(25): 2419-32.
7. Thiele H, Naidu SS, Henry TD, et al. American Heart Association Cardiogenic Shock Registry powered by Get with The Guidelines: Rationale, Design, and First Report. Circulation: Cardiovascular Quality and Outcomes. 2023;16(8):e009986.

Coronary LASER—Light at the End of the Tunnel: Expanding Indications

CHAPTER 18

Smit Shrivastava

INTRODUCTION

Excimer (excited dimer) LASER coronary atherectomy (ELCA) has evolved from a niche intervention to a front-line modality in managing complex coronary artery disease. Originally introduced for peripheral vascular applications in the 1980s, its coronary utility gained traction after the first clinical use in 1988 at the Cedars-Sinai Medical Center, Los Angeles.[1] In India, the transformative potential of Excimer LASER was first realized with the first commercial use at the Advanced Cardiac Institute, Pt JNM Medical College, Raipur **(Fig. 1)**. Over the past decade, technological improvements, expanded indications, and increasing familiarity have reignited interest in this versatile tool.

The US Food and Drug Administration approved excimer LASER coronary atherectomy for percutaneous coronary intervention (PCI) in 1992. ELCA utilizes a xenon-chloride excited dimer LASER to produce a fusillade of ultraviolet rays at 308 nm, at pulse repetition rates from 25 to 80 Hz with effective incursion depth (<10–50 µm), from one of concentric-type 0.9, 1.4, 1.7, and 2.0 Fr and eccentric-type 1.7 and 2.0 Fr catheters.[2]

The action of ELCA relies on the molecular bond dissociation by the larger energy delivered by a 308-nm photon (photochemical effect),[3] vaporization of water into steam (photothermal effect),[4] and finally steamed ejection of debris (photomechanical effect).[1]

ADVANTAGE OVER OTHER PLAQUE MODIFICATION TOOLS

Unlike mechanical atherectomy, excimer LASER causes photochemical decomposition to disrupt molecular bonds; photomechanical action to generate shock waves; and photothermal energy to soften fibrotic and thrombotic materials. The excimer LASER is exclusive among all the atheroablative tools for avoiding plaque abruption, platelet activation experienced in other plaque modification tools—whether percutaneous transluminal coronary angioplasty (PTCA) balloon, directional (DCA), or rotational atherectomy (RA). Excimer LASER energy ablates inorganic material without the generation of excessive heat and prevents immediate elastic recoil, distal embolization, and platelet activation witnessed in PTCA and rotablative techniques. The DCA and RA pose additional risks of ischemia and perforations with the use of an 8-Fr guiding catheter and dedicated wire.

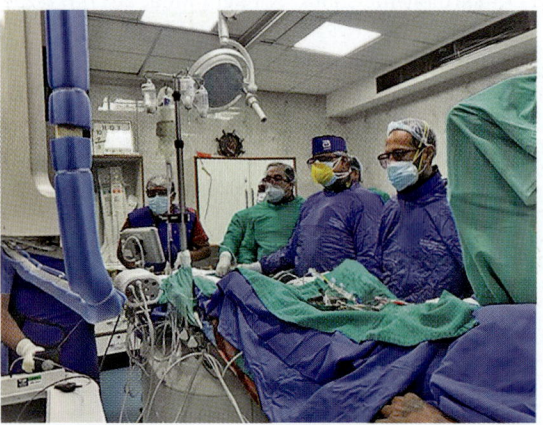

Fig. 1: First commercial LASER in India.

Balloon-uncrossable Lesions

Balloon-uncrossable lesions are frequently encountered in CTO, with approximately 6.4–9% of cases primarily due to calcification (82%) and tortuosity (61%).[5,6] ELCA catheters are compatible with any standard 0.014-inch coronary guidewire and even with a "buddy wire" support. ELCA modifies the plaque composition, selectively acting on the hard-calcified components by creating cracks and dissection flaps, to promote stent expansion. The LAVA multicenter registry reported that balloon-uncrossable lesions as the most common indication for ELCA (43.8%), reporting high success rates from 81.6% to 96.8%.[6] ELCA can be effective even if the catheter cannot fully cross the lesion, by sufficiently modifying the proximal cap plaque **(Figs. 2A and B)**.

Balloon-undilatable Lesions

These are defined as coronary artery lesions that fail to expand adequately despite high-pressure balloon inflation, usually due to severe calcification and/or fibrosis. ELCA has demonstrated high technical and procedural success rates in treating such lesions. In one multicenter registry, undilatable lesions were the second most common indication for LASER use (40.8%), with 94.3% technical success and 93.8% procedural success rates.[7] The LEONARDO study reported a 93.7% LASER success rate in balloon failure cases without major complications.[8] A significant advantage of ELCA here is its compatibility with any standard 0.014-inch guidewire, unlike RA or orbital atherectomy (OA), which require specialized wires and larger catheters **(Figs. 3A to D)**.

Stent Thrombosis

Excimer LASER coronary atherectomy is a viable and effective treatment for acute stent thrombosis (AST), particularly as a "bail-out" strategy for massive thrombus burden. It is often used when initial attempts at thrombus aspiration or balloon angioplasty fail to restore proper blood flow. The ULTRAMAN registry demonstrated a high technical and procedural success rate for ELCA in patients with massive thrombus and ACS, with a lower rate of in-hospital major adverse cardiac events (MACE) and distal embolization with ELCA compared to conventional methods. ELCA has been shown to successfully restore thrombolysis

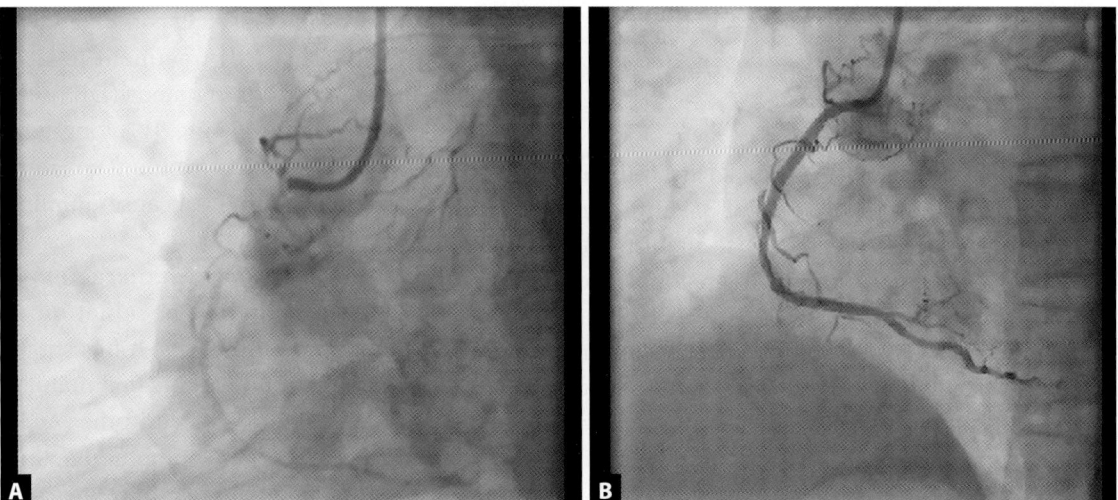

Figs. 2A and B: (A) Uncrossable lesion and (B) Uncrossable lesion result.

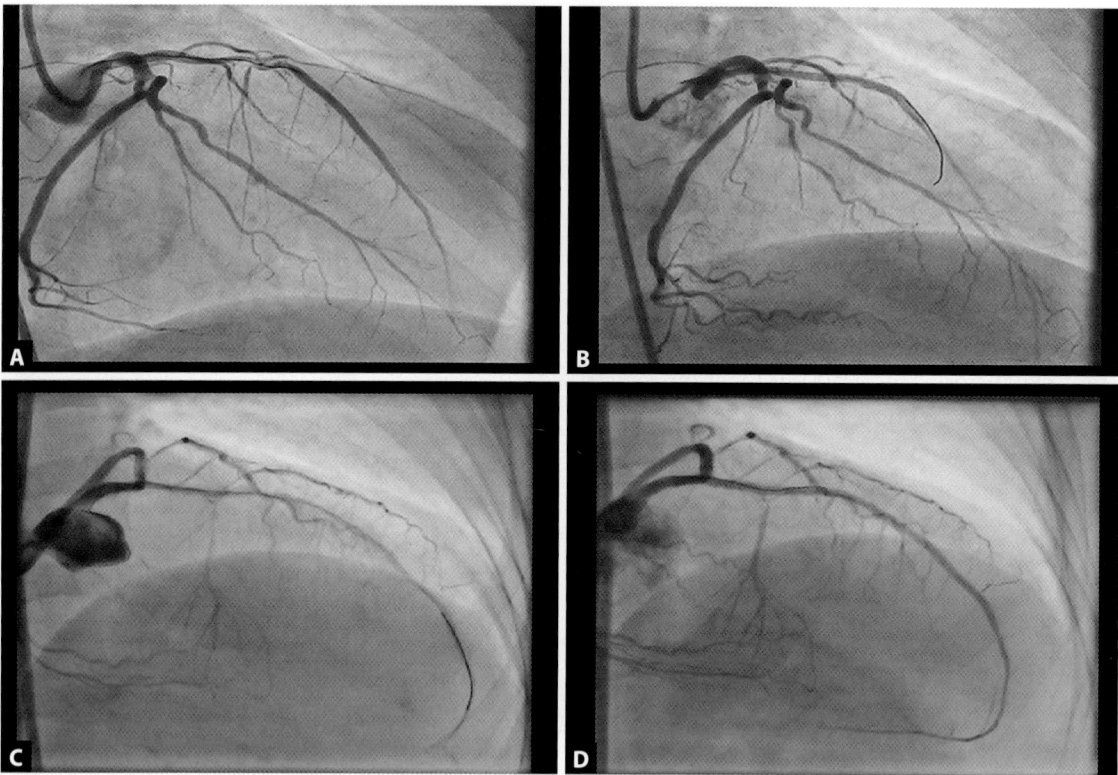

Figs. 3A to D: (A) Undilatable lesion—ELCAtripsy; (B) Undilatable lesion result; (C) Undilatable lesion—ELCA-OPN; and (D) Undilatable lesion after ELCA-OPN.

in myocardial infarction (TIMI) flow and improve myocardial blush grade[9] **(Figs. 4A and B)**.

In-stent Restenosis (Calcific Neoatheroma)

In-stent restenosis (ISR) is caused by intimal hyperplasia (IH) and can be focal or diffuse in distribution. ELCA aims to reduce neointimal tissue, improve final lumen dimensions, and decrease clinical recurrence. Intravascular ultrasound (IVUS) studies indicate that lumen enlargement after ELCA for ISR is primarily due to tissue ablation. ELCA alone reduced plaque area by 34%, with adjunctive PTCA further reducing it by 65%. High procedural success rates (91–100%) are reported for ELCA plus adjunctive PTCA in ISR treatment.[10] It can also crack calcium behind stent struts. ELCA is increasingly combined with drug-coated balloon (DCB) treatment for ISR, especially in the drug-eluting stent (DES) era, with the DERIST study showing 91% long-term success.[11] A key advantage is avoiding collateral damage to stents, as saline-ELCA causes minimal damage to DES polymer coatings.

Excimer LASER coronary atherectomy's unique attributes facilitate the ablation of neoatherosclerosis and thrombus. It has shown successful ablation of eruptive calcified nodules, particularly in acute coronary syndrome (ACS), where it can reduce the risk of hemodynamic compromise and slow reflow. ELCA-treated lesions show larger minimum lumen area (MLA)

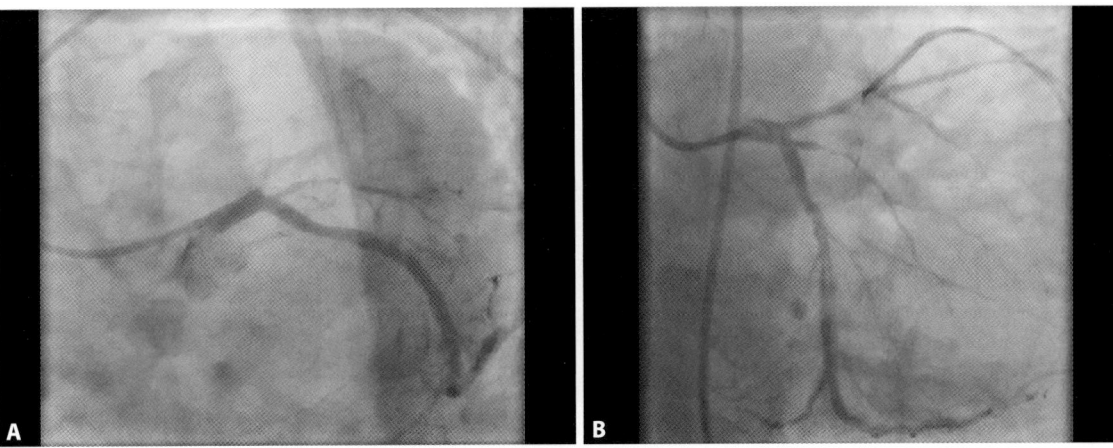

Figs. 4A and B: (A) Acute stent thrombosis (post-COVID) and (B) Acute stent thrombosis results.

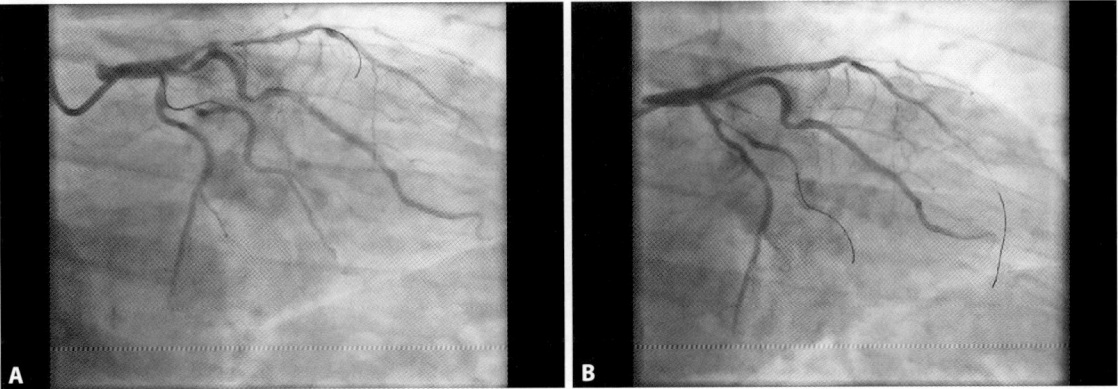

Figs. 5A and B: (A) In-stent restenosis (due to excessive neointimal proliferation) and (B) In-stent restenosis after lasing and drug-coated balloon angioplasty.

and minimum stent area (MSA) compared to non-ELCA-treated lesions. Using contrast flush during ELCA is associated with more frequent and thicker calcium fractures. ELCA is noted for having a low no-reflow rate as generated particles are small and easily filtered **(Figs. 5A and B)**.

Chronic Total Occlusion

Chronic total occlusions (CTOs) are complete vessel occlusions (TIMI flow grade 0) for over three months. ELCA is primarily used in CTO-PCI when standard techniques fail, particularly for balloon-uncrossable and undilatable lesions, or for modifying the proximal cap of highly calcified or fibrotic lesions. It has a major advantage with standard 0.014-inch guidewire compatibility and the small crossing profile of the 0.9 mm ELCA catheter. ELCA has shown high success rates (86–100%) in CTO interventions, with registries reporting higher technical and procedural success rates when ELCA is used in balloon-uncrossable or undilatable CTOs[6] **(Figs. 6A and B)**.

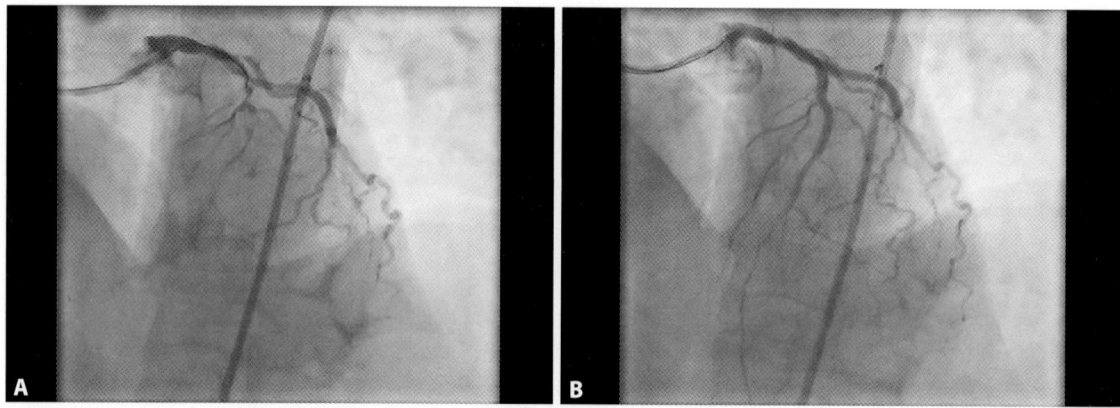

Figs. 6A and B: (A) CTO and (B) CTO after lasing and stent.

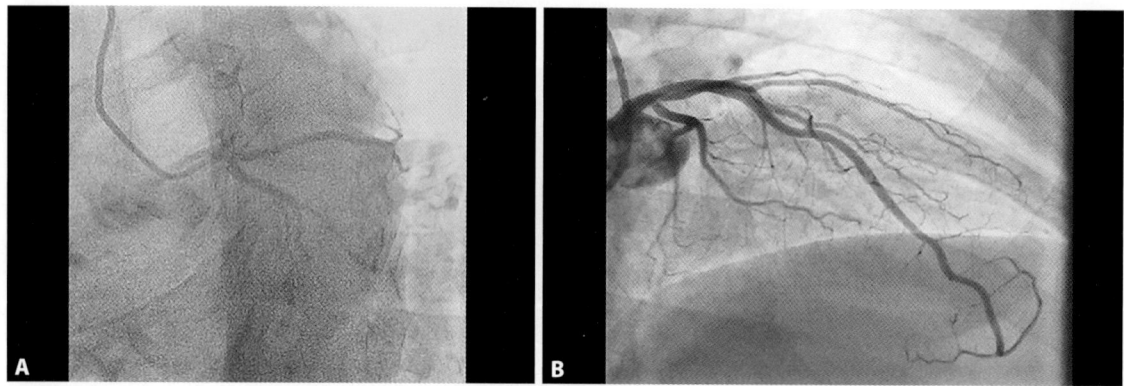

Figs. 7A and B: (A) Primary percutaneous coronary intervention with large thrombus burden and (B) Primary percutaneous coronary intervention results with lasing and thrombus aspiration.

Thrombus-laden Vessels in Primary Percutaneous Coronary Intervention

Excimer LASER coronary atherectomy vaporizes atherosclerotic plaques and thrombotic material through photomechanical and photothermal processes, producing debris particles typically <10 µm, with minimal risk of distal embolization. It also causes a dose-dependent suppression of platelet aggregation, known as the "stunned platelet phenomenon." Studies comparing ELCA to manual aspiration for ACS found ELCA to be superior in lesion crossability, attainment of TIMI 3 flow, blush score 3, and reduced distal embolization. Benefits include rapid thrombus removal, reduced distal embolization, concomitant plaque debulking, facilitation of further interventions, antithrombogenic effects, and avoidance of systemic lysis[12] **(Figs. 7A and B)**.

Saphenous Vein Graft Restenosis and Thrombosis

Excimer LASER coronary atherectomy is an established and FDA-approved therapeutic modality for SVG lesions, which are prone to distal embolization and myocardial infarction. It is primarily used to debulk and vaporize

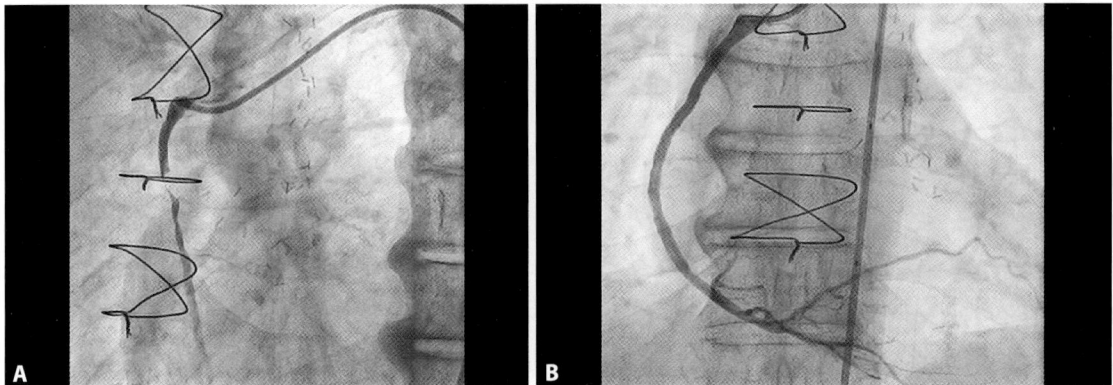

Figs. 8A and B: (A) Thrombus/restenosis in SVG graft and (B) Thrombus/restenosis in SVG graft results.

atherosclerotic plaque and thrombus in SVGs, especially for multifocal, diffuse, and thrombotic lesions. A major advantage is its potential to reduce distal embolization and periprocedural myocardial infarction by converting thrombus into microscopic, easily cleared particles. ELCA is indicated for complex SVG lesions, including occluded or degenerated SVGs, and ostial SVG lesions. It can also serve as an adjunctive tool when distal protection devices (DPDs) cannot be deployed and can create a channel for their delivery. Success rates for ELCA in SVG lesions range as high as 100% in some studies, and overall, between 82 and 97%[13] **(Figs. 8A and B)**.

Underexpanded Stents (without Obvious Thrombus)

Stent underexpansion (SU) is a significant challenge contributing to ISR and stent thrombosis. ELCA can modify the underlying resistant plaque and calcium without significantly damaging stent architecture, creating calcium cracks and dissection flaps to improve stent expansion. The ELLEMENT registry demonstrated high success (96.4%) in LASER-assisted stent dilation in underexpanded stents, with acceptable complication rates.[14] Contrast-enhanced ELCA can be used as an "explosion technique" to generate powerful pressure pulses, disrupting resistant plaque and calcium behind stent struts, especially for thick, extensive, and resistant peri-stent calcium **(Figs. 9A to D)**.

Ostial and Bifurcation Lesions

Ostial coronary artery stenoses are historically challenging for balloon angioplasty due to lower success rates, higher complication risks (acute vessel closure, late restenosis), rigidity, increased elastic recoil, and potential heavy calcification. ELCA is considered better suited for ostial lesions due to its minimal thermal injury and ability to ablate calcified plaque, without the high risks of perforations, acute closures, or major dissections seen with compression techniques. ELCA has shown high procedural success rates (90%) in aorto-ostial procedures, with the majority of acute lumen gain attributed to ELCA itself.[15] It is particularly well-suited for calcified, aorto-ostial, left main coronary artery (LMCA) and thrombus-containing lesions, as it minimizes the risk of side branch occlusion and provides a stentless alternative in some cases. ELCA offers advantages over kissing balloon angioplasty, rotablation, and directional atherectomy by reducing plaque shifting, spasm, and distal embolization **(Figs. 10A and B)**.

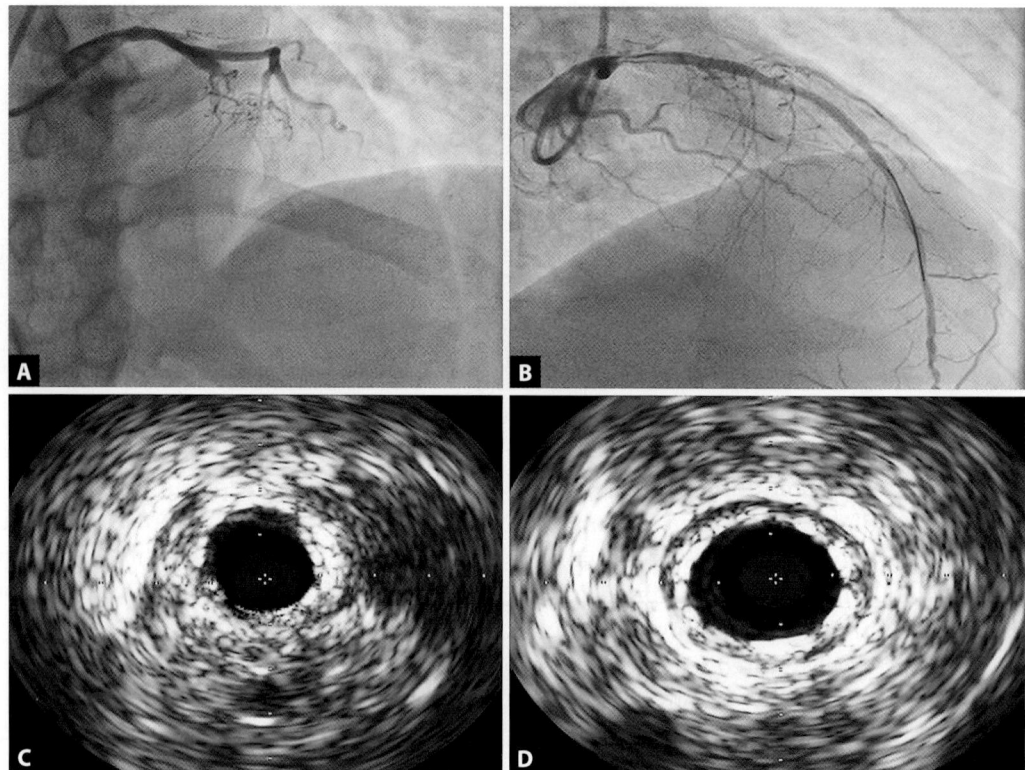

Figs. 9A to D: (A) Underexpanded stent; (B) Underexpanded stent results; (C) Underexpanded stent IVUS; and (D) Underexpanded stent IVUS result.

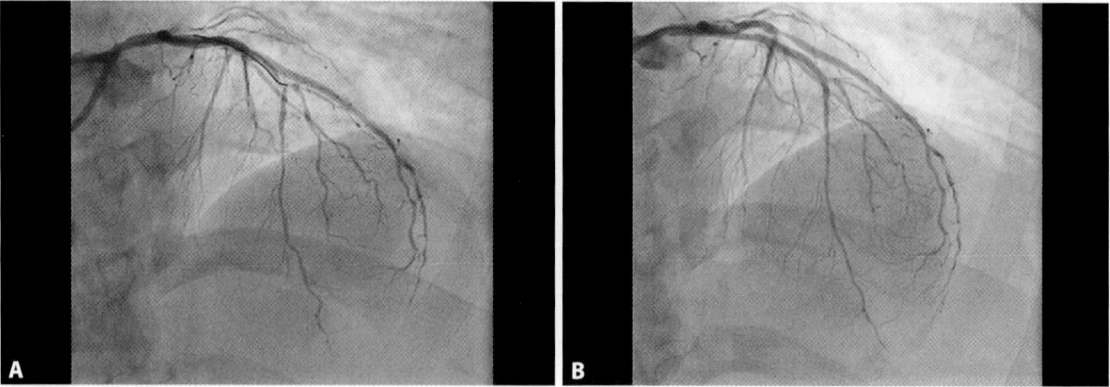

Figs. 10A and B: (A) Ostial or bifurcation lesions and (B) Ostial or bifurcation lesions results.

Pacemaker and Implantable Cardiodefibrillator Lead Extraction

LASER sheaths are critical for removing chronically adherent leads, particularly complex types like dual-coil ICD leads or coronary sinus leads, where extensive fibrous ingrowth makes extraction challenging **(Fig. 11)**.

Calcified Lesions

Although the success of LASER therapy shows an inverse relationship with the degree of calcification (79% in calcified lesions vs. 96% in noncalcified lesions; $p < 0.05$), in most cases, the LASER is able to ablate at least the proximal calcified cap sufficiently to allow subsequent successful PCI. Bilodeau reported a procedural success rate of 93% and a clinical success rate of 86% with excimer LASER in a subgroup of patients with highly complex lesions[16] **(Figs. 12A and B)**.

Expanding Indications

Beyond these established uses, ELCA's versatility is highlighted in its application across numerous other complex scenarios:

- *Takayasu aortoarteritis:* ELCA facilitates revascularization in severe arterial occlusion, serving as an "important bail out strategy" for near-total, balloon-noncrossable occlusions, such as in middle aortic syndrome[17] **(Figs. 13A and B)**.
- *LASER-assisted fenestration of aortic dissection flaps:* LASER in situ fenestration (LISF) using excimer or diode LASERs creates deliberate holes in endograft fabric to preserve blood flow into critical vessels during TEVAR or to bridge true and false lumens in aortic dissection.[18]
- *Coronary embolic events—embolus vaporization:* ELCA vaporizes obstructing material into microparticles and gas to restore distal flow, particularly effective for soft embolic material in tortuous or small vessels resistant to aspiration.[12]
- *LASER in below-the-knee arterial disease:* ELCA has been used to photoablate atherosclerotic tissue, thrombus, fibrous plaque, or neointimal tissue, creating a pilot channel and debulking occlusive material[19] **(Figs. 14A and B)**.
- *Endovenous LASER ablation:* A minimally invasive technique for varicose veins, using thermal LASER energy to collapse vein walls.[20]
- *LASER for arteriovenous (AV) fistula thrombectomy/LASER in peripheral vein*

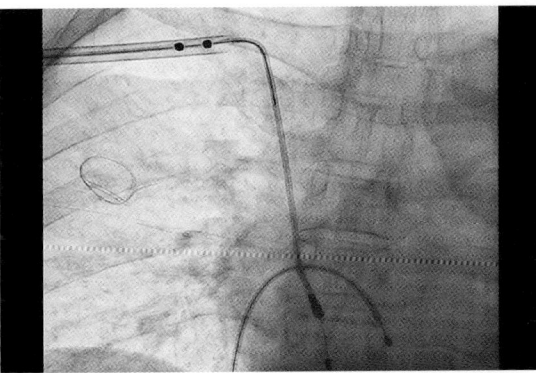

Fig. 11: Pacemaker lead extraction.

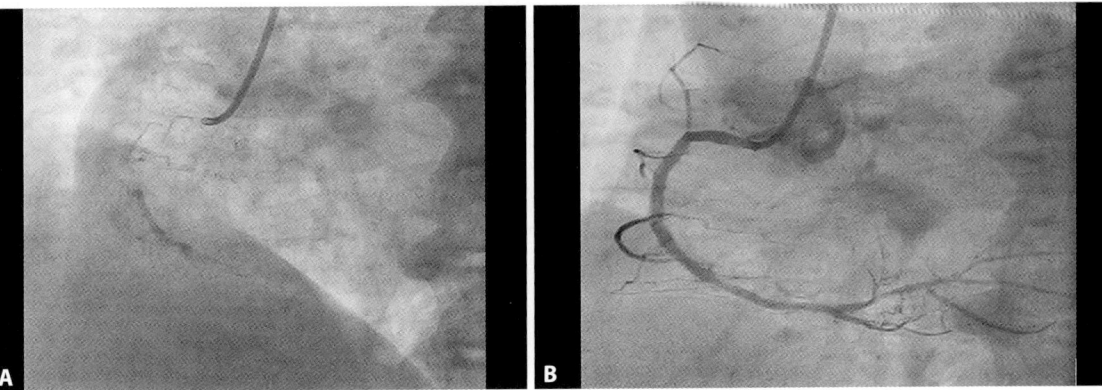

Figs. 12A and B: (A) Severe fibrocalcific lesion and (B) Severe fibrocalcific Lesion.

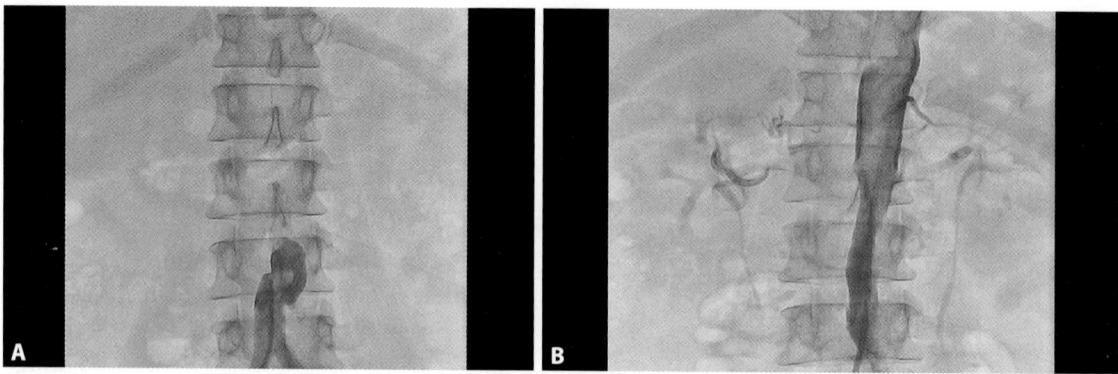

Figs. 13A and B: (A) Takayasu aortoarteritis and (B) Takayasu aortoarteritis results.

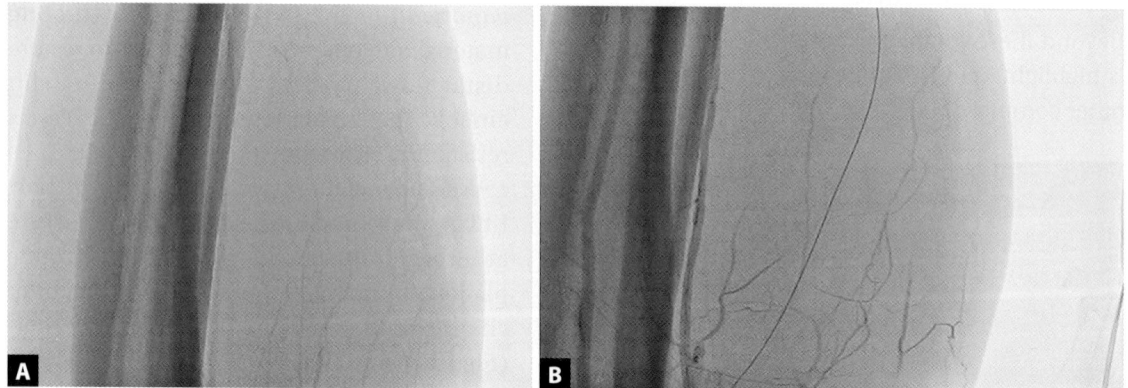

Figs. 14A and B: (A) Below-knee intervention and (B) Below-knee intervention results.

stenosis or occlusion: LASERs are being explored for chronic peripheral venous occlusion as an adjunct to balloon venoplasty.[21]
- *LASER in pulmonary artery chronic thromboembolism (experimental):* Investigational use for fibrotic webs or organized material is difficult to cross or dilate with balloon angioplasty, aiming to debulk or create a channel.[22]
- *Drug delivery facilitation via vascular LASER:* LASER-assisted drug delivery (LADD) creates microscopic channels for enhanced drug penetration, while site-specific pharmacoLASER therapy (SSPLT) uses LASERs to trigger local drug releases from liposomes.[23]
- *Treatment of endoluminal infections (infected thrombus/fibrin sheaths)/LASER decontamination of infected or biofilm-laden leads and catheters:* While not standard for in-situ sterilization, excimer LASER sheaths aid in the removal of infected or biofilm-laden leads by ablating fibrous adhesions and biofilm, reducing the mechanical traction needed for removal and subsequent infection.
- *LASER-assisted thrombolysis in acute stroke or cerebral venous thrombosis (experimental):* Experimental use, primarily for photoacoustic disruption of thrombus, potentially enhancing thrombolytic drug penetration or reestablishing flow in resistant cases.[24,25]

- *Crossing or debulking organized thrombus in prosthetic valve thrombosis:* ELCA may be utilized during recrossing a previously implanted bioprosthetic valve for PCI in TAVI.
- *Lampoon (laceration of the anterior mitral leaflet to prevent outflow obstruction) procedure in transcatheter mitral valve replacement (TMVR):* In the author's belief, ELCA can be utilized to "burn" or split safely and precisely the anterior mitral leaflet over a single catheter than the practiced electrified wire requiring two catheters.
- *Testing vascular grafts or endografts:* Not only LISF is used to create holes through endograft fabric for accessing branch vessels, and excimer LASERs recanalize occluded stents and grafts, it is utilized in ex vivo and bench testing for variable effects on graft material, tear patterns, and heat/irradiation effects—important when planning biopsy/transgraft punctures (risk of fabric tearing, embolic material, or thermal injury).
- *LASER to facilitate delivery of intravascular imaging catheters or pressure wires:* LASERs clear or modify lesions, especially calcified or occluded vessels, to allow subsequent passage of IVUS/optical coherence tomography (OCT) intravascular Imaging catheters or pressure wires.
- *Recanalization of occluded hemodialysis catheters and central venous occlusions:* Excimer LASERs are used as a sharp-recanalization adjunct to create a channel through organized fibrotic occlusions when conventional methods fail.[21]
- *Plaque modification prior to lithotripsy or intravascular brachytherapy:* ELCA improves device crossing and facilitates subsequent calcium-fracturing with intravascular lithotripsy (IVL) or delivery of brachytherapy catheters by debulking neointima/organized tissue **(Figs. 3A and B).**

- *Coronary vein occlusion during cardiac resynchronization therapy (CRT) implantation/LASER-assisted coronary sinus recanalization for CRT upgrade:* LASERs are primarily used to restore central venous access by facilitating lead extraction and traversing fibrotic occlusions, enabling new CRT lead placement.
- *Modification of polymer-coated or covered stents (e.g., Viabahn and PK Papyrus):* LISF has been performed to revascularize branch vessels or recover jailed branches through the fabric of stent grafts.
- *Vascular access in transcatheter aortic valve implantation (TAVI) or endovascular procedures:* ELCA ablates native obstructive plaque, fibrotic tissue, or occluded stent-grafts to enable safe sheath insertion in challenging iliofemoral arteries.
- *LASER to treat early stent thrombosis resistant to thrombectomy:* ELCA is a rescue option when aspiration/manual thrombectomy and ballooning fail for thrombus-laden or underexpanded stents, ablating thrombus and modifying plaque/calcium beneath stent struts **(Figs. 7A and B).**
- *Facilitating rotational/OA by creating a microchannel:* ELCA photoablates a small depth of tissue to open a microchannel or modify the proximal cap of noncrossable lesions, allowing passage of subsequent atherectomy devices (e.g., "RASER," ELCA-Tripsy, ELCA-OPN, and ELCA-Cut technique) **(Figs. 3 and 9).**
- *LASER-assisted management of iatrogenic coronary dissection:* ELCA vaporizes thrombus and creates a microchannel through an obstructing flap, facilitating restoration of flow or passage of equipment when the true lumen cannot be rewired.
- *Creating fenestrations in iatrogenic aortic occlusion post-TAVI or endovascular aortic repair (EVAR):* ELCA can theoretically provide

- a safe modality to recanalize iatrogenic aortic occlusions during such procedures.
- *Off-label neurovascular intervention (e.g., carotid webs or fibromuscular dysplasia):* Excimer LASER-assisted nonocclusive anastomosis (ELANA) is a neurosurgical bypass technique, but direct endovascular intraluminal LASER treatment for carotid webs or FMD is largely unestablished.[26,27]
- *Use in pediatric congenital heart disease interventions:* Applications include LASER perforation/valvotomy of atretic valves, LASER-assisted balloon dilation, recanalization of occluded central veins/shunts, and modification of tough lesions.[28]
- *Facilitating valve-in-valve procedures:* While LASER valvotomy exists for native valves, for valve-in-valve, electrosurgical techniques like CLEVE are clinically validated.[29]
- *Recanalizing occluded or jailed side branches through stent struts:* While direct evidence is limited, LASER techniques have proven effective in analogous in-stent occlusions and venous stent recanalization **(Figs. 10A and B)**.
- *LASER-assisted recanalization of peripheral chronic vein occlusion in May–Thurner syndrome:* Useful for chronic, fibrotic iliac/iliocaval occlusions or occluded venous stents when conventional methods fail.[30]
- *Biofilm sterilization in cardiovascular implant infections (theoretical/in vitro):* LASERs can disrupt biofilms in vitro by thermal, photoacoustic, and photochemical mechanisms, and enhance killing with photosensitizers or nanoparticles, but clinical cardiovascular applications are limited.
- *Pulmonary vein occlusion postablation therapy:* LASER is not a routine therapy, but excimer/ablative LASERs are used investigationally for selected chronic total pulmonary vein occlusions after pulmonary vein isolation for atrial fibrillation in expert centers.
- *Dural sinus thrombosis:* LASER-based interventions are not commonly used; mechanical thrombectomy and catheter-directed thrombolysis are established treatments.
- *LASER crossing of long-segment peripheral bypass graft occlusion:* Excimer LASER ablates blockages to create a channel for subsequent angioplasty and stenting, particularly for long, complex occlusions.
- *Treatment of stent edge restenosis in bifurcations:* ELCA is a viable option for ISR at stent edges, especially with SU.
- *LASER-assisted removal of embedded IVC filters:* High success rates reported for removing filters are difficult to retrieve with standard methods.[31]
- *Research into excimer LASER-induced endothelial regeneration:* Excimer LASER photoablation preserves vessel media, potentially allowing normal endothelial migration and coverage.
- *Kawasaki aneurysm:* ELCA has been used to vaporize massive thrombus in restenosis within coronary artery aneurysms in Kawasaki disease patients.[32,33]
- *Free entrapped guidewire:* Guidewire entrapment (GE) occurs in 0.1–0.2% of PCI cases, increasing to 0.2–0.5% in CTO patients. Prolonged manipulation or retention of guidewires increases the risk of coronary thrombosis. Retained guidewire fragments can cause complications, such as thrombosis, dissection, vessel occlusion, embolization, and perforation. A registry analysis showed that retrieval of entrapped or fractured guidewires was attempted in 71.4% of cases, but the success rate was only 26.7%. ELCA has been used to free guidewires entrapped between a newly deployed stent and a calcified vessel wall.[6]
- *Septal collateral atherectomy:* Useful for enlarging tiny septal collaterals to

facilitate retrograde guidewire and balloon advancement in CTOs.[34]

- *Ablation of conductive pathways:* The Nd:YAG LASER is frequently employed for endoscopic ablation used for the treatment of atrial fibrillation by pulmonary vein isolation. A multicenter study demonstrated significant success rates of pulmonary vein isolation (PVI) using excimer-assisted systems (EAS), reporting that the 1-year success rate (approximately 63%) was comparable to that achieved with conventional PVI techniques.[35]

CONCLUSION

In conclusion, ELCA has firmly established itself as an indispensable tool for a wide array of complex coronary and peripheral lesions, and its applications continue to expand into novel and challenging cardiovascular interventions.

REFERENCES

1. Litvack F, Eigler N, Margolis J, et al. Percutaneous excimer laser coronary angioplasty: results in the first consecutive 3,000 patients. The ELCA Investigators. J Am Coll Cardiol. 1994;23(2):323-9.
2. Nakabayashi K, Sunaga D, Kaneko N, et al. Simple percutaneous coronary interventions using the modification of complex coronary lesion with excimer laser. Cardiovasc Revasc Med. 2019;20(4):293-302.
3. Appelman YE, Piek JJ, Strikwerda S, et al. Randomised trial of excimer laser angioplasty versus balloon angioplasty for treatment of obstructive coronary artery disease. Lancet. 1996;347(8994):79-84.
4. Deckelbaum LI, Natarajan MK, Bittl JA, et al. Effect of intracoronary saline infusion on dissection during excimer laser coronary angioplasty: a randomized trial. The Percutaneous Excimer Laser Coronary Angioplasty (PELCA) Investigators. J Am Coll Cardiol. 1995;26(5):1264-9.
5. Patel SM, Pokala NR, Menon RV, et al. Prevalence, Presentation and Treatment of 'Balloon Undilatable' Chronic Total Occlusions: Insights from a Multicenter US Registry. J Invasive Cardiol. 2015;https://doi.org/10.1002/ccd.27510.
6. Karacsonyi J, Armstrong EJ, Truong HTD, et al. Contemporary Use of Laser During Percutaneous Coronary Interventions: Insights from the Laser Veterans Affairs (LAVA) Multicenter Registry J Invasive Cardiol. 2018;30(6):195-201.
7. Tajti P, Karmpaliotis D, Alaswad K, et al. Prevalence, Presentation and Treatment of 'Balloon Undilatable' Chronic Total Occlusions: Insights from a Multicenter US Registry. Catheter Cardiovasc Interv. 2018;91(4):657-66.
8. Ambrosini V, Sorropago G, Laurenzano E, et al. Early outcome of high energy Laser (Excimer) facilitated coronary angioplasty ON hARD and complex calcified and balloOn-resistant coronary lesions: LEONARDO Study. Cardiovasc Revasc Med. 2015;16(3):141-6.
9. Nishino M, Mori N, Takiuchi S, et al. Indications and outcomes of excimer laser coronary atherectomy: Efficacy and safety for thrombotic lesions-The ULTRAMAN registry. J Cardiol. 2017;69(1):314-9.
10. Bardooli FK, Hussain T, Amin H, et al. Case Series and Brief Review Report: Excimer Laser Coronary Atherectomy, Facilitating Daily Complex Interventional Challenges. Heart Views. 2021;22(3):206-11.
11. Ambrosini V, Golino L, Niccoli G, et al. The combined use of Drug-eluting balloon and Excimer laser for coronary artery Restenosis In-Stent Treatment: The DERIST study. Cardiovasc Revasc Med. 2017;18(3):165-8.
12. Dahm JB, Topaz O, Woenckhaus C, et al. Laser-facilitated thrombectomy: a new therapeutic option for treatment of thrombus-laden coronary lesions. Catheter Cardiovasc Interv. 2002;56(3):365-72.
13. Tsutsui RS, Sammour Y, Kalra A, et al. Excimer laser atherectomy in percutaneous coronary intervention: A contemporary review. Cardiovasc Revasc Med. 2021;25:75-85.
14. Latib A, Takagi K, Chizzola G, et al. Excimer Laser LEsion modification to expand non-dilatable stents: the ELLEMENT registry. Cardiovasc Revasc Med. 2014;15(1):8-12.
15. Eigler NL, Weinstock B, Douglas Jr JS, et al. Excimer laser coronary angioplasty of aorto-ostial

stenoses. Results of the excimer laser coronary angioplasty (ELCA) registry in the first 200 patients. Circulation. 1993;88(5 Pt 1):2049-57.
16. Bilodeau L, Fretz EB, Taeymans Y, et al. Novel use of a high-energy excimer laser catheter for calcified and complex coronary artery lesions. Catheter Cardiovasc Interv. 2004;62(2):155-61.
17. Shrivastava S. Excimer LASER in middle aorta syndrome in Takayasu aortoarteritis: A case report. IHJ Cardiovasc Rep. 2024;8(3):90-1.
18. Murphy EH, Dimaio JM, Dean W, et al. Endovascular repair of acute traumatic thoracic aortic transection with laser-assisted in-situ fenestration of a stent-graft covering the left subclavian artery. J Endovasc Ther. 2009;16(4):457-63.
19. Zhou M, Qi L, Gu Y. Cool Excimer Laser-Assisted Angioplasty vs. Percutaneous Transluminal Angioplasty for Infrapopliteal Arterial Occlusion: A Meta-Analysis and Systematic Review. Front Cardiovasc Med. 2022;8:783358.
20. Teter KA, Kabnick LS, Sadek M. Endovenous laser ablation: A comprehensive review. Phlebology. 2020;35(9):656-62.
21. Çildağ BM, Köseoğlu KÖ. Percutaneous treatment of thrombosed hemodialysis arteriovenous fistulas: use of thromboaspiration and balloon angioplasty. Clujul Med. 2017;90(1):66-70.
22. Tang H, Gan H, Yang H, et al. Exciter laser coronary atherectomy (ELCA) can be a powerful weapon in the treatment of chronic thromboembolic pulmonary hypertension (CTEPH). Medical Hypotheses. 2022;160(18):110779.
23. Shangguan H, Gregory KW, Casperson LW, et al. Enhanced laser thrombolysis with photomechanical drug delivery: An in vitro study. Lasers Surg Med. 1998;23(3):151-60.
24. Jo J, Forrest ML, Yang X. Ultrasound-assisted laser thrombolysis with endovascular laser and high-intensity focused ultrasound. Med Phys. 2021;48(2):579-86.
25. Singh R, Jo J, Riegel M, et al. The feasibility of ultrasound-assisted endovascular laser thrombolysis in an acute rabbit thrombosis model. Med Phys. 2021;48(8):4128-38.
26. van Doormaal TP, van der Zwan A, Redegeld S, et al. Patency, flow, and endothelialization of the sutureless Excimer Laser Assisted Non-occlusive Anastomosis (ELANA) technique in a pig model. J Neurosurg. 2011;115(6):1221-30.
27. Crocker M, Walsh D, Epaliyanage P, et al. Excimer laser-assisted non-occlusive cerebral vascular Anastomosis (ELANA): Review of the first UK experience. Br J Neurosurg. 2010;24(2):148-55.
28. Riemenschneider TA, Lee G, Ikeda RM, et al. Laser irradiation of congenital heart disease: potential for palliation and correction of intracardiac and intravascular defects. Am Heart J. 1983;106(6):1389-93.
29. McCandless M, Otto S, Elmariah S, et al. A comparison of laser, electrosurgical, and mechanical transcatheter traversal of calcified aortic valve leaflets. JTCVS Struct Endovasc. 2025;6:100054.
30. Smeds MR, Jacobs DL. Treatment of Chronic Venous Stent Occlusion With a Wildcat Catheter. Vasc Endovascular Surg. 2011;45(5):453-6.
31. Desai KR, Kaufman J, Truong P, et al. Safety and Success Rates of Excimer Laser Sheath-Assisted Retrieval of Embedded Inferior Vena Cava Filters. JAMA Netw Open. 2022;5(12):e2248159.
32. Kawamura I, Komiyama K, Fukamizu S, et al. Combination of drug-coated balloon angioplasty and excimer laser coronary angioplasty ablation for coronary restenosis of Kawasaki disease: A case report. J Cardiol Cases. 2016;15(1):18-21.
33. Yamamoto H, Takaya T, Oishi S, et al. Combined therapy with excimer laser coronary atherectomy and intracoronary thrombolysis for the management of massive thrombi in coronary aneurysms of post-Kawasaki disease myocardial infarction. Eur Heart J Case Rep. 2022;6(5):ytac186.
34. Ohlow MA, Lotze U, Lauer B. Excimer laser coronary atherectomy in septal collaterals during retrograde recanalization of a chronic total occlusion. Heart Int. 2011;6(2):e20.
35. Metzner A, Wissner E, Schmidt B, et al. Acute and Long-Term Clinical Outcome After Endoscopic Pulmonary Vein Isolation: Results from the First Prospective, Multicenter Study. J Cardiovasc Electrophysiol. 2013;24(1):7-13.

Indian Perspective in Chronic Total Occlusion Management and Algorithmic Approach

CHAPTER 19

Pravin K Goel, Ankit Kumar Sahu, B Hilbert Sahoo

INTRODUCTION

Chronic total occlusion (CTO) is defined as 100% obstruction to antegrade flow in the coronary arteries for at least 3 months duration.[1] CTO represents one of the most challenging lesion subsets in patients undergoing percutaneous coronary intervention (PCI).[2] Historically, CTO-PCI had been associated with significantly lower success rates and increased adverse events compared with PCI for other lesion subsets.[3] Recently, there has been a rapid and continuous evolution of CTO hardware and techniques that has driven greater procedural success and improved clinical outcomes.[2] CTOs are encountered in 18–52% coronary artery disease (CAD) patients undergoing coronary angiography (CAG).[4-7] In the past decade, the field of CTO intervention has rapidly developed, with several significant breakthroughs.[8] The introduction of the retrograde technique in 2006 opened up an alternative approach that has proven to improve CTO PCI success rates.[9]

The landmark work by Brilakis et al.[10] describing a percutaneous treatment algorithm for crossing CTO, commonly referred to as the hybrid algorithm emphasizes on the importance of dual injections for CTO PCI angiography, careful review and a standardized approach to the evaluation of the coronary angiogram, used the angiographic characteristics to guide selection of the initial strategy, and encouraged early conversion to an alternative crossing strategy if the initial crossing strategy failed. The algorithm has been shown to enhance success rates in complex CTO lesions and to be reproducible and teachable. Although there are many excellent recommendations within the hybrid algorithm, there has been infrequent adoption of the hybrid algorithm in the Asia Pacific region, where most of the world's population resides. This is caused in part by the traditional wire-based CTO teaching that is dominant in the region, and limited access to the CrossBoss® and Stingray™ system (Boston Scientific Corp, Marlborough, MA, USA), which eliminates the antegrade dissection reentry arm of the hybrid algorithm.[2] Other factors, such as lower rates of coronary artery bypass grafting, have also likely contributed to the differences in CTO-PCI approaches seen in the Asia Pacific region.[11,12]

WHY IS THERE A NEED FOR CHANGE IN APPROACH IN THE INDIAN POPULATION?

Canadian multicentric data reported CTO prevalence of 14.7% in the general population and 18.4% among CAD patients.[4] In the US veteran cohort, nearly one in three (≈31%) patients with significant CAD had a CTO.[7] Comparatively, Indian patients differ in many aspects compared to Western and other Asian countries. A study conducted by Vemuri et al.[13] in North India, CTO was identified in 16.3% ($n = 1,968$) patients undergoing CAG and in 24.4% of all patients with hemodynamically significant CAD, with a male preponderance ($n = 8724$, 72.5%). Exclusively, every CTO-PCI was initially attempted by an antegrade approach only. Increasing age, male sex, CTO in left circumflex (LCX) arterial territorial distribution, multivessel involvement, and higher J CTO score were associated with poorer outcomes in CTO PCI. Traditional risk factors like diabetes mellitus (DM), hypertension (HT), smoking, and family history of CAD were seen in 44.6%, 51.6%, 24%, and 13.9% patients, respectively. In all patients with CTO, PCI was attempted at 456 (23.1%) patients and was successful in 340 (74.6%) patients. However, CTO-PCI accounted for only 10% of all PCIs performed. Almost all the cases (99.3%) were performed by antegrade wire escalation or parallel wire technique, and only three (0.65%) patients underwent retrograde technique. Radial artery access (for performing PCI or for contralateral artery engagement) was obtained in 164 (36%) of cases only. There were only four (0.9%) procedure-related deaths during the index hospitalization in the entire cohort.

Indian CTO patients are shown to be younger (59–60 years) compared to western counterparts (median age ~64 years) as seen in the RECHARGE-CTO registry. Males are commonly affected in both the Indian and Western population (80% vs. 85–98%).[13-15] Diabetes is more commonly prevalent (53%) in the Indian population with CTO as compared to the US population (19%). US data show higher rates of obesity, HTN, dyslipidemia, past PCI/CABG, and comorbidities.[16] In the OPEN-CTO registry, patients were predominantly male (80%), frequently diabetic (41%), and more than one-third had undergone a prior CABG (37%).[17] 72% of those presenting with stable angina were classified as having severe (Canadian Classification System class III or IV) angina.[17]

CLINICAL PRESENTATION

In India, CTOs are often detected incidentally as nonculprit lesions during angiography done for acute coronary syndrome (ACS) evaluation. This may reflect late-stage presentation or referral patterns to tertiary centers. Globally, CTOs more commonly manifest as chronic stable angina that is refractory to medical therapy, with fewer presenting as acute emergencies—except when complicated by myocardial infarction (MI) with shock. Differences reflect healthcare access variations, patient help-seeking behavior, and referral thresholds—leading to more acute, ACS-dominant presentations in India, versus more elective, symptom-driven recognition in Western settings.[18,19]

ECHOCARDIOGRAPHIC FEATURES

Preprocedural echocardiographic evaluation plays a crucial role in assessing left ventricular ejection fraction (LVEF), regional wall motion abnormalities (RWMA), myocardial viability, and the presence of ischemic cardiomyopathy. Differences in these echo parameters between Indian and global CTO patients arise due to varied disease presentation, referral patterns, access to imaging modalities, and comorbidities **(Table 1)**. Average LVEF in Indian CTO patients undergoing PCI ranges from 40 to 45%, which is quite lower than in Western cohorts. Many patients present late with established ischemic cardiomyopathy and heart failure with reduced ejection fraction (HFrEF). In one tertiary Indian center study,[20] 62% had anterior and/or apical hypokinesia, with nearly 25–35% of patients having LVEF <40%. Apical dyskinesia is not uncommon due to long-standing ischemia and aneurysm formation. Diastolic dysfunction (grade I–III) is commonly seen due to long-standing ischemia, especially in diabetics and hypertensives. Eccentric left ventricular (LV) hypertrophy and remodeling are frequently observed in patients with inferior or multivessel CTO. LV thrombus is seen in a small percentage of cases, particularly in anterior infarcts with aneurysmal changes.

TABLE 1: Key differences observed in various observational and registry-based studies regarding echocardiographic features seen in CTO patients in India and the rest of the global population.

ECHO parameters	Indian CTO population	Global CTO population
Mean LVEF	40–45%	47–55%
Presence of RWMA	High (~60–70%)	Moderate (~40–50%)
Modality of viability assessment	Low use (DSE only in a few centers)	High use (DSE, CMR, and PET)
Presence of diastolic dysfunction	Common; underreported	Systematically graded
Use of strain imaging (GLS)	Rarely used	Frequently used
LV Aneurysm or Thrombus	Seen in anterior infarcts	Rare due to early PCI
Use of CMR/nuclear imaging	Limited access	Routinely available
Pre-PCI Echo Guided Decisions	Often empirical	Imaging-guided (LVEF+ viability + GLS)

(CMR: cardiac magnetic resonance; CTO: chronic total occlusion; DSE: dobutamine stress echocardiography; ECHO: echocardiographic; GLS: global longitudinal strain; LV: left ventricular; LVEF: left ventricular ejection fraction; PCI: percutaneous coronary intervention; PET: positron emission tomography; RWMA: regional wall motion abnormality)

CORONARY ANGIOGRAPHIC FEATURES

In the Indian population, CTOs are predominantly found in LAD (48.1%), followed by RCA (42.9%) and LCX (25.2%) arterial distribution.[13] Compared with Indian data, in the OPEN-CTO registry majority of lesions were de-novo (89.3%), in RCA (61.5%), with almost half of them being complex CTO, as defined by a J-CTO score >2. The mean occlusion length was 29 mm, and calcification was present in 33% of lesions.[17] In the RECHARGE-CTO registry, the most common vessels involved were RCA (61%), followed by LAD (23%), LCX (16%), and LM coronary artery (0.3%).[15]

CHRONIC TOTAL OCCLUSION SCORES

Chronic total occlusion scoring systems were created to predict the result of the procedure. Procedures with a higher CTO score are technically more complex and have with lower success rate.[21] As the first scoring system, the J-CTO score was proposed in 2006. The system was designed to predict the possibility of CTO antegrade crossing with a wire within 30 minutes.[11] Since 2006, coronary intervention techniques have changed, and the J-CTO scoring system has been criticized for containing subjective and biased factors. Several attempts have been made to create a better scoring system. Nevertheless, the prognostic value of the J-CTO score remains high, which is also confirmed by various studies. J-CTO score contains mainly factors that cannot in themselves worsen the patient's prognosis (CTO stump, occluded segment length, occluded artery tortuosity, previous PCI attempt), which could be the reason why it has less impact on long-term outcome than other scores.[21] At the same time, analyzing cases with PROGRESS-CTO score and CASTLE score, more complex patients had a statistically worse long-term prognosis. Some risk factors are included in several scoring systems, but some are unique.

PROGRESS-CTO score differs from others as it is based on four angiographic-only variables, among which there are collateral estimation and CTO localization in the left circumflex artery, which are not included in other scores. These two factors obviously make the procedure more difficult, and the long-term results worsen. In terms of the maximal number of points, the PROGRESS-CTO score has the smallest possible sum of points (only four), with patient apportionment being not as wide as in other scores. The CASTLE score differs as it contains as risk factors patient age and MI in the past as risk factors.[20] All four CTO scoring systems had moderate ability to predict procedural success. More complex CTO-PCI patients assessed by PROGRESS-CTO and CASTLE scores had worse all-cause survival in 6–7 years after a successful procedure, whereas J-CTO and Clinical and Lesion-related (CL) scores had no association with survival.[21]

The *weighted CTO (W-CTO) score* is a scoring model developed from 404 CTO cases in an Indian single-center study.[22] It specifically predicts the likelihood of antegrade wire crossing success during CTO-PCI. The total weighted score thus derived, with a maximum of 6.5 (W-CTO score), is then segregated into three levels of difficulty as per predefined criteria in methodology. The difficulty levels thus derived ascribe a low level of difficulty to 0–2, an intermediate level of difficulty to 2.5–4, and a high level of difficulty to >4 **(Table 2)**. The success rate of CTO-PCI was 98%, 74.2% and 42.5%, in low, intermediate, and high levels of difficulty W-CTO scores, respectively.[22]

Unlike the J-CTO score (equal points per factor), the W-CTO scoring system assigns statistical weights, reflecting the true predictive strength of each factor **(Table 3)**. As it is developed from an Indian population database, it remains more representative for South Asian lesion profiles, which often have more calcification, tortuosity, and diffuse disease. However, as the majority of the cases in the study were successfully revascularized by the antegrade strategy, this score focuses specifically on antegrade strategy success prediction rather than retrograde strategy outcomes.

■ PREDICTORS OF SUCCESS

A recent study from PGIMER, Chandigarh, reported CTO-PCI being attempted in 23.1% of CTO cases, with 74.6% success achieved using antegrade-only approaches.[13] Advanced age, male sex, increasing J-CTO score, and CTO in LCX distribution were found to be independently associated with poor procedural success of CTO-PCI.[13] Similarly, the overall success rate was 71.9% as reported by Mehta et al.[23] Presence of blunt stump, bridging collaterals, side branch at occlusion site, severe tortuosity, and multivessel disease had a significant impact on the short-term and intermediate-term procedural outcomes of CTO-PCI.[23]

A study from South India reported procedural success of 85.5%, with unsuccessful cases showing significantly higher MACE rates (36.7% vs. 8.9%) and greater residual symptoms, with predictors of failure including higher J-CTO scores, long and/or calcified lesions.[14] However, a successful wiring yields ~97% procedural success rates once the CTO segment is crossed.[23] On the contrary, according to a Canadian registry, only 30% of CTO patients underwent PCI, with NCDR (USA) figures being much lower (~3.2–4.8% of all PCI).[13] European data (Cardio-ARSIF registry) reports CTO-PCI procedural success to be ~75.7%, which is notably lower than non-CTO PCI (97.1%).[24]

In the PROGRESS-CTO registry, Western patients had more complex lesions, with higher

TABLE 2: Weighted CTO (W-CTO) score.

Parameter	Score	Weight (β coefficient)
Blunt stump	2	2.12
Lesion length >20 mm	1.5	1.71
Severe tortuosity	1	1.06
Heavy calcification	1	0.72
Collateral circulation (Rentrop grade <2)	1	Weighted according to grade

TABLE 3: Comparative analysis of commonly used scores for CTO-PCI.

Feature	W-CTO score	J-CTO score	PROGRESS-CTO score
Origin	India (*Asia Intervention*, 2022)	Japan (*Circ Cardiovasc Interv*, 2011)	USA (*JACC Cardiovasc Interv*, 2016)
Purpose	Predict antegrade guidewire crossing success	Predict guidewire crossing ≤30 min	Predict overall technical success (any approach)
Parameters	• Blunt stump • Lesion length >20 mm • Severe tortuosity • Heavy calcification • Collateral difficulty (weighted Rentrop grade)	• Blunt stump • Lesion length >20 mm • Severe tortuosity • Heavy calcification • Prior failed attempt	• Ambiguous proximal cap • No interventional collaterals • Lesion length >20 mm • Location in RCA
Scoring method	Weighted β-coefficients based on logistic regression	Equal weight (1 point each)	Equal weight (1 point each)
Score range	Variable (continuous)	0–5	0–4
Difficulty stratification	• Low (0–2) • Intermediate (2–4) • High (>4)	• Easy (0) • Intermediate (1) • Difficult (2) • Very Difficult (≥3)	• Low (0–1) • Intermediate (2) • High (≥3)
Population base	Indian cohort	Japanese cohort	North American multicenter
Special strengths	Adjusted for the actual statistical impact of each variable; tailored to Indian/South Asian lesions	Simple, widely used, validated internationally	Emphasizes collateral availability and vessel location
Limitations	Single-center derivation, limited retrograde applicability	Does not weigh variables by strength	Less predictive for antegrade-only cases
Success rates for low scores	~98%	~88–90%	~92–94%

J-CTO scores, calcification (53% vs 20.6%), tortuosity, and more use of retrograde or antegrade dissection re-entry (ADR) techniques, whereas non-North American centers (including some of the Asian centers) leaned more on antegrade strategies for procedural success.[16]

In the RECHARGE-CTO registry, success was achieved in 1,075 of 1,253 procedures (86%). Patients in whom CTO-PCI failed had a significantly higher frequency of prior MI (48% vs. 38%; $p = 0.011$), prior coronary artery bypass graft surgery (35% vs. 15%; $p < 0.001$), and prior CABG on the CTO target vessel (25% vs.11%; $p < 0.001$).[15] Patients with negative angiographic characteristics (blunt cap, lesion length ≥20 mm, tortuosity ≥45°, presence of calcification, proximal cap ambiguity, proximal cap side branch ≥2 mm, lack of interventional collaterals, and diseased distal landing zone) were associated with high failure rates. More patients in the failure group were included for a second or third attempt (27% vs. 21%). The high prevalence of negative angiographic characteristics corresponded to a significantly higher J-CTO lesion complexity score in the failure group compared with the successful group (3.0 ± 1.1 vs. 2.0 ± 1.2; $p < 0.001$). The average PROGRESS-CTO score was significantly higher in the failure group (1.6 ± 1.0 vs. 1.0 ± 1.0; $p < 0.001$).[15]

TREATMENT APPROACH IN THE INDIAN SUBSET

Indian patients often opt for PCI over CABG due to surgical waitlists, economic considerations, and angina burden, leading to a CTO-PCI rate of 23.1% of detected CTOs, significantly higher than US data (~3–5%) but aligned with Canadian rates (~30%).[13] Indian centers predominantly use antegrade wire escalation, with modest success rates (~74–85%), with the retrograde approach being used <1% of CTO-PCI cases as compared to Japanese centers (30).[25]

Contrastingly, in Japanese or Western centers, where a retrograde or hybrid approach is more common, the success rates have improved to 86–90%.[13] Utilization, availability, and technical advancement adoption, such as intravascular ultrasound (IVUS)-guided subintimal tracking or stingray/cross-boss techniques, is low in the Indian subset. Only ~1% of all PCI procedures used IVUS in one public hospital study.[26] In India, intravascular imaging (IVUS/OCT) is limited to a minority of high-volume public and private sector hospitals. Owing to the additional financial burden, microcatheters are also used less frequently when compared to the global practice, for example, only ~66% microcatheter use in published Indian data.[27] STEMI reperfusion rates are low in many of the Indian states, with only ~53,416 primary PCIs against 3 million STEMIs reported. Resource-diverse practices across rural and urban areas affect treatment strategies and patient presentation profiles.[27]

CHRONIC TOTAL OCCLUSION-PERCUTANEOUS CORONARY INTERVENTION COMPLICATION RATES

In the Indian population, direct complication rates related to CTO-PCI are often underreported.[25] However, unsuccessful PCIs in the Malabar study[14] were associated with significantly worse MACE and persistent symptoms. Meta-analysis shows CTO-PCI improves long-term outcomes (cardiac death, nonfatal MI, and target vessel revascularization) versus medical therapy alone.[28] European populations have low (~2–3%) CTO PCI complication rates, though in registries (OPEN-CTO), having high CTO complexity, in-hospital major adverse cardiovascular events (MACE), and coronary perforation rates reach up to 7% and ~8.8%, respectively.[29]

CONCLUSION

Recent advancements in the contemporary interventional tools, along with top-notch operator expertise, have significantly raised success rates, making these procedures more effective, predictable, and safe. Indians, by virtue of being overtly diabetic and obese, demonstrate an increasing incidence of significant calcium deposits as well as diffusely diseased distal vessel in patients having CTO lesions. Indian CTO patients tend to be younger with higher rates of diabetes and tobacco-related habits. In contrast, Western patients carry more comorbidities related to metabolic syndrome and prior interventions. The hybrid CTO-PCI algorithm is currently the basis of discussion and reference for CTO PCI worldwide.

REFERENCES

1. Tajti P, Burke MN, Karmpaliotis D, et al. Update in the percutaneous management of coronary chronic total occlusions. JACC Cardiovasc. Intern. 2018;11(7):615-25.

2. Harding SA, Wu EB, Lo S, et al. A new algorithm for crossing chronic total occlusions from the Asia Pacific chronic total occlusion club. JACC Cardiovasc Interv. 2017;10(21):2135-43.
3. Safley DM, House JA, Rutherford BD, et al. Success rates of percutaneous coronary intervention of chronic total occlusions and long-term survival in patients with diabetes mellitus. Diab Vasc Dis Res. 2006;3(1):45-51.
4. Fefer P, Knudtson ML, Cheema AN, et al. Current perspectives on coronary chronic total occlusions: the Canadian Multicenter Chronic Total Occlusions Registry. J Am Coll Cardiol. 2012;59(11):991-7.
5. Werner GS, Gitt AK, Zeymer U, et al. Chronic total coronary occlusions in patients with stable angina pectoris: impact on therapy and outcome in present day clinical practice. Clin Res Cardiol. 2009;98(7):435-41.
6. Christofferson RD, Lehmann KG, Martin GV, et al. Effect of chronic total coronary occlusion on treatment strategy. Am J Cardiol. 2005;959(9):1088-91.
7. Jeroudi OM, Alomar ME, Michael TT, et al. Prevalence and management of coronary chronic total occlusions in a tertiary veterans affairs hospital. Catheter Cardiovasc Interv. 2014;84(4):637-43.
8. Wu EB, Tsuchikane E, Lo S, et al. Chronic total occlusion wiring: A State-of-the-art guide from the Asia Pacific chronic total occlusion club. Heart Lung Circ. 2019;28(10):1490-500.
9. Surmely JF, Tsuchikane E, Katoh O, et al. New concept for CTO recanalization using controlled antegrade and retrograde subintimal tracking: the CART technique. J Invasive Cardiol. 2006;18(7):334-8.
10. Brilakis ES, Banerjee S, Karmpaliotis D, et al. Procedural outcomes of chronic total occlusion percutaneous coronary intervention: a report from the NCDR (National Cardiovascular Data Registry). JACC Cardiovasc. Interv. 2015;8(2):245-53.
11. Morino Y, Kimura T, Hayashi Y, et al. In-hospital outcomes of contemporary percutaneous coronary intervention in patients with chronic total occlusion insights from the J-CTO Registry (Multicenter CTO Registry in Japan). JACC Cardiovasc. Interv. 2010;3(2):143-51.
12. Kim BK, Shin S, Shin DH, et al. Clinical outcome of successful percutaneous coronary intervention for chronic total occlusion: results from the multicenter Korean Chronic Total Occlusion (K-CTO) registry. J Invasive Cardiol. 2014;26(6):255-9.
13. Vemuri KS, Sihag BK, Sharma Y, et al. Real world perspective of coronary chronic total occlusion in third world countries: A tertiary care centre study from northern India. Indian Heart J. 2021;73(2):156-60.
14. Deshmukh V, Phutane MV, Munde K, et al. Clinical profile of patients with chronically occluded coronary arteries: a single center study. Cardiol Res. 2018;9(5):279-83.
15. Maeremans J, Walsh S, Knaapen P, et al. The hybrid algorithm for treating chronic total occlusions in Europe: The RECHARGE Registry. J Am Coll Cardiol. 20165;68(18):1958-70.
16. Alexandrou M, Rempakos A, Mutlu D, et al. Geographic diversity in chronic total occlusion percutaneous coronary intervention: insights from the PROGRESS-CTO registry. J Invasive Cardiol. 2024;36(9).
17. Sapontis J, Salisbury AC, Yeh RW, et al. Early Procedural and Health Status Outcomes After Chronic Total Occlusion Angioplasty: A Report From the OPEN-CTO Registry (Outcomes, Patient Health Status, and Efficiency in Chronic Total Occlusion Hybrid Procedures). JACC Cardiovasc Interv. 2017;10(15):1523-34.
18. Umar HK, Murtaza RP, Shabir A, et al. The clinical and coronary angiographic profile of 601 older adult patients with acute coronary syndrome treated at a tertiary hospital in North India and complications of percutaneous coronary intervention with the 30-day mortality. J. Indian Acad Geriatr. 2020;16(4):139-44.
19. Vallabhajosyula S, Prasad A, Gulati R, et al. Contemporary prevalence, trends, and outcomes of coronary chronic total occlusions in acute myocardial infarction with cardiogenic shock. IJC Heart Vasc. 2019;24:100414.
20. Gawande GDR, Shaikh S, Bansal NO. Clinical and etiological profile of patients with chronically occluded coronary arteries (CTO): a single

center study from Mumbai. Indian Heart J. 2020;72(S1):S19-20.
21. Kalnins A, Strele I, Lejnieks A. Comparison among Different Scoring Systems in Predicting Procedural Success and Long-Term Outcomes after Percutaneous Coronary Intervention in Patients with Chronic Total Coronary Artery Occlusions. Medicina (Kaunas). 2019;55(8):494.
22. Khanna R, Pandey CM, Bedi S, et al. A weighted angiographic scoring model (W-CTO score) to predict success of antegrade wire crossing in chronic total occlusion: analysis from a single centre. AsiaIntervention. 2018;4(1):18-25.
23. Mehta AB, Mehta N, Chhabria R, et al. Predictors of success in percutaneous coronary intervention for chronic total occlusion. Indian Heart J. 2018;70 Suppl 3(Suppl 3):S269-74.
24. Boukantar M, Teiger E, Cardio-Arsif investigators. P3637Contemporary perspectives on coronary chronic total occlusion: data from a vast French registry (Cardio-ARSIF). Eur Heart J. 2018; 39(Suppl 1).
25. Vinayakumar D, Raikar MP, Mohanan KS. Percutaneous Coronary Interventions in Chronic Total Occlusion - Profile, Technique and Outcome-The Malabar Experience. J Saudi Heart Assoc. 2020;32(2):274-83.
26. Pillai AA, Ramasamy S, Jagadheesan KS, et al. Procedural and follow-up clinical outcomes after chronic total occlusion revascularization: data from an Indian public hospital. Indian Heart J. 2019;71(1):65-73.
27. Arramraju SK, Koganti S, Janapati R, et al. The report on the Indian coronary intervention data for the year 2017-National Interventional Council. Indian Heart J. 2019;71(2):146-8.
28. Khanra D, Mishra V, Jain B, et al. Percutaneous coronary intervention provided better long term results than optimal medical therapy alone in patients with chronic total occlusion: A meta-analysis. Indian Heart J. 2020;72(4): 225-31.
29. Konstantinidis NV, Werner GS, Deftereos S, et al. Temporal trends in chronic total occlusion interventions in Europe: 17 626 procedures from the European registry of chronic total occlusion. Circ Cardiovasc Interv. 2018;11(10): e006229.

CHAPTER 20

Drug-eluting Balloon: Coming of Age

Siddarth Varshney, Deepti Yadav, Tanu Chaudhary, Praveen Chandra

INTRODUCTION

Percutaneous coronary intervention (PCI) has undergone a remarkable transformation since the pioneering work of Andreas Grüntzig in 1977, when the first percutaneous transluminal coronary angioplasty (PTCA) was performed using a balloon catheter. While balloon angioplasty demonstrated that coronary atherosclerotic stenosis could be mechanically dilated, the procedure was limited by acute vessel recoil, abrupt closure, and high rates of restenosis approaching 30–40%.[1] This led to the development of bare-metal stents (BMS), which provided permanent scaffolding and significantly reduced the incidence of acute vessel occlusion. However, BMS were soon found to be plagued by neointimal hyperplasia and subsequent in-stent restenosis (ISR), requiring repeat interventions in a substantial proportion of patients.

The introduction of drug-eluting stents (DES) in the early 2000s represented a major advance, as the elution of antiproliferative drugs from stent platforms dramatically reduced ISR rates compared with BMS. Over successive generations, DES technology improved with thinner struts, more biocompatible polymers, and more predictable drug release, establishing DES as the standard of care in coronary revascularization. Nonetheless, challenges persisted: Late-stent thrombosis, the requirement for prolonged dual antiplatelet therapy (DAPT), limitations in small-vessel disease and bifurcation lesions, and the fundamental issue of permanent metallic caging within the vessel wall.

In this context, the drug-eluting balloon (DEB) emerged as an elegant alternative: A semi-compliant angioplasty balloon coated with an antiproliferative agent, capable of delivering a high local concentration of drug into the arterial wall during brief balloon inflation, but without leaving a permanent implant behind. Paclitaxel, due to its lipophilic properties and rapid tissue uptake, was the first drug to be successfully employed in DEBs. Initial randomized trials such as PEPCAD II ISR and ISAR-DESIRE 3 demonstrated the efficacy of DEBs in the treatment of ISR, establishing proof of concept.[2,3]

Over the past decade, the use of DEBs has expanded beyond ISR to include small-vessel disease (BELLO trial, BASKET-SMALL 2),[4,5] bifurcation lesions, and select de novo lesions. Real-world registry data and meta-analyses have further validated their role in contemporary PCI practice.[6,7] More recently, technological innovations have enabled the development of sirolimus-coated balloons (SCBs), overcoming earlier challenges related to drug transfer and providing more durable antiproliferative effects.

Reflecting this body of evidence, the 2023 European Society of Cardiology (ESC) guidelines on acute coronary syndromes (ACS) and European revascularization guidelines endorse DEBs as a Class I recommendation for ISR and as a reasonable option in small-vessel disease.[8] These endorsements signal that DEBs are no longer confined to niche applications, but have matured into a recognized and guideline-supported therapy in interventional cardiology.

Thus, the journey of PCI has come full circle: From plain old balloon angioplasty, to decades of reliance on metallic scaffolds, and back again to a balloon-based approach—now armed with modern pharmacology and refined technology. With growing trial evidence, registry data, and broader clinical experience, DEBs can rightfully be considered to be "coming of age".

EVIDENCE FOR DRUG-ELUTING BALLOONS

In-stent Restenosis: The Strongest Evidence Base

The earliest and most compelling data for DEBs comes from the treatment of ISR.

- *PEPCAD II ISR (2009):* This landmark randomized trial compared paclitaxel-coated balloon (PCB) angioplasty with paclitaxel-eluting stents in BMS restenosis. PCB significantly reduced late lumen loss (0.38 mm vs. 0.74 mm) and binary restenosis rates at 6 months.[2]
- *ISAR-DESIRE 3 (2013):* In patients with DES-ISR, PCB was noninferior to repeat paclitaxel-eluting stent implantation and superior to plain balloon angioplasty, with similar 12-month target lesion revascularization rates.[3]
- *RIBS IV and V (2014–2015):* These Spanish multicenter trials compared DEB with everolimus-eluting stents in BMS-ISR and DES-ISR. Both demonstrated similar efficacy between DEB and contemporary DES, although DES showed a slight angiographic advantage in DES-ISR.[9,10]
- *Meta-analyses:* Pooled data confirm that DEB is superior to POBA and comparable to repeat DES for both BMS-ISR and DES-ISR, with durable outcomes up to 3–5 years.[6,7]

Guidelines: The 2023 ESC guidelines for ACS and 2018 ESC/EACTS revascularization guidelines both assign DEB a Class I recommendation for ISR.[8,11]

Small-vessel Disease

Stenting in vessels <2.5–3.0 mm is associated with higher restenosis risk due to small luminal area and higher metal-to-artery ratio.

- *BELLO trial (2012):* The first randomized comparison of PCB versus everolimus-eluting stent in small coronary vessels. At 6 months, late lumen loss was lower with PCB (0.08 mm vs. 0.29 mm), with comparable major adverse cardiac events (MACE).[4]
- *BASKET-SMALL 2 (2018):* A large, pragmatic, noninferiority RCT of DEB versus DES in vessels <3.0 mm; at 12 months, MACE rates were identical (7.5% vs. 7.3%), establishing DEB as a valid alternative to DES.[5]
- *Registry data:* Long-term outcomes from the German SeQuent Please registry and others confirm low rates of restenosis and TLR in small vessels.[12]

Guidelines: DEB is recommended as an alternative to DES in small-vessel PCI, particularly when multiple stents or overlapping scaffolds should be avoided.

Bifurcation Lesions

Side branch treatment in bifurcations often risks stent protrusion and restenosis. DEBs, when used after adequate lesion preparation, can deliver drug effectively without leaving a stent.

- *PEPCAD-BIF (2013):* It showed feasibility of DEB in side branches, with lower restenosis than POBA.[13]
- Subsequent registries confirm safety and efficacy, although randomized data remain limited.

De Novo Lesions in Larger Vessels

The role of DEBs in de novo disease is under investigation.

- *DEB-AMI (2013):* Early studies in STEMI showed higher restenosis with DEB compared to DES, highlighting the importance of lesion preparation and careful selection.[14]
- *Recent SCB trials (2020–2023):* These show improved outcomes in de novo lesions, suggesting that next-generation balloons may expand indications.[15,16]
- Current data remain less robust than ISR/SVD, and DES is still preferred in most de novo lesions.

Peripheral Artery Disease

Drug-eluting balloons have also shown strong evidence in femoropopliteal lesions, where they reduce restenosis compared to plain balloon angioplasty. The IN.PACT SFA and LEVANT 2 trials established their role in lower-limb PAD.[17,18]

INDICATIONS FOR DRUG-ELUTING BALLOONS

The clinical applications of DEBs have evolved considerably since their first use in coronary interventions. While the initial indication was limited to ISR, subsequent randomized trials, registries, and guideline endorsements have expanded their role into small-vessel disease, bifurcations, and selected de novo lesions. Beyond the coronary circulation, DEBs also have established indications in peripheral artery disease (PAD).

Coronary In-stent Restenosis

- Primary and guideline-supported indication
- Both BMS-ISR and DES-ISR can be effectively treated with DEBs.
- Multiple randomized controlled trials (PEPCAD II ISR, ISAR-DESIRE 3, RIBS IV/V) and meta-analyses have established DEB as superior to plain balloon angioplasty and comparable to repeat DES implantation.[2,3,9,10]
- *Guidelines:* The ESC 2018 Revascularization Guidelines and 2023 ACS Guidelines recommend DEB as a Class I, Level A therapy for ISR.[8,11]

Small-vessel Disease

- Stenting in vessels <2.5–3.0 mm is challenging due to increased restenosis risk and greater metal burden.
- Trials such as BELLO and BASKET-SMALL 2 confirmed that DEBs are noninferior to contemporary DES, while avoiding additional stent layers.[4,5]
- *Guidelines:* ESC consensus documents acknowledge DEB as an attractive option in small-vessel PCI, particularly when stent implantation is undesirable or technically challenging.

Bifurcation Lesions (Side Branches)

- Side branch stenting often increases procedural complexity and restenosis risk.
- DEBs can be applied after adequate lesion preparation to deliver antiproliferative drug to the side branch, avoiding stent protrusion.
- PEPCAD-BIF trial and registries demonstrate feasibility and reduction in side branch restenosis compared with POBA.[13]
- Not yet a guideline Class I indication, but increasingly used in practice for side branch protection.

Ostial Lesions

- DEBs may be advantageous in de novo ostial disease, where precise stent placement is technically challenging and geographic miss frequently leads to restenosis.
- By avoiding the need for permanent scaffolding, DEBs minimize mechanical complications, though evidence remains largely observational and randomized data are awaited.

De Novo Lesions in Larger Vessels

- Initial data (DEB-AMI) showed inferior outcomes compared to DES, especially in ACS, likely due to inadequate lesion preparation.[14]
- With newer SCBs, outcomes in de novo lesions are improving.[16]
- *Current role:* Considered in patients at high bleeding risk (HBR) requiring shorter DAPT, in long diffuse disease, or where additional stents are undesirable (e.g., long overlapping lesions).
- *Guidelines:* Not yet universally endorsed for de novo large vessels—considered an emerging indication

Acute Coronary Syndromes

- Early studies using DEBs in STEMI had mixed results, with higher rates of restenosis compared to DES.[14]
- Recent registry data with sirolimus balloons show promising outcomes, particularly in NSTEMI patients at HBR.
- Still considered investigational in ACS, results are awaited of ongoing large-scale RCTs.

Peripheral Artery Disease

- DEBs have strong evidence in femoropopliteal disease.
- Trials such as IN.PACT SFA and LEVANT 2 confirmed superiority over plain balloon angioplasty in reducing restenosis and target lesion revascularization.[17,18]
- Endorsed in European and US PAD guidelines as a frontline therapy.

Special Populations

- *HBR:* Since DEBs do not require long-term DAPT, they are particularly advantageous in elderly, frail, or anticoagulated patients.[6]
- *Patients with diffuse ISR or multiple layers of stents:* DEB avoids additional metal layers, reducing risk of stent thrombosis and neoatherosclerosis.
- *Patients with tortuous or calcified vessels:* Where stent delivery is difficult, DEB offers a feasible treatment alternative.

■ TECHNICAL CONSIDERATIONS

Choice of Drug-coated Balloon

In India, there are many different drug-coated balloons (DCBs) available for treating coronary artery disease **(Table 1)**. Paclitaxel remains the most commonly used drug, with typical doses ranging from 2 to 3.5 µg/mm^2 on the balloon surface. The effectiveness of drug transfer depends heavily on the coating formulation and

TABLE 1: Drug-eluting balloons available in India.

Drug and device	Company	Additive	Dose (µg/mm^2)	Arterial tissue concentration
Paclitaxel				
Essential	iVascular	Undisclosed	3	212 pg/g after 15–30 minutes
Protégé	Blu Medical	Butyryl trihexyl citrate	3	NA
Prevail	Medtronic	Urea	3.5	NA
Sirolimus				
Selution	Med Alliance	Biodegradable polymer	1	NA
Magic Touch	Concept Medical	NA	1.28	140.6 ng/mg after 1 day
Mozec SEB	Meril Life Sciences	Solid nano particle	3	NA

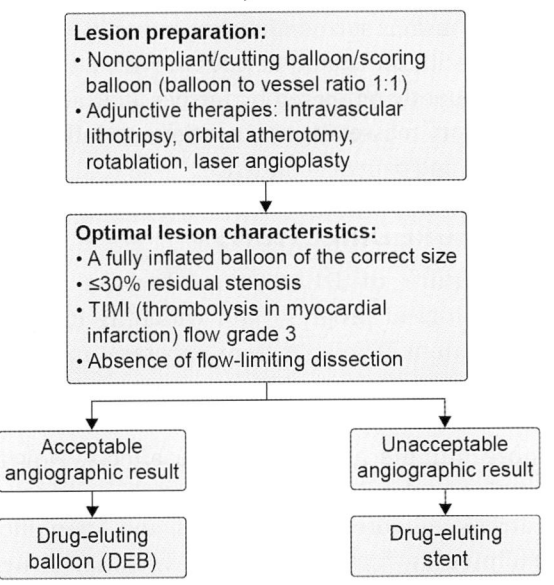

Flowchart 1: DEB strategy for PCI in coronary artery disease.

(PCI: percutaneous coronary intervention)

the technique used to apply it, which can lead to varying pharmacokinetic profiles.

Lesion Preparation

- *Uncomplicated lesions:* A semi- or non-compliant balloon with a balloon-to-artery ratio of 1:1 is recommended **(Flowchart 1)**.
- *Difficult cases:* If there are concerns about balloon delivery or vessel sizing, starting with a smaller balloon is advisable. Reassess the vessel size after administering vasodilators.
- *Balloon expansion failure:* High-pressure noncompliant balloons or cutting and scoring balloons should be used if a standard semicompliant balloon fails to expand.
- *ISR:* Aggressive predilation with high pressures is recommended to address severe stent underexpansion. Scoring balloons may improve outcomes in ISR and possibly de novo lesions.
- *Adjunctive therapies:* If balloon angioplasty is inadequate, consider rotablation, laser or orbital atherectomy, lithotripsy, or prolonged dilation to achieve optimal results before DCB intervention.

Optimal Balloon Angioplasty Result

- *Ensure the following before DCB delivery:*
  - A fully inflated balloon of the correct size
  - ≤30% residual stenosis
  - Thrombolysis in myocardial infarction (TIMI) flow grade 3
  - Absence of flow-limiting dissection
- *Angiography considerations:* It must exclude delayed contrast clearance from the vessel lumen, wall, and any dissection plane. Dissections of type A and B are usually safe post-balloon angioplasty. Type C dissections, however, should generally be treated with stent implantation, although recent data suggest some type C dissections may have good outcomes without significant neointimal hyperplasia.

Balloon Delivery Aids

- *Tools:* A guiding catheter with good support, a guide extension, a buddy wire, or deep guide engagement can facilitate balloon delivery.
- *Handling of DCBs:* Care is essential, as some DCB brands may shed drugs or carriers upon handling or contact with liquid. Each brand has specific instructions regarding maximum transit time and minimum inflation time to ensure proper drug delivery.

Drug-coated Balloon Application

- The DCB should cover the lesion and extend at least 2 mm proximally or distally beyond the lesion.
- Reinserting the same DCB after a failed delivery is generally not recommended by most manufacturers.

This comprehensive approach to lesion preparation and DCB application is aimed at optimizing outcomes and minimizing complications in interventional procedures.

LIMITATIONS OF DRUG-ELUTING BALLOONS

Despite their growing importance in contemporary PCI, DEBs continue to face several limitations when compared with DES. Their efficacy is critically dependent on meticulous lesion preparation, as residual stenosis, recoil, or flow-limiting dissections can markedly reduce drug transfer and increase restenosis risk, whereas DES maintain luminal patency through their metallic scaffold. Another inherent challenge is the lack of immediate scaffolding; since DEBs provide no mechanical support, bailout stenting is often required in cases of recoil or major dissection, undermining the "leave nothing behind" strategy that defines this technology.

Although robust randomized evidence exists for ISR and small-vessel disease, the data supporting DEB use in more complex settings—such as bifurcation lesions, large epicardial vessels, and ACS—remain primarily registry-based, with few large-scale, head-to-head comparisons against new-generation DES. Additionally, heterogeneity in drug-coating technologies complicates interpretation of outcomes across different trials and platforms. Early PCBs offered favorable drug uptake due to lipophilicity but raised safety concerns in PAD, while SCBs have shown encouraging results though with variability in coating methods and release kinetics.

Further challenges include less predictable outcomes in diffuse, calcified, or long lesions, where DES often provide superior results owing to their combination of sustained drug release and mechanical scaffolding. Limited geographic availability, cost concerns in certain healthcare systems, and the operator learning curve regarding lesion preparation, dissection management, and bailout strategies also restrict widespread adoption. Finally, ongoing apprehensions surrounding late mortality signals with paclitaxel-coated devices in PAD, although subsequently tempered by further analyses and regulatory reassessments, continue to influence clinical and patient confidence.

FUTURE DIRECTIONS

The future of DEBs is marked by rapid technological progress and widening clinical applications. The shift from paclitaxel to SCBs represents a pivotal advance, offering improved safety, a broader therapeutic index, and more durable antiproliferative effects. Novel coating technologies—including nanoparticle carriers, microreservoir systems, and lipophilic excipients—further enhance vascular drug transfer and retention. While DEBs are well established in ISR and small-vessel disease, ongoing research is expanding their use to de novo coronary lesions, bifurcation disease (particularly for side branch treatment), and ACS, where a stentless approach may reduce risks associated with late stent thrombosis and prolonged DAPT. In addition, hybrid strategies that combine DEBs with DES in selected complex anatomies could redefine lesion-specific therapy algorithms.

Beyond coronary interventions, DEBs are also gaining renewed interest in the peripheral vasculature, particularly with the emergence of sirolimus-based platforms supported by vessel preparation tools such as intravascular lithotripsy and atherectomy. Intravascular imaging modalities like OCT and IVUS are expected to play an increasing role in optimizing lesion preparation, confirming adequate vessel expansion, and ensuring effective drug delivery. Future innovations—including nanotechnology-based coatings, polymer-free matrices, and dual-drug delivery systems combining sirolimus with anti-inflammatory or antithrombotic agents—are poised to broaden therapeutic potential even further. Importantly, DEBs are uniquely suited to HBR patients requiring short-duration DAPT, where the "leave nothing behind" concept aligns directly with precision medicine. Collectively, these advances suggest that DEBs are evolving from a niche solution to a central pillar of contemporary PCI, heralding their true "coming of age".

CONCLUSION

Drug-eluting balloons have progressed from a specialized tool to a mature, guideline-supported modality within contemporary percutaneous coronary intervention. Their most robust evidence lies in the treatment of in-stent restenosis and small-vessel disease, where multiple randomized trials and long-term registries have demonstrated outcomes comparable to modern drug-eluting stents while avoiding the long-term limitations of permanent metallic scaffolding. The evolution from paclitaxel- to sirolimus-coated platforms has further enhanced safety and drug-delivery durability, strengthening their role across broader clinical scenarios. Nevertheless, the effectiveness of DEBs remains dependent on optimal lesion preparation, careful procedural technique, and appropriate patient selection, and evidence in complex lesions, bifurcations, large de novo disease, and acute coronary syndromes continues to develop. With ongoing technological refinement, integration of advanced imaging, and the increasing relevance of "leave-nothing-behind" strategies—particularly in high-bleeding-risk patients—DEBs are positioned to become an essential component of modern coronary intervention, underscoring their true arrival into clinical maturity.

REFERENCES

1. Gruentzig AR, King SB, Schlumpf M, et al. Long-term follow-up after percutaneous transluminal coronary angioplasty. The early Zurich experience. N Engl J Med. 1987;316:1127-32.
2. Unverdorben M, Vallbracht C, Cremers B, et al. Paclitaxel-Coated Balloon Catheter Versus Paclitaxel-Coated Stent for the Treatment of Coronary In-Stent Restenosis. Circulation. 2009; 119(23):2986-94.
3. Byrne RA, Neumann FJ, Mehilli J, et al. Paclitaxel-eluting balloons, paclitaxel-eluting stents, and balloon angioplasty in patients with restenosis after implantation of a drug-eluting stent (ISAR-DESIRE 3): a randomised, open-label trial. Lancet. 2013;381(9865):461-7.
4. Latib A, Colombo A, Castriota F, et al. A randomized multicenter study comparing a paclitaxel drug-eluting balloon with a paclitaxel-eluting stent in small coronary vessels: the BELLO (Balloon Elution and Late Loss Optimization) study. J Am Coll Cardiol. 2012;60(24):2473-80.
5. Jeger RV, Farah A, Ohlow MA, et al. Drug-coated balloons for small coronary artery disease (BASKET-SMALL 2): an open-label randomised non-inferiority trial. Lancet. 2018; 392(10150):849-56.
6. Refaat H, Arab M. Long term outcomes of drug-coated balloons versus drug-eluting stents in patients with small vessel coronary artery disease. Indian Heart J. 2025;77(4):267-74.
7. Rittger H, Waliszewski M, Brachmann J, et al. Long-Term Outcomes After Treatment With a Paclitaxel-Coated Balloon Versus Balloon Angioplasty: Insights From the PEPCAD-DES Study (Treatment of Drug-eluting Stent [DES] In-Stent Restenosis With SeQuent Please Paclitaxel-Coated Percutaneous Transluminal Coronary Angioplasty [PTCA] Catheter). JACC Cardiovasc Interv. 2015;8(13):1695-700.
8. Byrne RA, Rossello X, Coughlan JJ, et al. 2023 ESC Guidelines for the management of acute coronary syndromes. Eur Heart J. 2023;44(38):3720-826.
9. Alfonso F, Pérez-Vizcayno M, Cuesta J, et al. 3-Year Clinical Follow-Up of the RIBS IV Clinical Trial: A Prospective Randomized Study of Drug-Eluting Balloons Versus Everolimus-Eluting Stents in Patients With In-Stent Restenosis in Coronary Arteries Previously Treated With Drug-Eluting Stents. JAAC Cardiovasc Interv. 2018; 11(10):981-91.

10. Alfonso F, Pérez-Vizcayno MJ, Cárdenas A, et al. A randomized comparison of drug-eluting balloon versus everolimus-eluting stent in patients with bare-metal stent-in-stent restenosis: the RIBS V Clinical Trial (Restenosis Intra-stent of Bare Metal Stents: paclitaxel-eluting balloon vs. everolimus-eluting stent). J Am Coll Cardiol. 2014; 63(14):1378-86.
11. Neumann FJ, Sousa-Uva M, Ahlsson A, et al. 2018 ESC/EACTS Guidelines on myocardial revascularization. Eur Heart J. 2019;40(2):87-165.
12. Wöhrle J, Zadura M, Möbius-Winkler S, et al. SeQuentPlease World Wide Registry: clinical results of SeQuent please paclitaxel-coated balloon angioplasty in a large-scale, prospective registry study. J Am Coll Cardiol. 2012;60(18): 1733-8.
13. Kleber FX, Rittger H, Ludwig J, et al. Drug eluting balloons as stand alone procedure for coronary bifurcational lesions: results of the randomized multicenter PEPCAD-BIF trial. Clin Res Cardiol. 2016;105(7):613-21.
14. Belkacemi A, Agostoni P, Nathoe HM, et al. First results of the DEB-AMI (Drug Eluting Balloon in Acute ST-Segment Elevation Myocardial Infarction) trial: a multicenter randomized comparison of drug-eluting balloon plus bare-metal stent versus bare-metal stent versus drug-eluting stent in primary percutaneous coronary intervention with 6-month angiographic, intravascular, functional, and clinical outcomes. J Am Coll Cardiol. 2012;59:2327-37.
15. Ahmad WAW, Nuruddin AA, Abdul Kader MASK, et al. Treatment of Coronary De Novo Lesions by a Sirolimus- or Paclitaxel-Coated Balloon. JACC Cardiovasc Interv. 2022;15(7):770-9.
16. Massaro G, Maffi V, Russo D, et al. 'Leave Nothing Behind' Strategy in Coronary and Peripheral Artery Disease: An Insight into Sirolimus-Coated Balloons. EMJ Interventional Cardiol. 2022;10(1): 60-71.
17. Tepe G, Laird J, Schneider P, et al. Drug-coated balloon versus standard percutaneous transluminal angioplasty for the treatment of superficial femoral and popliteal peripheral artery disease: 12-month results from the IN.PACT SFA randomized trial. Circulation. 2015;131(5): 495-502.
18. Jaff MR, Rosenfield K, Scheinert D, et al. Drug-coated balloons to improve femoropopliteal artery patency: Rationale and design of the LEVANT 2 trial. Am Heart J. 2015;169(4):479-85.

CHAPTER 21

A Primary Approach Moving Toward Early Catheter Directed Interventions in Acute Pulmonary Embolism

Rajiv Parakh, Siddhartha Paturi

INTRODUCTION

Pulmonary embolism (PE) constitutes a critical cardiovascular emergency marked by pulmonary arterial obstruction from thrombotic material, predominantly originating from thrombosis in the lower extremities and pelvic venous systems. This condition represents a significant manifestation of venous thromboembolism (VTE), contributing substantially to global morbidity and mortality burden. Contemporary recognition and management of PE remain inadequate despite advances in diagnostic imaging and therapeutic options.

The management landscape for PE has undergone profound transformation in recent years. Traditional approaches centered exclusively on medical anticoagulation have evolved toward multimodal strategies incorporating early catheter-based interventions designed to restore hemodynamic stability and preserve right ventricular (RV) function. This treatment philosophy parallels the success of primary percutaneous coronary intervention (PCI) in acute myocardial infarction, where time-sensitive reperfusion salvages myocardial tissue. In PE management, analogous principles apply—early thrombus removal and hemodynamic restoration can prevent RV dysfunction progression and potentially reduce long-term sequelae.[1,2]

This current chapter explores the evolving epidemiology and pathophysiology of PE, contemporary diagnostic approaches, conventional management strategies, and the emerging evidence supporting early catheter laboratory-based interventions as either alternatives to or complementary approaches with medical therapy.

EPIDEMIOLOGY AND CLINICAL BURDEN

Pulmonary embolism ranks among the leading causes of cardiovascular mortality globally. Annual VTE incidence in developed nations approximates 1–2 cases per 1,000 individuals, with PE accounting for 30–40% of these events.[1] The consequences of diagnostic delay and inadequate treatment are severe—in-hospital PE mortality may exceed 30% when untreated, whereas appropriately managed PE reduces in-hospital mortality to approximately 8% or lower.[2]

Submassive and massive PE presentations carry particularly grave prognoses, frequently progressing to acute RV failure and cardiogenic shock. These presentations demand urgent intervention to prevent hemodynamic collapse and end-organ dysfunction **(Fig 1)**.

Key mechanisms include:
- *Vascular obstruction:* Direct thrombus-mediated blockade of pulmonary arterial vessels increases pulmonary vascular resistance and acutely elevates RV afterload.
- *Neurohumoral activation:* Endothelial and platelet activation releases vasoconstrictor substances including serotonin and thromboxane A2, further amplifying pulmonary vascular impedance beyond mechanical obstruction.

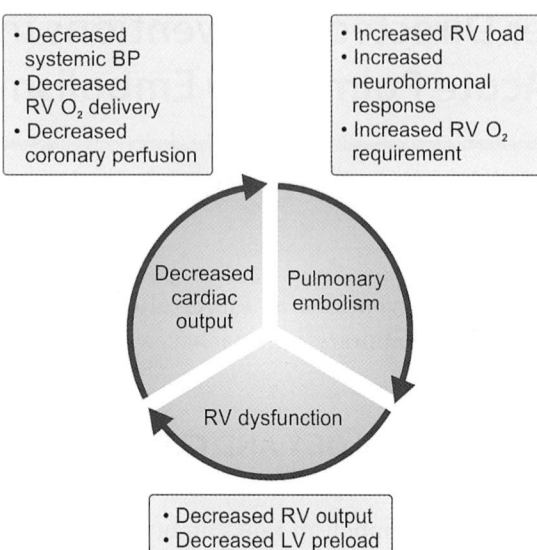

Fig. 1: Pulmonary embolism pathophysiology showing thrombus migration from deep veins to pulmonary arteries, RV strain, and impaired oxygenation. (BP: blood pressure; LV: left ventricular; RV: right ventricular)

- *Right ventricular dysfunction:* Sudden afterload elevation precipitates progressive RV dilation, interventricular septal deviation, and compromised left ventricular filling, ultimately reducing systemic cardiac output.
- *Oxygenation impairment:* Ventilation-perfusion mismatch develops distal to occluded vessels, producing characteristic hypoxemia and reduced arterial oxygen saturation.[1]

CLINICAL MANIFESTATIONS AND RISK STRATIFICATION

Clinical presentation of PE demonstrates substantial heterogeneity, ranging from asymptomatic peripheral emboli to rapidly fatal massive PE. Presentation severity depends on thrombus burden, location, and individual cardiopulmonary reserve capacity. Symptomatic patients commonly present with:

- Sudden-onset dyspnea
- Pleuritic or substernal chest pain
- Hemoptysis
- Syncope or presyncope
- Tachypnea and tachycardia.

RISK STRATIFICATION FRAMEWORK

Current guidelines stratify PE into risk categories to guide therapeutic decision-making. The European Society of Cardiology (ESC) and American Heart Association (AHA) recommend three-tiered classification:[1]

- *Risk stratification is essential for guiding therapy. The ESC divides PE into:*
  - *High risk (massive):* With shock or persistent hypotension.
  - *Intermediate risk (submassive):* RV dysfunction or myocardial injury without hypotension
  - *Low risk:* Hemodynamically stable with no RV strain. Risk assessment tools
- *Systematic risk assessment includes:*
  - Cardiac biomarkers (high-sensitivity troponin and brain natriuretic peptide)
  - Imaging markers (RV/LV diameter ratio >0.9 on computed tomography or echocardiography).

DIAGNOSTIC EVALUATION

Early and accurate diagnosis is critical in effective PE management.

Diagnostic Modalities

- *D-dimer:* This fibrin degradation product demonstrates high sensitivity and effectively excludes VTE when negative in low-risk populations, though limited specificity restricts use as a definitive diagnostic test.
- *Computed tomography pulmonary angiography (CTPA):* Currently, it serves as the reference diagnostic standard, permitting precise identification of thrombus location, distribution assessment, and evaluation of associated complications.

- *Echocardiography:* Particularly valuable in hemodynamically unstable patients, providing real-time visualization of RV structure, function, and septal position. Echocardiography enables rapid risk stratification in clinical emergencies.
- *Venous ultrasound:* It confirms deep venous thrombosis and identifies potential thrombus source when present in lower extremities.
- *Point-of-care ultrasound (POCUS):* Increasingly integrated into emergency department protocols to expedite diagnostic evaluation, particularly in hemodynamically unstable presentations where diagnostic delays risk further deterioration.[1]

CONVENTIONAL MANAGEMENT APPROACHES

- *Anticoagulation:* Unfractionated heparin, low-molecular-weight heparin derivatives, and direct oral anticoagulants constitute the foundational therapy for PE management, preventing thrombus propagation and reducing recurrence risk.
- *Systemic fibrinolytic therapy:* Reserved for hemodynamically unstable massive PE, systemic thrombolytic administration achieves rapid clot dissolution but carries substantial morbidity. Major hemorrhagic complications occur in 6–20% of treated patients, with intracranial hemorrhage occurring in 1–3% of cases.[3]
- *Surgical embolectomy:* Indicated for patients with absolute contraindications to thrombolytic therapy or documented failure of medical/catheter-based interventions, surgical embolectomy provides definitive clot removal but requires operative capability and carries inherent surgical risks.
- *Mechanical circulatory support:* Extracorporeal membrane oxygenation (ECMO) provides rescue cardiopulmonary support for patients experiencing cardiogenic shock refractory to medical and interventional therapies, serving as a bridge to recovery or definitive intervention.

RATIONALE FOR EARLY CATHETER-BASED INTERVENTIONS

Accumulating clinical evidence and outcomes data have motivated systematic reconsideration of catheter-based intervention roles in PE management. The conceptual foundation rests on several key observations:

- *Rapid hemodynamic restoration:* Similar to acute coronary syndromes, PE outcomes improve substantially with early reperfusion. Rapid thrombus removal limits progressive RV dilation, prevents myocardial ischemic injury, and potentially reduces chronic thromboembolic pulmonary hypertension (CTEPH) sequelae.
- *Targeted therapeutic delivery:* Catheter-directed approaches enable concentrated therapy at the thrombus site, permitting substantial dose reduction and decreased systemic medication exposure compared to full-dose systemic fibrinolysis, thereby reducing bleeding complications in vulnerable populations.
- *Restoration of RV function:* Beyond hemodynamic stabilization, catheter-based interventions aim to restore RV function, improve pulmonary perfusion, and prevent long-term cardiopulmonary dysfunction.

CATHETER-BASED THERAPEUTIC INTERVENTIONS

A Catheter-directed Thrombolysis

Catheter-directed thrombolysis (CDT) represents a localized therapeutic strategy wherein thrombolytic medications are delivered directly into pulmonary arterial thrombus through specialized infusion catheters. This targeted approach fundamentally differs from systemic administration by concentrating fibrinolytic activity at the obstruction site.

Technical Approach

The procedure begins with femoral venous access (typically under ultrasound guidance), followed by advancement of multiside hole infusion catheters into main or lobar pulmonary arteries under fluoroscopic visualization. Catheters are positioned to interface with thrombus burden, permitting direct medication delivery. Recombinant tissue plasminogen activator (alteplase) or urokinase undergoes infusion at controlled rates over 12-24 hours.

The localized delivery approach permits substantial dose reduction. Whereas systemic PE protocols employ 50-100 mg alteplase, CDT protocols typically utilize 8-24 mg total. This dose reduction correlates with reduced bleeding complications while maintaining therapeutic efficacy through concentrated drug concentration at the target site.

Ultrasound-accelerated Catheter-directed Thrombolysis

A significant technological advancement incorporates high-frequency, low-intensity ultrasonic energy to enhance fibrinolytic activity. The EKOS Endovascular System exemplifies this approach, integrating an ultrasonic transducer core within the infusion catheter generating acoustic pressure waves at 2.2 MHz frequency.

Ultrasound enhancement operates through multiple mechanisms—acoustic energy creates microstreaming within thrombus, facilitating deeper penetration of thrombolytic agents; ultrasonic vibration reversibly disrupts fibrin network architecture, exposing additional plasminogen receptor sites; and mechanical disruption accelerates enzymatic clot dissolution. Laboratory studies demonstrate that ultrasound-assisted delivery achieves approximately 48% greater medication absorption within 1 hour and 84% enhancement by 2 hours relative to standard infusion alone.[4,5]

Clinical implementation typically involves bilateral catheter placement spanning treatment zones of 6-50 cm. Continuous cooled saline perfusion prevents thermal injury from the ultrasound generator. This combined approach enables effective thrombolysis using modest total doses (typically 12-24 mg alteplase over 12-15 hours).

Clinical Advantages

Catheter-directed approaches confer several advantages over systemic thrombolysis. Substantially reduced lytic medication dosing correlates with intracranial hemorrhage rates below 1% compared to 2-3% with systemic administration.[6] Hemodynamic and RV functional improvements typically manifest within 24-48 hours of intervention initiation.

However, CDT implementation requires specialized equipment, experienced operators, and continuous hemodynamic monitoring. Patients require serial coagulation parameter assessment (fibrinogen, prothrombin time, and platelet counts) every 4-6 hours during infusion **(Fig. 2)**.

MECHANICAL THROMBECTOMY

Mechanical thrombectomy devices physically remove or disrupt thrombus without reliance on fibrinolytic medications. This approach provides particular utility for patients with absolute fibrinolytic contraindications including recent intracranial surgery, active hemorrhage, or severe coagulopathy.

Large-bore Aspiration Systems

Contemporary mechanical thrombectomy platforms employ high-volume aspiration for

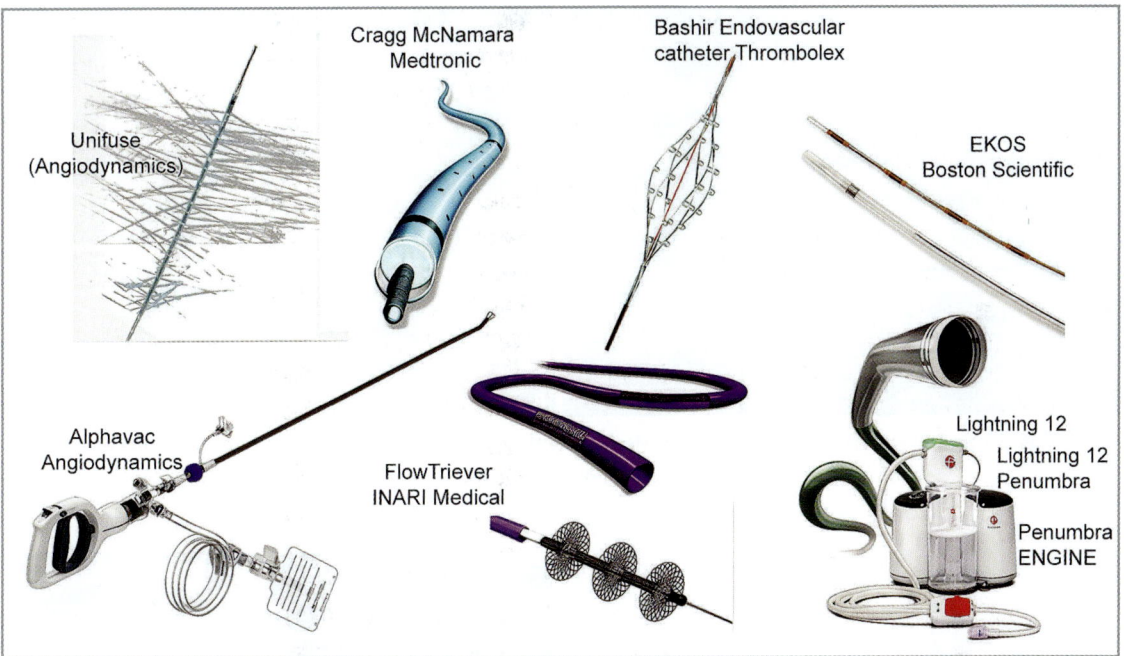

Fig. 2: The major mechanical thrombectomy and catheter-directed thrombolysis devices currently used in pulmonary embolism treatment.

direct clot extraction. The FlowTriever® system (Inari Medical) pioneered this approach, combining large-lumen aspiration guidance catheters (16–24 French) with self-expanding nitinol mesh retrieval disks and manual aspiration capabilities.

Procedurally, femoral venous access permits advancement of the aspiration guide catheter proximal to target thrombus under fluoroscopic guidance. Initial aspiration creates sustained negative pressure withdrawing thrombus into a collection reservoir. For organized or adherent clot, the FlowTriever® retrieval catheter extends distally, with three self-expanding nitinol disks deploying within and around thrombus. Operator retraction causes these mesh disks to engage clot mechanically, disrupting attachment to vessel walls while delivering fragmented material into the aspiration guide. This synchronized retraction-aspiration mechanism achieves substantial clot removal frequently in single passes **(Figs. 3A and B)**.[7]

Aspiration-based Mechanical Systems

The Penumbra Indigo System represents an alternative mechanical approach utilizing continuous negative pressure aspiration derived from neurovascular stroke intervention technology. The system comprises flexible aspiration catheters with large internal lumens (0.088–0.131 inches), an external pump unit generating sustained vacuum (-29 inHg), and separator devices facilitating thrombus clearance from catheter tips.

The newest Indigo Lightning Iteration incorporates microprocessor-controlled algorithms with dual pressure sensors enabling automated differentiation between thrombus and blood. When the catheter encounters clot, aspiration continues; in patent vascular flow, aspiration

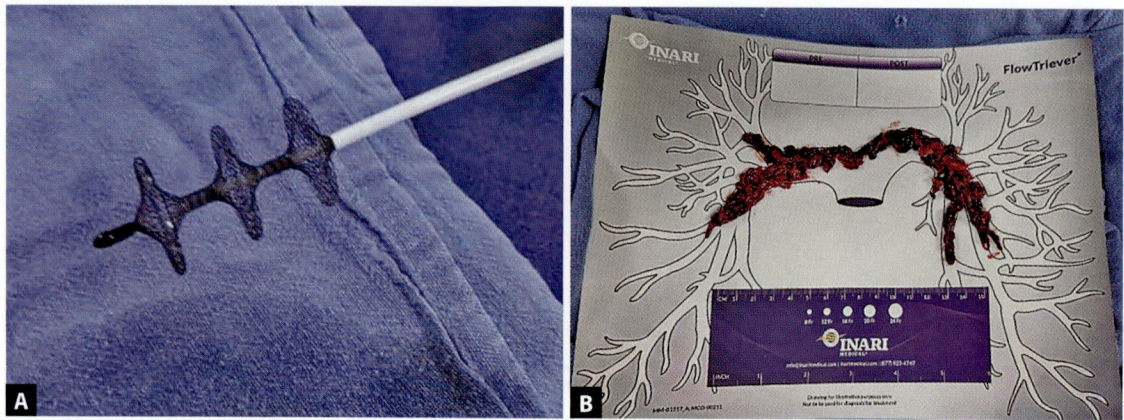

Figs. 3A and B: FlowTriever® system (Inari Medical) with self-expanding nitinol mesh retrieval disks and clot load retrieved.

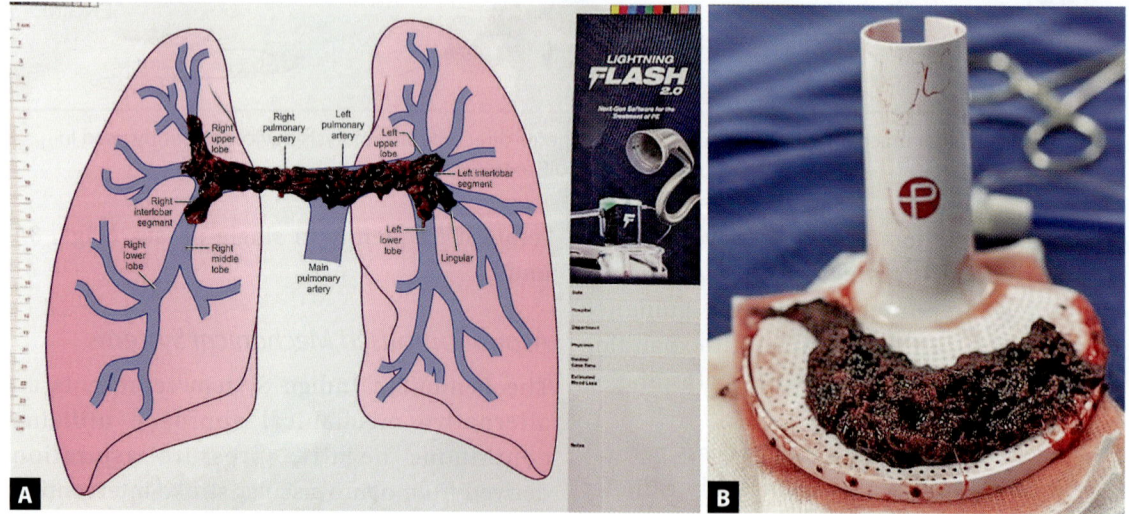

Figs. 4A and B: Clot burden aspirated using the Penumbra Indigo system.

switches to intermittent mode, substantially reducing blood extraction. Real-time audio and visual alerts notify operators to thrombus location, optimizing catheter positioning **(Figs. 4A and B)**.[8]

Comparative Mechanical Approach Features

Mechanical thrombectomy offers immediate clot removal with angiographic visualization of procedural success. Procedure duration ranges from approximately 37 minutes (Indigo) to 94 minutes (FlowTriever), substantially shorter than 12–24 hour CDT regimens.[7,8] Most patients experience rapid symptomatic improvement, with many avoiding intensive care unit admission.

Elimination of thrombolytic drug requirements eliminates associated bleeding risks in vulnerable populations including postoperative patients, those with recent trauma, or individuals with prior intracranial pathology. Published data indicate that 98-99% of patients treated with these devices avoid adjunctive fibrinolytic therapy.[7,8]

Hybrid and Multimodal Strategies

Pharmacomechanical Approach

Contemporary practice increasingly combines pharmacological and mechanical techniques. One strategy involves brief initial thrombolytic infusion (2-4 hours) to "soften" organized thrombus, followed by mechanical extraction. This combined approach may optimize thrombus clearance relative to either technique independently while using minimal lytic medication (4-8 mg alteplase total).

Treatment Selection Algorithms

Institutional protocols increasingly define algorithmic treatment selection based on PE severity, thrombus characteristics, and individual patient factors. Intermediate-high-risk PE with substantial proximal thrombus and no bleeding contraindications may be managed with ultrasound-accelerated CDT as first-line therapy. Conversely, intermediate-high-risk patients with recent surgery or hemorrhagic risks receive primary mechanical thrombectomy. High risk massive PE typically necessitates immediate mechanical intervention for expedited hemodynamic stabilization, potentially supplemented by brief adjunctive fibrinolysis if bleeding risk permits.

Mechanical Circulatory Support

A minority of massive PE patients develop refractory cardiogenic shock despite reperfusion attempts, requiring temporary mechanical circulatory support to maintain systemic perfusion during RV recovery.

Extracorporeal Membrane Oxygenation

Venoarterial ECMO provides comprehensive cardiopulmonary support by draining venous blood, oxygenating it through an external membrane lung, and returning oxygenated blood to the arterial system. ECMO implementation typically involves femoral venoarterial cannulation with large-bore (19-23 French) catheters, with circuit flow (3-6 L/min) completely bypassing the failing RV and obstructed pulmonary circulation, immediately stabilizing hemodynamics.

Right Ventricular Assist Devices

Emerging devices like the Impella® RP provide isolated RV assistance by positioning the device across the tricuspid valve with inflow in the inferior vena cava and outflow in the pulmonary artery, actively propelling blood forward. This targeted RV unloading addresses primary pathophysiology while potentially avoiding certain ECMO-related complications, though PE experience remains limited to select specialized centers.

CLINICAL EVIDENCE FROM TRIALS AND REGISTRIES

ULTIMA Trial: Establishing Early Proof-of-concept

The Ultrasound Accelerated Thrombolysis of Pulmonary Embolism (ULTIMA) trial represented the first randomized controlled investigation specifically evaluating ultrasound-assisted CDT in intermediate-risk PE populations.

Study Design

ULTIMA compared ultrasound-facilitated CDT combined with anticoagulation versus anticoagulation monotherapy in patients with acute submassive PE. Participants demonstrated CT-confirmed PE, echocardiographic evidence of RV dysfunction (RV/LV diameter ratio 0.9), and hemodynamic stability. The trial enrolled 59 participants across multiple European centers, with 30 randomized to intervention and 29 to anticoagulation control.[6]

Treatment Protocol and Results

Intervention participants received bilateral placement of EKOS ultrasound-enabled infusion catheters positioned in main or lobar pulmonary arteries, receiving 10–20 mg recombinant tissue plasminogen activator administered over 15 hours with continuous ultrasound energy application.

Primary efficacy assessment evaluated RV/LV diameter ratio change from baseline to 24 hours. Ultrasound-assisted CDT produced significantly greater ratio reduction compared to anticoagulation alone, with treatment-group mean reduction of 0.30 ± 0.20 versus control-group reduction of 0.03 ± 0.20 (between-group difference 0.27; 95% CI 0.17–0.36; $p < 0.001$).[6]

Secondary outcomes revealed sustained improvement in RV/LV ratios at 90-day follow-up and functional status trends favoring intervention. Notably, no major bleeding occurred in either group during hospitalization.

SEATTLE II Study: Large-scale Validation

The Study of Endovascular System (EKOS) for Submassive and Massive Pulmonary Embolism (SEATTLE II) expanded the evidence base through prospective, single-arm, multicenter evaluation of ultrasound-facilitated CDT in both intermediate and high-risk PE populations.

SEATTLE II enrolled 150 participants across 22 U.S. institutions, including both submassive ($n = 119$) and massive PE ($n = 31$) patients. Participants required proximal PE confirmation via CT angiography and RV dilation (RV/LV diameter ratio ≥0.9 on baseline imaging).[9]

Participants received 24 mg tissue (EKOS) plasminogen activator administered via ultrasound system over 12–24 hours.

The overall cohort demonstrated substantial RV/LV ratio improvement, decreasing from baseline mean 1.55–48-hour mean 1.13 (mean reduction 0.42; 95% CI 0.35–0.49; $p < 0.0001$), representing 27% relative improvement.[9] Mean pulmonary artery systolic pressure declined from 51.4 to 36.9 mm Hg (28% reduction; $p < 0.0001$). Thrombus burden assessment via modified Miller Index decreased from 22.5 to 15.8 ($p < 0.0001$).

Subgroup analysis of 31 massive PE participants revealed particularly notable outcomes: all survived to 30-day follow-up, with RV/LV ratio reduction from baseline 1.79 to 1.20.

Major bleeding occurred within 72 hours in 15 patients (10%), with notably zero intracranial hemorrhage events. Single 30-day mortality occurred, unrelated to PE or intervention.[9] SEATTLE II's robust dataset substantially influenced clinical adoption of ultrasound-facilitated CDT.

EXTRACT-PE Trial: Mechanical Aspiration Effectiveness

The EXTRACT-PE investigation provided the first rigorous prospective evaluation of mechanical aspiration thrombectomy administered without concomitant fibrinolytic therapy.

This prospective, single-arm, multicenter investigational device exemption trial was conducted at 22 U.S. sites. The study enrolled 119 participants with symptomatic submassive PE diagnosed within 14 days, systolic blood pressure >90 mm Hg, and RV/LV diameter ratio >0.9.[8]

All participants underwent mechanical thrombectomy using the Penumbra Indigo Aspiration system. Median procedural time was 37 minutes (interquartile range 23.5–60 minutes). Only two participants (1.7%) required intraprocedural fibrinolytic supplementation, demonstrating that aspiration thrombectomy alone achieved adequate results in 98.3% of the cohort.[8]

Primary efficacy endpoint demonstrated mean RV/LV ratio reduction of 0.43 (95% CI 0.38–0.47; $p < 0.0001$), corresponding to 27.3% relative decrease. Major adverse events occurred in only two patients (1.7%), with major bleeding in 1.7% and device-related death in 0.8%.[8] These outcomes led to FDA clearance of the Indigo Aspiration System in December 2019.

FLARE Trial: Large-bore Thrombectomy Validation

The FlowTriever Pulmonary Embolectomy Clinical Study (FLARE) was a prospective, multicenter investigation enrolling 106 participants at 18 U.S. sites. All participants underwent thrombectomy using the FlowTriever system combining large-bore aspiration with mechanical clot retrieval via self-expanding nitinol mesh disks.[7]

Procedural metrics demonstrated mean duration of 94 minutes, with mean intensive care unit stay of 1.5 days and 41.3% requiring no ICU admission. Only 1.9% received adjunctive fibrinolytic therapy.[7]

Primary efficacy endpoint showed mean RV/LV ratio reduction of 0.38 (25.1% decrease; $p < 0.0001$). Major adverse events occurred in four participants (3.8%), with 1% major bleeding and 1% mortality unrelated to PE intervention.[7]

FLASH Registry: Real-world Evidence

The FlowTriever All-Comer Registry (FLASH) provided extensive real-world clinical evidence, enrolling 800 participants across the United States and Europe. The population encompassed 76.7% intermediate–high-risk PE, 7.9% high-risk PE, and 32.1% with fibrinolytic contraindications.[10]

Intraprocedural hemodynamic assessment revealed mean pulmonary artery pressure reduction of 7.6 mm Hg (23% reduction; $p < 0.0001$). At 48-hour follow-up, RV/LV ratio decreased from baseline 1.23Â ± 0.36 to 0.98Â ± 0.31 ($p < 0.0001$). Severe dyspnea declined from 66.5% at baseline to 15.6% at follow-up ($p < 0.0001$).[10]

Major adverse events occurred in only 1.8% of participants. All-cause mortality measured 0.3% at 48 hours and 0.8% at 30-day follow-up, with zero device-related deaths reported. Notably, 62.6% of participants required no overnight intensive care unit admission.[10]

PEITHO Trial: Risk-benefit of Systemic Thrombolysis

The Pulmonary Embolism Thrombolysis (PEITHO) trial was a multicenter, double-blind, placebo-controlled randomized investigation conducted at 76 sites across 13 countries, enrolling 1,006 participants with intermediate-risk PE. Participants received either single-bolus tenecteplase (30–50 mg) plus anticoagulation or placebo plus anticoagulation.[3]

Primary efficacy endpoint (death or hemodynamic decompensation within 7 days) occurred in 2.6% receiving tenecteplase versus 5.6% receiving placebo ($p = 0.02$), demonstrating efficacy in reducing acute deterioration.[3]

However, treatment-associated bleeding complications proved substantial—major extracranial bleeding occurred in 6.3% versus 1.2% of tenecteplase versus placebo recipients ($p < 0.001$), and intracranial hemorrhage in 2.0% versus 0.2% ($p = 0.003$).[3] PEITHO crystallized the fundamental therapeutic dilemma, whereas systemic fibrinolysis prevents hemodynamic deterioration, it carries unacceptable bleeding risk in substantial patient subsets, thereby motivating investigation of alternative catheter-based approaches.

PEERLESS Trial: Comparative Intervention Analysis

The PEERLESS trial represented the first randomized controlled investigation directly comparing two catheter-based interventional strategies. This prospective, multicenter trial enrolled 550 participants with intermediate-risk PE, randomized 1:1 to FlowTriever mechanical thrombectomy versus CDT.[9]

Primary endpoint employed hierarchical win ratio methodology assessing mortality, intracranial hemorrhage, major bleeding, clinical deterioration requiring rescue therapy, and intensive care unit resource utilization. Mechanical thrombectomy demonstrated superiority with win ratio of 5.01 (95% CI 3.68–6.97), driven primarily by threefold reduction in clinical deterioration events, substantially decreased ICU resource requirements, and shortened hospitalization duration with lower 30-day readmission rates.[11]

No significant differences emerged in mortality, intracranial hemorrhage, or major bleeding between intervention strategies, with both achieving mortality rates below 1%.[11]

STORM-PE Trial: A Landmark Randomized Controlled Trial

The trial enrolled 100 patients across 22 international sites with acute intermediate–high-risk PE (symptom onset ≤14 days, proximal thrombus on CT angiography, RV/LV ratio ≥1.0, and elevated cardiac biomarkers). Patients were randomized 1:1 to receive either anticoagulation plus computer-assisted vacuum thrombectomy (CAVT) using the Penumbra Lightning Flash system or anticoagulation alone. Primary Results (48-hour primary endpoint):

- *Significantly greater RV/LV ratio reduction:* Mean reduction of 0.52 with CAVT versus 0.24 with anticoagulation alone ($p < 0.001$)—a 2.3-fold improvement in right heart recovery
- *Higher proportion achieving RV normalization:* Nearly 80% of CAVT-treated patients achieved RV/LV ratio decrease >0.2 versus 52% on anticoagulation alone ($p = 0.001$).
- *Faster thrombus burden reduction:* 2.7-fold greater reduction in modified Miller score with CAVT (42.1% vs. 15.6% relative reduction).

The STORM-PE findings represent a paradigm shift in PE management, supporting the evolution from mechanical thrombectomy as a rescue therapy to its consideration as upfront therapy for appropriately selected intermediate–high-risk patients.

CURRENT GUIDELINES AND RECOMMENDATIONS

- *According to 2024 ESC and 2023 AHA guidelines:* Catheter-based therapies receive Class IIa recommendation (reasonable to consider) for intermediate–high-risk PE with RV dysfunction and low bleeding risk.[1,12]
- *STORM-PE Trial Evidence (October 2025):* The landmark STORM-PE randomized controlled trial, presented at Transcatheter Cardiovascular Therapeutics (TCT) 2025 in October, provides the first level 1 prospective evidence supporting mechanical thrombectomy for acute intermediate-high-risk PE.

PULMONARY EMBOLISM RESPONSE TEAMS: INSTITUTIONAL COLLABORATION MODELS

The complexity of PE management spanning risk stratification, treatment selection across multiple modalities, and coordination among diverse subspecialties have driven institutional adoption of multidisciplinary pulmonary embolism response teams (PERT). These collaborative programs represent systematic approaches to optimizing care delivery for intermediate and high-risk PE through rapid expert consultation, shared decision-making, and coordinated resource mobilization.

The Genesis and Rationale of PERT Programs

The PERT model emerged from recognition that optimal PE management requires integrated expertise from cardiology, interventional radiology, vascular surgery, pulmonary/critical care medicine, hematology, and emergency medicine. The Massachusetts General Hospital established a pioneering PERT program in October 2012, creating a 24/7 rapid-response consultation service for complex PE evaluation. Since program inception, this institution has managed over 1,200 activations.[13,14]

Core program objectives encompass enabling rapid, standardized risk stratification; ensuring balanced treatment-option consideration through multidisciplinary input; facilitating immediate access to advanced therapies; and generating institutional databases for quality improvement and research.

Program Structure and Operations

Team Composition

Core PERT membership generally comprises vascular surgeons, cardiologists, interventional radiologists, cardiac surgeons, pulmonary/critical care specialists, and hematologists. Additional specialists may include emergency medicine, and pharmacy representatives. Programs designate a PERT director for administrative oversight with rotating on-call structures ensuring 24/7 availability.[13]

Activation Mechanisms

The PERT activation typically occurs via dedicated hotline accessible to any clinician managing a PE patient. Activation criteria generally include confirmed or suspected PE with high-risk features (hemodynamic instability, shock, and cardiac arrest) or intermediate-risk features (imaging evidence of RV dysfunction and elevated cardiac biomarkers). Upon activation, the on-call responder performs initial assessment and convenes the full team via group communication platforms.[13]

The PERT team meetings occur in real-time via telephone or video conference, permitting simultaneous specialist input. This parallel assessment structure accelerates decision-making from sequential consultations (typically hours) to integrated assessment (minutes). The team renders a unified recommendation based on collective expertise, then mobilizes necessary resources for indicated interventions.[13]

Risk Stratification and Treatment Algorithms

The PERT programs typically employ standardized risk stratification frameworks aligned with ESC and AHA guidelines, incorporating both PE severity classification and individual bleeding risk assessment.

Treatment Selection Algorithm

- *For high-risk massive PE:* Systemic thrombolysis if no contraindications, otherwise mechanical thrombectomy or surgical embolectomy; ECMO for refractory shock
- *For intermediate-high risk PE:* Consider catheter-directed low-dose thrombolysis if low bleeding risk and large proximal thrombus, or mechanical thrombectomy if bleeding contraindications
- *For lower-risk categories:* Therapeutic anticoagulation with close monitoring and early mobilization.

Clinical Impact

Accumulating evidence demonstrates that PERT implementation improves multiple PE care dimensions. Process improvements include increased biomarker testing (rising from 47%

to 80%; $p = 0.005$) and echocardiographic evaluation (from 55% to 97%; $p = 0.0001$) rates.[15] Comparative effectiveness research correlates PERT availability with reduced 30-day mortality, with greatest benefit in intermediate-high and high-risk cohorts.[15] Meta-analysis of 16 studies (3,827 PERT-era and 3,967 control patients) noted mortality reduction despite PERT cohorts demonstrating more acute presentations, with increased advanced therapy utilization but no increase in bleeding complications.[16]

National PERT Consortium

The success of pioneering PERT programs catalyzed broader adoption, culminating in National PERT Consortium formation in 2015. This collaborative network encompasses over 100 member institutions across six continents. The Consortium provides implementation guidance for nascent programs, maintains educational resources and protocols, operates the Consortium Registry (the largest international complex PE database), and advocates for PE care advancement at medical societies and guideline committees.[16,17]

Implementation Challenges and Future Evolution

Despite rapid dissemination, PERT programs encounter implementation barriers including substantial resource requirements (dedicated personnel, specialist availability, and catheterization laboratory access) and operational challenges in smaller or resource-limited institutions. Future PERT evolution will likely incorporate telemedicine for "virtual PERT" consultations extending expertise to underserved regions, artificial intelligence algorithms for automated risk assessment, and integration with regional acute coronary syndrome and stroke response networks.[18]

KNOWLEDGE GAPS AND RESEARCH NEEDS

Despite substantial progress, multiple knowledge gaps persist in PE management:

- *Patient selection criteria:* Ideal candidate characteristics for early catheter-based intervention remain incompletely defined, with ongoing controversy regarding optimal risk-benefit thresholds for intervention.
- *Intervention timing:* Optimal window for intervention and consequences of delayed presentation require clarification.
- *Resource accessibility:* High procedural costs and equipment requirements limit widespread access in resource-limited healthcare settings.
- *Operator expertise:* Catheter-based PE intervention requires specialized training and 24/7 catheterization laboratory availability, restricting implementation to centers with substantial interventional capabilities.
- *Long-term functional outcomes:* Limited randomized data directly compare catheter-based approaches with anticoagulation monotherapy regarding long-term functional status, CTEPH prevention, and quality of life.[19]

Emerging Research Directions

- *Device refinement:* Development of smaller-profile, safer thrombectomy systems designed for easier deployment in patients with anatomical constraints
- *Biomarker-guided intervention:* Integration of biomarker trajectories with imaging findings to tailor intervention timing, optimizing outcomes while minimizing complications
- *Artificial intelligence-assisted imaging:* Implementation of machine learning algorithms for automated high-risk PE identification and clinical deterioration prediction

- *Network expansion:* Continued PERT network growth with telemedicine-enabled decision support extending expertise beyond quaternary centers
- *Outcome validation:* Ongoing randomized trials (PEERLESS II, HI-PEITHO, and PE-TRACT) expected to define long-term outcome benefits of interventional approaches versus medical management.[20]

CONCLUSION

Pulmonary embolism remains a substantial global health challenge requiring timely recognition and appropriate therapeutic intervention. The evolution from conventional anticoagulation monotherapy to early catheter-based interventional approaches represents a significant paradigm shift in PE management, mirroring the transformative impact of primary PCI in acute myocardial infarction.

Successful PE management integration requires adoption of structured PERT systems enabling rapid multidisciplinary assessment, adherence to contemporary evidence-based guidelines, and continued research defining optimal interventional strategies. These elements collectively will shape PE care evolution prioritizing early intervention guided by risk assessment, multidisciplinary collaboration, and improved patient outcomes.

REFERENCES

1. Konstantinides SV, Meyer G, Becattini C, Bueno H, Geersing GJ, Harjola VP, et al. 2019 ESC Guidelines for the diagnosis and management of acute pulmonary embolism developed in collaboration with the European Respiratory Society (ERS). Eur Heart J. 2020;41(4):543-603.
2. Vyas V, Goyal A. Acute Pulmonary Embolism. In: StatPearls. Treasure Island (FL): StatPearls Publishing; 2024.
3. Meyer G, Vicaut E, Danays T, Agnelli G, Becattini C, Beyer-Westendorf J, et al. Fibrinolysis for patients with intermediate-risk pulmonary embolism. N Engl J Med. 2014;370(15):1402-11.
4. Owens CA. Ultrasound-enhanced thrombolysis: EKOS EndoWave infusion catheter system. Expert Rev Med Devices. 2008;5(5):567-75.
5. Ariëns RAS, Lai TS, Weisel JW, Duval C. Ultrasound-mediated catheter delivery of tissue plasminogen activator enhances thrombolysis through reversible modification of clot architecture. Haematologica. 2025;110(3):756-70.
6. Kucher N, Boekstegers P, Müller OJ, Kupatt C, Beyer-Westendorf J, Heitzer T, et al. Randomized, controlled trial of ultrasound-assisted catheter-directed thrombolysis for acute intermediate-risk pulmonary embolism. Circulation. 2014;129(4):479-86.
7. Tu T, Toma C, Tapson VF, Adams C, Jaber WA, Silver M, et al. A prospective, single-arm, multicenter trial of catheter-directed mechanical thrombectomy for intermediate-risk acute pulmonary embolism: the FLARE study. JACC Cardiovasc Interv. 2019;12(9):859-69.
8. Sista AK, Horowitz JM, Tapson VF, Rosenberg M, Elder MD, Schiro BJ, et al. Indigo aspiration system for treatment of pulmonary embolism: results of the EXTRACT-PE trial. JACC Cardiovasc Interv. 2021;14(3):319-29.
9. Piazza G, Hohlfelder B, Jaff MR, Ouriel K, Engelhardt TC, Sterling KM, et al. A prospective, single-arm, multicenter trial of ultrasound-facilitated, catheter-directed, low-dose fibrinolysis for acute massive and submassive pulmonary embolism: the SEATTLE II study. JACC Cardiovasc Interv. 2015;8(10):1382-92.
10. Toma C, Jaber WA, Weinberg MD, Bunte MC, Khandhar S, Stegman B, et al. Acute outcomes for the full US cohort of the FLASH mechanical thrombectomy registry in pulmonary embolism. EuroIntervention. 2023;18(13):1090-9.
11. Jaber WA, McDaniel MC, Moser KM. Primary results of the PEERLESS randomized controlled trial: large-bore mechanical thrombectomy versus catheter-directed thrombolysis for treatment of intermediate-risk pulmonary embolism. Circulation. 2025;151(5):381-91.
12. Jaff MR, McMurtry MS, Archer SL, Cushman M, Goldenberg N, Goldhaber SZ, et al. Management of massive and submassive pulmonary embolism,

iliofemoral deep vein thrombosis, and chronic thromboembolic pulmonary hypertension: a scientific statement from the American Heart Association. Circulation. 2011;123(16):1788-830.
13. Kabrhel C, Rosovsky R, Channick R, Jaff MR, Weinberg I, Sundt T, et al. A multidisciplinary pulmonary embolism response team: initial 30-month experience with a novel approach to delivery of care to patients with submassive and massive pulmonary embolism. Chest. 2016;150(2):384-93.
14. Provias T, Dudzinski DM, Jaff MR, Rosenfield K, Channick R, Baker J, et al. The Massachusetts General Hospital Pulmonary Embolism Response Team (MGH PERT): creation of a multidisciplinary program to improve care of patients with massive and submassive pulmonary embolism. Hosp Pract (1995). 2014;42(1):31-7.
15. Rosovsky R, Chang Y, Rosenfield K, Channick R, Jaff MR, Weinberg I, et al. Changes in treatment and outcomes after creation of a pulmonary embolism response team (PERT), a 10-year analysis. J Thromb Thrombolysis. 2019;47(1):31-40.
16. Hobohm L, Farmakis IT, Keller K, Scibior B, Mavromanoli AC, Sagoschen I, et al. Pulmonary embolism response team (PERT) implementation and its clinical value: a scoping review and meta-analysis. Clin Res Cardiol. 2023;112(2):172-86.
17. Rivera-Lebron B, McDaniel M, Ahrar K, Alrifai A, Dudzinski DM, Fanola C, et al. Diagnosis, treatment and follow up of acute pulmonary embolism: consensus practice from the PERT Consortium. Clin Appl Thromb Hemost. 2019;25:1076029619853037.
18. Secemsky E, Chang Y, Jain CC, Beckman JA, Giri J, Jaff MR, et al. Contemporary management and outcomes of patients with massive and submassive pulmonary embolism. Am J Med. 2018;131(12):1506-14.
19. Giri J, Sista AK, Weinberg I, Kearon C, Kumbhani DJ, Desai ND, et al. Interventional therapies for acute pulmonary embolism: current status and principles for the development of novel evidence: a scientific statement from the American Heart Association. Circulation. 2019;140(20):e774-801.
20. Gottlieb M, Bailitz J, Christian E. Epidemiology of pulmonary embolism diagnosis and outcomes in the emergency department. Am J Emerg Med. 2024;86:54-8.

Heart Transplant and Left Ventricular Assist Device: Chennai Experience

Jagadish A, Suresh Rao KG, Balakrishnan KR

INTRODUCTION AND CURRENT LANDSCAPE

The management of advanced heart failure has undergone significant transformation since the early 2020s. While heart transplantation remains the gold standard therapy for eligible patients with end-stage heart failure, the field has witnessed a paradigm shift with the increasing adoption of LVADs. These mechanical circulatory support systems now serve dual purposes as a bridge to transplantation for patients awaiting donor hearts and as destination therapy for those who are ineligible for transplantation.

According to the International Society for Heart and Lung Transplantation (ISHLT) registry data, approximately 5,000 heart transplants are performed annually worldwide.[1] In India, however, this number represents only a fraction of patients who could benefit from transplantation, as donor organ availability remains a critical limiting factor. The shortage of donor hearts has catalyzed the development and refinement of LVAD technology. Current survival statistics reflect remarkable improvements in both modalities. 1-year survival following heart transplantation now exceeds 90% at experienced centers, with 5-year survival rates approaching 80%.

Similarly, contemporary continuous-flow LVADs have dramatically improved outcomes compared to earlier generations of devices, with 1-year survival rates now exceeding 85% and 2-year rates approaching 80% in appropriately selected patients. Global trends indicate regional variations in the adoption of these therapies. While North America, Western Europe, and Australia have robust programs for both heart transplantation and LVAD therapy, middle-income countries are increasingly developing transplant capabilities and exploring more cost-effective LVAD solutions. Low-income regions continue to face significant challenges in implementing these advanced therapies due to infrastructure limitations and financial constraints.

EPIDEMIOLOGY OF ADVANCED HEART FAILURE

Advanced heart failure represents the final common pathway of numerous cardiovascular conditions and constitutes a growing public health concern. According to the American Heart Association (AHA) and American College of Cardiology (ACC) 2022 guidelines, approximately 6.2 million Americans are living with heart failure, with projections suggesting this number will increase to >8 million by 2030.[2] Of these, roughly 5–10% have advanced (Stage D) heart failure, the population most likely to benefit from heart transplantation or LVAD therapy.

Ischemic cardiomyopathy: Remains the leading cause (40–50%) of advanced heart failure requiring transplant or LVAD. Characterized by myocardial damage due to coronary artery disease and prior myocardial infarction.

Dilated cardiomyopathy: Accounts for approximately 30–40% of advanced heart failure cases. Includes idiopathic, familial, viral, alcohol-induced, and chemotherapy-related subtypes.

OTHER ETIOLOGIES

Hypertrophic cardiomyopathy, restrictive cardiomyopathy, congenital heart disease, valvular heart disease, and other rare conditions collectively represent 10–20% of cases.

Our Center Experience

In Tamil Nadu, the maximum number of heart transplants performed annually is around 90.[3] Our center independently conducts an average of 70 heart transplants each year, positioning us among the most experienced teams in both heart transplantation and LVAD implantation **(Table 1)**.

The demographic profile of patients with advanced heart failure has evolved significantly over the past decade. The median age of heart transplant recipients has increased from 54 years in 2010 to 58 years in 2022, reflecting broader acceptance of older candidates with good physiologic status. Similarly, LVAD recipients are increasingly older, with a median age now exceeding 60 years. Gender disparities persist, with men representing approximately 75% of both transplantation and LVAD recipients, despite heart failure affecting both sexes.

Comorbidity patterns have shifted in the contemporary era, with increasing prevalence of obesity, diabetes, renal dysfunction, and frailty among advanced heart failure patients. These comorbidities significantly impact eligibility for transplantation and LVAD therapy, as well as postintervention outcomes. Notably, pulmonary hypertension, previously a contraindication to heart transplantation, can now often be managed with pulmonary vasodilators or temporary mechanical circulatory support as a bridge to candidacy.

INDICATIONS AND PATIENT'S SELECTION

The determination of candidacy for heart transplantation versus LVAD therapy represents one of the most complex clinical decisions in cardiovascular medicine. The 2022 ACC/AHA/HFSA Guidelines for the Management of Heart Failure provide updated consensus recommendations for patient's selection, emphasizing a personalized approach that considers multiple factors beyond hemodynamic alone.

Perioperative Management of Heart Transplantation

Heart Transplant Candidacy

A subset of patients with chronic heart failure will progress to advanced disease despite maximally tolerated guideline directed medical and device therapies. The most common indications for heart transplantation are highly symptomatic heart failure, cardiogenic shock, or uncontrolled ventricular arrhythmias. Other less common etiologies encompass restrictive cardiomyopathies (RCMs), including hypertrophic cardiomyopathy (HCM) and complex CHD after surgical palliation has failed. The first essential step in evaluation is to determine if the patient's clinical situation is limited enough to warrant transplantation consideration, which requires confirmation that all attempts to optimize cardiac function—using

TABLE 1: Number of heart transplantation with diagnosis from our series in the last 5 years.

S. No.	Diagnosis	Count
1.	Ischemic cardiomyopathy	102
2.	Dilated cardiomyopathy	280
3.	Hypertrophic cardiomyopathy	13
4.	Congenital heart disease	36
5.	Post LVAD status	4
6.	Postpartum cardiomyopathy	2

OMT and interventions, such as CRT and transcatheter mitral valve repair, as indicated—have been exhausted. Measures to identify advanced heart failure include clinical indicators, CPET, right heart catheterization (RHC), and heart failure prognosis scores.

Markers of Advanced Heart Failure

Parameter description: "I NEED HELP".

I: Inotropes
Previous or ongoing requirement for dobutamine, milrinone, dopamine, or levosimendan

N: New York Heart Association class/Natriuretic peptides
Persisting NYHA class III or IV and/or persistently high BNP or NT-pro-BNP

E: End-organ dysfunction
Worsening renal or liver dysfunction in the setting of heart failure

E: Ejection fraction
Very low LVEF <20%

D: Defibrillator shocks
Recurrent appropriate defibrillator shocks

H: Hospitalizations
More than 1 hospitalization with heart failure in the last 12 months

E: Edema/Escalating diuretics
Persisting fluid overload and/or increasing diuretic requirement

L: Low blood pressure
Consistently low blood pressure with systolic <90–100 mm Hg

P: Prognostic medication
Inability to uptitrate (or need to decrease/cease) GDMP[1]

Contraindications to heart transplantation have evolved significantly, with many former absolute contraindications now considered relative. Active malignancy remains a contraindication, though patients with cancer in remission may be considered after an appropriate disease-free interval. Advanced age alone is no longer an absolute contraindication, with carefully selected patients in their 70s now receiving transplants at some centers. Irreversible pulmonary hypertension (pulmonary vascular resistance >5 Wood units unresponsive to vasodilators) remains a contraindication, as it significantly increases the risk of right heart failure after transplantation.

Special Considerations

Pediatric Patients

Heart transplantation remains the preferred strategy for end-stage heart failure in children, with excellent long-term outcomes. Size-matched donor hearts represent the primary limitation. LVAD options for pediatric patients have expanded, with the Berlin Heart EXCOR® specifically designed for children and increasing experience using adult continuous-flow devices in adolescents with appropriate body surface area.

Adult Congenital Heart Disease

The growing population of adults with congenital heart disease (ACHD) presents unique challenges for both transplantation and LVAD therapy. Complex anatomy may necessitate extensive reconstruction during transplantation or preclude standard LVAD implantation. These patients require evaluation at centers with specific expertise in ACHD and advanced heart failure.

Management

Most commonly encountered complications are as follows:
- Hemodynamic instability
- Transfusion and hemostatic disorders

- Immunosuppression
- Infectious complications
- Acute kidney injury and renal replacement therapy

Hemodynamic Profiles in Perioperative Period of Heart Transplantation

Cardiogenic shock can be present in various subtypes that can be broadly classified into the following:

- Preshock normotensive hypoperfusion
- Preshock hypotensive normoperfusion
- Left ventricle dominant shock
- Right ventricle dominant shock
- Biventricular shock

Determining type of shock is of vital importance in managing patients in the perioperative period, above-mentioned shock can be differentiated based upon the following parameters:

Systolic blood pressure (SBP), central venous pressures (CVP), pulmonary capillary wedge pressures (PCWP), CVP/PCWP ratio, pulmonary artery pulsatility index (PAPi), cardiac index (CI), systemic vascular resistance (SVR), cardiac power output (CPO).

In preshock normotensive hypoperfusion systolic blood pressure will be >90 mm Hg with variable CVP, PCWP, and CPO. One definitive parameter can diagnose this condition is cardiac index will be <2.2 (L/min/m^2). In case of preshock hypotensive normoperfusion systolic blood pressure will be <90 mm Hg with cardiac index ≥2.2. In left ventricular (LV) shock, PCWP will be >18, pulmonary artery pulsatility index (PAPi) >1.5. In predominant right ventricular failure shock central venous pressure will be >14, and PAPi <1.5.

Primary Graft Dysfunction[4]

Risk Factors

See **Table 2**.

Primary Graft Dysfunction (Left Ventricle vs. Right Ventricle)[4]

Classification of Left Ventricle Primary Graft Dysfunction

See **Flowchart 1**.

Indicators for Right Ventricle Primary Graft Dysfunction

- RAP >15 mm Hg
- PCWP <15 mm Hg
- Cardiac index <2.0 L/min/m^2
- Tricuspid pressure gradient <15 mm Hg

TABLE 2: Primary graft dysfunction—donor, recipient, and surgical procedural risk factors.

Donor risk factors	Recipient risk factors	Surgical procedural risk factors
• Age • Trauma • Cardiac dysfunction • Inotropic support • Diabetes mellitus • Hypertension	• Age • Weight • Mechanical support • Congenital heart disease • Redo surgery • Comorbidities renal or liver dysfunction • Pulmonary hypertension • Allosensitization • Infection • Retransplant	• Ischemia time • Donor—recipient sex mismatch • Noncardiac organ donation • Blood transfusion requirement

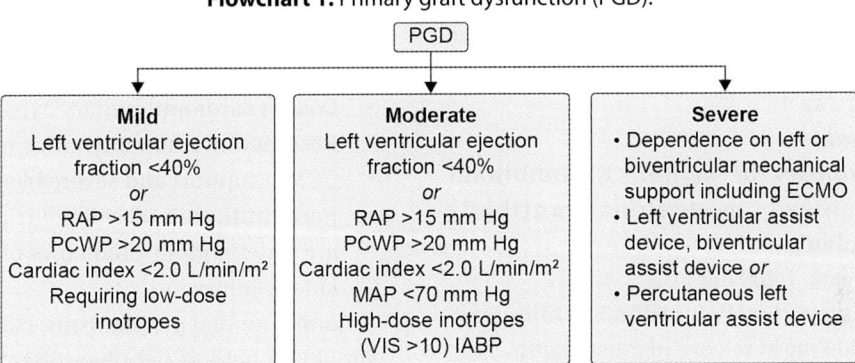

Flowchart 1: Primary graft dysfunction (PGD).

- Systolic PAP <50 mm Hg, or
- Need for right ventricular assist device

Management

- *Inotropic drugs and vasopressors* (including dobutamine, dopamine, milrinone, epinephrine, and norepinephrine) remain the first-line treatment for primary graft dysfunction.
- When cardiac output remains inadequate despite high doses of inotropes and/or vasopressors, the use of temporary mechanical circulatory support is needed to provide systemic perfusion and oxygenation, allowing the graft to recover and maintaining the other organs.
- For patients needing a temporary mechanical circulatory support, venoarterial ECMO seems to be associated with shorter assistance duration, lower incidence of major bleeding, lower incidence of renal failure requiring renal replacement therapy, and reduced mortality compared with patients supported with a continuous-flow external ventricular assist device.[4]
- Venoarterial ECMO implantation appears to be an efficient strategy for the management of severe primary graft dysfunction, in spite of a significant impact on long-term quality of life.

Perioperative Management of Immunosuppression

Induction Therapy

- The principle of an induction therapy is to induce a profound and rapid immunosuppression to lower the risk of rejection.
- Three approaches are widely used (sorted by the level of immunosuppression required):
  1. No induction therapy
  2. Nondepletive monoclonal induction using IL-2 receptor antagonists
  3. Polyclonal induction with antithymocyte globulins (T-cell depletion therapy)[4]
- No study ever proved a survival benefit of one strategy over another at the population level.
- The benefit–risk ratio of each approach should be discussed for every patient at the time of listing.

List of Drugs Used as Immunosuppressants

- *Antithymocyte globulin:*
  - *Mechanism of action:* Depletion of T cells (Polyclonal)
  - *Dose:* 1.25 mg/kg
  - *Administration:* Slow IV >4 hours
- *Basiliximab:*
  - *Mechanism of action:* Inhibition of IL-2 (monoclonal antibody)

- *Dose:* 20 mg
- *Administration:* IV bolus or 20–30 minutes infusion, 20 mg day of transplant, and 20 mg day-4
■ *Eculizumab:*
- *Mechanism of action:* Recombinant humanized monoclonal antibody C-inhibitor
- *Dose:* 900–1,200 mg
- *Administration:* IV infusion >35 minutes
  - 1,200 mg at release of cross clamp
  - 900 mg on day-1 then weekly for 3 weeks
  - 1,200 mg at weeks 4, 6, and 8
■ *Mycophenolate mofetil:*
- *Mechanism of action:* Inhibition of cell cycle
- *Dose:* 500–1,000 mg twice per day
- *Administration:* Oral or IV (over 2 hours)
■ *Tacrolimus:*
- *Mechanism of action:* Calcineurin inhibitor
- *Dose:* Oral—0.10–0.20 mg/kg/day, IV—0.01–0.05 mg/kg/day
- *Administration:* Oral—twice a day (every 12 hourly)
■ *IV immunoglobulin:*
- *Mechanism of action:* Primary humoral immunodeficiency, ITP
- *Dose:* 1–2 g/kg (maximum 80 kg)
- *Administration:* IV 4–6 hourly, total dose spread >2–4 days.

Acute Kidney Injury

- Early postoperative acute kidney injury is frequent in the first 7 days after heart transplantation, with an incidence between 40 and 76% according to kidney disease: Improving Global Outcomes classification.[5]
- Renal replacement therapy is required in 7–19% of patients.
- The preoperative factors independently associated with early acute kidney injury include:
  - Higher body mass index
  - Diabetes
  - Chronic kidney disease
  - Longer cardiopulmonary bypass time
  - Postoperative hemodynamic instability
  - ECMO support and severe bleeding
  - Early initiation of calcineurin inhibitors are independent predictors of early acute kidney injury.
- Among potential mechanisms, close attention should be paid to right heart hemodynamics, especially preoperative pulmonary hypertension, postoperative right ventricular failure, and renal congestion, which appears as a strong predictor of early acute kidney injury.
- There is no single pharmacologic treatment, heart transplant patients might benefit from early prediction and recognition of postoperative acute kidney injury and multimodal bundle implementation.
- Treating AKI in perioperative period includes postponing calcineurin inhibitors.
- Providing both left and right ventricle support (inotropes, pulmonary vasodilators, and circulatory support).

Infectious Complications

- A classic timeline describes three distinct periods of infection after solid organ transplantation:
  1. The postoperative period within the first month is characterized by nosocomial and donor-derived infections (cytomegalovirus, Epstein–Barr virus, or *Toxoplasma* species).
  2. The second period, up to 6 months after surgery, is characterized by opportunistic infections.
  3. After 6 months, community-acquired or rare infectious agents are expected.

Classification of Ventricular Assist Devices

VADs may be classified as first, second, or third generation. Third-generation devices use continuous flow centrifugal pumps. Examples include the HeartMate-3 LVAD and the HeartWare HVAD (Medtronic, Minneapolis, MN, USA). The HeartWare HVAD was withdrawn from the market in 2021 and currently the HeartMate-3 is the predominant device being implanted worldwide. The HeartMate-3 uses a magnetically driven, fully levitated, centrifugal pump. Compared with second-generation devices, the pump design of the HeartMate-3 minimizes friction and wear, and reduces the incidence of thrombotic and hemolytic complications.

Second-generation devices used continuous flow of axial pumps. Examples include the Jarvik-2000 (Jarvik Heart, Inc. New York, NY, USA) and the HeartMate-2.

While second-generation devices offered improved durability compared with first-generation VADs, thrombotic and hemolytic complications were common. Second-generation devices may still be encountered but are no longer being implanted. First-generation VADs used membrane pumps to generate pulsatile flow. First-generation devices were associated with high-complication rates and are no longer used **(Fig. 1)**.

Our Center Experience

See **Table 4**.

Left Ventricular Assist Device Candidacy

LVAD therapy is appropriate for patients with advanced heart failure who are either ineligible for transplantation or face extended waiting times. Contraindications include severe right ventricular failure unresponsive to medical therapy, severe

TABLE 3: Recommended drugs for common infectious agents.

Infectious agent	Recommended drugs
Pneumocystis jirovecii	Trimethoprim 80 mg/sulfamethoxazole 160 mg
Candida species (mucocutaneous infection)	Nystatin 4 times daily, clotrimazole lozenges after extubation
Skin flora	First or second generation cephalosporin
Cytomegalovirus	• High risk—valganciclovir 900 mg OD or ganciclovir 1,000 mg three times per day for 3 months • Intermediate risk—valganciclovir/ganciclovir for 3 months

- Among infectious agents, bacteria were the most frequently involved (>50%).
- Viruses were also frequent (30%).
- Fungal infection accounted for only 13–14% **(Table 3)**.

Perioperative Management of Left Ventricular Assist Device

The Ventricular Assist Device System

The various components of a VAD system consist of an inflow cannula in the LV apex drains blood to a pump. An outflow cannula (graft conduit) returns blood from the pump to the patient's ascending aorta. A driveline (percutaneous lead) connects the pump to a controller, providing power to the pump and transmitting information between the pump and the controller. The controller is connected to main power and an external battery pack. A touch screen monitor can be attached to the controller with different screens for viewing and changing the device settings and alarms, and for displaying trends. The driveline exits the patient's skin through the upper abdominal wall.

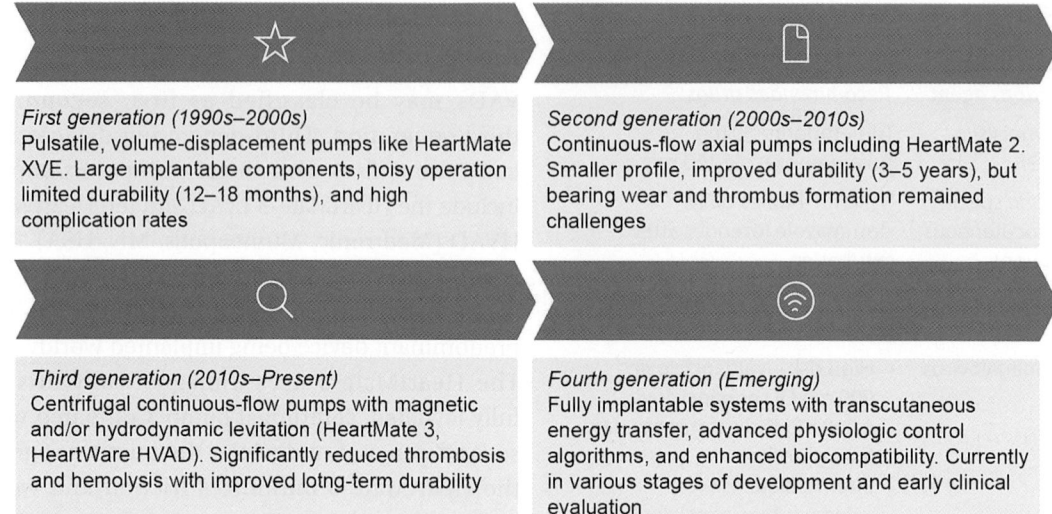

Fig. 1: Classification of ventricular assist devices (VADs).

TABLE 4: Our center experience.		
S. No	LVAD	Count
1.	HeartWare	23
2.	HeartMate-2	10
3.	HeartMate-3	21
4.	Berlin EXCOR BIVAD	1

TABLE 5: Bridging strategy in clinical scenarios.	
Bridging strategy	Clinical scenario
Bridge to decision	Acutely ill patients with uncertain recovery potential or transplant candidacy
Bridge to candidacy	Potentially reversible contraindications to transplant (e.g., pulmonary hypertension and recent malignancy)
Bridge to transplant	Eligible transplant candidates with high waiting list mortality risk
Bridge to recovery	Selected patients with potentially reversible cardiomyopathy (e.g., peripartum and myocarditis)

irreversible hepatic dysfunction, active systemic infection, severe coagulopathy, and inability to manage the device (with no available caregiver support). Psychosocial evaluation is particularly critical for LVAD candidates, as successful outcomes depend heavily on patient's adherence to a complex care regimen.

Bridging Strategies[6]

See **Table 5**.

Intraoperative Considerations

A review of patient's history and disease progression is essential. Optimization of therapy is key to a successful outcome. Assessment of fluid status and assessment of device compliance are important. A review of blood investigations, echocardiogram, pulmonary function testing, electrocardiogram/chest X-ray, and right heart catheter are mandatory. Appropriate fluid balance is important and if found in excess modifying diuretic therapy/fluid extraction by venovenous hemodialysis is mandatory. If extremely unstable usage of inotropes/intra-aortic balloon pump should be considered.

Consider full invasive monitoring. Use of a pulmonary artery catheter (PAC) is important. These patients invariably have an automated implantable circulatory device (AICD)/pacemaker in situ. The defibrillator if present needs to be turned off before surgery. Use of external defibrillator pads is prudent. Assessment of clotting profile by means of a baseline thromboelastogram (TEG) is useful.

Consider using cerebral oximetry as a pulse oximeter may not function well post bypass when the LVAD is operational. Limiting blood loss, usage of TEG to guide product replacement, use of cell salvage, and tranexamic acid are recommended. Transoesophageal echocardiography (TEE) is vital to obtain a good outcome. A comprehensive TEE study is routinely performed preoperatively to evaluate patients for LVAD insertion.

Surgical Approaches and Implantation Techniques

Parallel to device evolution, surgical techniques for LVAD implantation have advanced significantly. Traditional sternotomy remains the standard approach, but less invasive alternatives have emerged for appropriate candidates.

These include left thoracotomy approaches, which preserve sternal integrity and potentially reduce surgical trauma, particularly valuable for patients who may eventually undergo transplantation. Hybrid approaches combining thoracotomy for the pump with upper hemisternotomy for outflow graft placement offer balanced compromise between exposure and invasiveness.

Off-pump implantation techniques have gained traction at experienced centers, potentially reducing bleeding complications and right ventricular dysfunction associated with cardiopulmonary bypass. Additionally, concomitant procedures during LVAD implantation such as tricuspid valve repair for significant regurgitation or patent foramen ovale closure have become more common as their impact on outcomes has been better characterized.

Specialized Applications

The application of LVAD technology has expanded beyond traditional LV support to address specialized needs. Right ventricular assist devices (RVADs) using modified LVAD technology have been developed for isolated right heart failure or biventricular support. These systems, while still less evolved than LVADs, represent important options for the approximately 20–30% of LVAD recipients who develop significant right ventricular dysfunction.

Pediatric applications have advanced with the miniaturization of continuous-flow technology. While the Berlin Heart EXCOR remains the only FDA-approved device specifically for children, the HeartMate-3 and other compact adult devices are increasingly used off-label in adolescents with appropriate body surface area, and with promising results in specialized centers. Infection prevention has seen notable progress with antimicrobial driveline coatings, silver-impregnated velour, and novel exit site management protocols. These advances, combined with refined surgical techniques and postimplant care pathways, have reduced but not eliminated device-related infections, which remain among the most challenging complications of LVAD therapy.

Management of Cardiopulmonary Bypass and Postcardiopulmonary Bypass

- Ensure adequate de-airing.
- Evaluate inlet cannula position and blood flow velocity by continuous wave Doppler.
- Recheck for intracardiac shunts.
- In presence of any aortic regurgitation suture closure of aortic valve can be done to prevent any valvular regurgitation.

TABLE 6: Parameters assessed in postoperative period.

Device	Flow (L/min)	Speed (rpm)	Pulsatility
HeartMate-2	4–8	8,800–10,000 (minimum—8,600) (maximum—12,000)	4–6
HeartMate-3	3–6	5,200–5,800 (minimum—4,800) (maximum—6,200)	1–4

- Confirm proper LVAD function by evaluating LV decompression, presence of the outlet cannula in the aorta with appropriate flow, and a centered ventricular septum.

Inotropic support should be tailored to the TEE and PAC findings. Use of a combination of inotropes, inodilators, vasoconstrictors, and nitric oxide may be needed.

Postoperative Considerations

Aim for early extubation and weaning of inotropes and vasoconstrictor therapy. Maintain low right heart pressures with the aid of meticulous fluid and diuretic therapy. Postoperatively, physiotherapy and institution of anticoagulation for the device are crucial. A watchful eye for postoperative problems such as strokes, device thrombosis, infection, right ventricular failure, and timely intervention can ensure a possibility for a bridge to transplantation/destination therapy.

Parameters Assessed in Postoperative Period

See **Table 6**.

Hemodynamic Trouble Shooting of Left Ventricular Assist Device in Postoperative Period

Troubleshooting in Decreased Flow (Flowchart 2)

In decreased pulsatility either LVAD preload may be low or may be due to partial inflow obstruction.

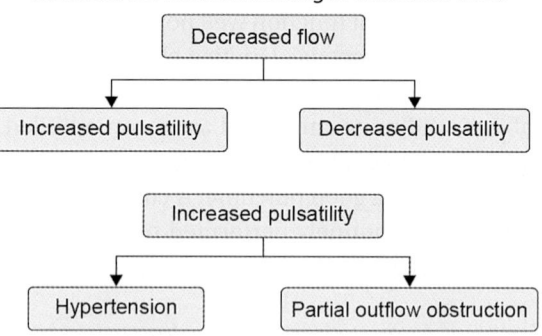

Flowchart 2: Troubleshooting in decreased flow.

Three main reasons for low LVAD preload are as follows:
1. Hypovolemia
2. Tamponade
3. Right ventricular failure

Troubleshooting in Increased Flow

In high pulsatility index flow may be increased due to either of two reasons:
1. Improved contractility
2. Hypervolemia

In low pulsatility index flow may be decreased due to following three reasons:
1. Vasodilation
2. Aortic insufficiency
3. High-speed operation

CONTEMPORARY OUTCOMES: HEART TRANSPLANT VERSUS LEFT VENTRICULAR ASSIST DEVICE

The comparison of outcomes between heart transplantation and LVAD therapy remains a cornerstone of clinical decision-making for patients with advanced heart failure. Contemporary data demonstrate significant improvements in both modalities, though important differences persist in survival, complications, quality of life, and functional recovery.

- 92.2%—2-year heart transplant survival (<65 years): Represents a 5% improvement over the previous decade, attributed to enhanced immunosuppression protocols and improved donor selection.[7]
- 88.8%—2-year LVAD survival (<65 years): Reflects dramatic improvement from 58% with first-generation devices, primarily due to continuous-flow technology and refined patient selection.
- 3.5%—survival gap: The narrowing difference between modalities has significant implications for allocation policy and clinical decision-making.

While survival outcomes have improved, both therapies continue to be associated with significant complications that impact quality of life and resource utilization. Heart transplant recipients face rejection (occurring in approximately 15–20% within the first year), infection related to immunosuppression, cardiac allograft vasculopathy (affecting up to 50% by 10 years of post-transplant), and malignancy (particularly post-transplant lymphoproliferative disorder and skin cancers).

LVAD recipients experience device-specific complications, including driveline infections (15–20% at 1 year), pump thrombosis (8–10% at 2 years with contemporary devices), stroke (10–15% at 2 years), right heart failure (20–25% requiring prolonged inotropic support), and gastrointestinal bleeding related to acquired von Willebrand syndrome (affecting up to 30% of patients). The most recent generation of magnetically levitated centrifugal flow pumps has demonstrated reduced rates of pump thrombosis and stroke compared to earlier devices.

QUALITY OF LIFE AND FUNCTIONAL OUTCOMES

Both heart transplantation and LVAD therapy significantly improve quality of life and functional capacity compared to medical therapy for advanced heart failure. Transplant recipients typically experience greater improvements in exercise capacity, with peak oxygen consumption (VO_2) increasing by 40–60% from baseline, compared to 20–30% improvements in LVAD recipients. This difference is attributed to the restoration of normal cardiac physiology and chronotropic competence with transplantation.

Quality of life metrics, including the Kansas City Cardiomyopathy Questionnaire (KCCQ)[8] and Minnesota Living with Heart Failure Questionnaire (MLHFQ),[9] demonstrates substantial improvements with both therapies. Transplant recipients report higher overall satisfaction and fewer limitations, though the gap has narrowed with contemporary LVADs. The persistent burden of external power supply and driveline management represents the most significant quality-of-life limitation for LVAD recipients.

READMISSION AND LONG-TERM CARE

Readmission rates differ significantly between the two therapies. LVAD recipients experience higher rates of rehospitalization, with approximately 65% requiring at least one readmission within the first-year postimplantation, compared to 40% for transplant recipients. The ISHLT registry data reveal that late mortality (beyond 5 years) for transplant recipients is approximately 3–4% annually, primarily due to cardiac allograft vasculopathy, malignancy, and renal failure.

Comparable long-term data for current-generation LVADs are still emerging, though technology-related failures and complications are expected to result in higher late mortality. This uncertainty regarding very long-term LVAD outcomes remains an important consideration in the selection process for younger patients.

TECHNOLOGICAL ADVANCES IN LEFT VENTRICULAR ASSIST DEVICE THERAPY

The evolution of LVAD technology represents one of the most remarkable success stories in modern cardiovascular medicine. From the bulky, pulsatile first-generation devices to today's compact, durable continuous-flow pumps, technological innovation has transformed outcomes and expanded the population of patients who can benefit from mechanical circulatory support.

UPDATES ON PRIORITIZATION AND ALLOCATION

The guidelines acknowledge recent changes in the UNOS heart allocation system, which now prioritizes critically ill patients requiring temporary mechanical circulatory support or inotropic therapy with evidence of end-organ dysfunction. This revised system has implications for LVAD candidates, as those with highest urgency status (Status 1-2) may proceed directly to transplantation when suitable donors are available, while those with lower urgency (Status 3-6) may benefit from LVAD as a bridge to transplantation during extended waiting periods. For patients receiving LVAD therapy, the guidelines outline criteria for subsequent transplant listing, including demonstration of good device outcomes, adherence to therapy, and absence of major complications. The guidelines specifically address the challenge of "prioritization penalty" for stable LVAD recipients, who typically receive lower allocation priority despite demonstrated compliance and favorable post-transplant outcomes. The guidelines emphasize the importance of longitudinal planning, with regular reassessment of goals and strategies throughout the patient's journey. This dynamic approach acknowledges the evolving nature of advanced heart failure and the potential for changes in patient's status, preferences, and therapeutic options over time.

Finally, the guidelines highlight the need for ongoing research to address critical knowledge gaps, particularly regarding optimal patient's selection for specific device types, strategies to minimize adverse events, and approaches to improve long-term outcomes for both transplant and LVAD recipients.

PERSONALIZED APPROACHES TO THERAPY SELECTION

The dichotomous choice between transplantation and LVAD therapy is evolving toward more nuanced, personalized decision-making. The PREDICT-HF trial is developing and validating a machine learning algorithm that integrates over 200 clinical, laboratory, imaging, and social variables to predict individual patient outcomes with each therapeutic approach.[10] Preliminary validation suggests the model achieves 85% accuracy in identifying patients who would derive greater survival benefit from one modality versus the other.

This personalized approach extends to the selection of specific LVAD systems based on individual patient's characteristics. The RIGHT-PUMP study is evaluating whether right ventricular function measurements can guide selection between axial and centrifugal flow devices to optimize biventricular interactions and reduce right heart failure.[11] Similarly, the ANTHROPOMORPHIC trial is examining whether body habitus and chest dimensions can predict optimal pump positioning to minimize thrombus formation and optimize flow dynamics.

Persistent Challenges

Despite remarkable progress, significant challenges remain in the field of advanced heart failure therapy. Donor organ availability continues to limit heart transplantation, with approximately 50% of listed patients receiving transplants within 1 year. Efforts to expand the donor pool through donation after circulatory death (DCD), extended criteria donors, and ex vivo perfusion have shown promise but require further refinement and validation.

For LVAD therapy, driveline infections remain the most persistent complication, affecting 15–20% of recipients by 2 years despite improved exit site management and antimicrobial strategies. Cerebrovascular events, although reduced with contemporary devices, continue to impact approximately 10% of patients by 2 years. Right ventricular failure after LVAD implantation affects 20–25% of recipients and significantly impacts survival and quality of life.

Perhaps most concerning are the persistent disparities in access to these life-saving therapies. Geographic, socioeconomic, racial/ethnic, and gender factors continue to influence who receives advanced heart failure interventions, with downstream effects on outcomes and quality of life.

Patient-centered Perspective

Perhaps the most important evolution in advanced heart failure therapy has been the shift toward patient-centered approaches that prioritize individual goals, preferences, and quality of life rather than focusing exclusively on survival.

This perspective recognizes that the "best" therapy varies based on patient's age, comorbidities, social support, lifestyle priorities, and personal values. Shared decision-making tools have been developed to facilitate these complex discussions, helping patients and families understand the implications of each therapeutic option within the context of their unique circumstances.

Palliative care integration, even for patients pursuing life-extending interventions, ensures that symptom management and quality of life remain priorities throughout the disease trajectory.

The measure of success in advanced heart failure therapy is no longer simply survival, but rather survival with acceptable quality of life and the ability to pursue meaningful activities consistent with each patient's values and priorities.

- 2022 AHA/ACC/HFSA Guidelines for the Management of Heart Failure[2]

As the field continues to advance, this patient-centered focus must remain the guiding principle, ensuring that technological innovation, policy development, and clinical practice evolution all serve the ultimate goal of improving the lives of individuals with advanced heart failure. Through continued collaboration among clinicians, researchers, industry partners, policymakers, patients, and caregivers, the remarkable progress of recent decades will undoubtedly continue, offering hope to the growing population affected by this challenging condition.

Critical Resources for Advanced Heart Failure Management

This appendix compiles essential resources for clinicians, researchers, patients, and caregivers involved in advanced heart failure management, heart transplantation, and LVAD therapy. These references provide detailed guidance, data repositories, educational materials, and support networks that complement the information presented in this review.

Clinical Guidelines and Consensus Documents

- 2022 AHA/ACC/HFSA Guidelines for the Management of Heart Failure
- ISHLT Guidelines for the Care of Heart Transplant Recipients (2021)
- Mechanical Circulatory Support: ISHLT Evidence Based Review (2020) American Society of Transplantation: Cardiac Transplantation Practice Guidelines (2023)
- CCS/CHFS Guidelines for the Management of Heart Failure with Reduced Ejection Fraction (2021)

Registries and Data Resources

- International Society for Heart and Lung Transplantation Registry (ISHLT)
- Interagency Registry for Mechanically Assisted Circulatory Support (INTERMACS)
- United Network for Organ Sharing (UNOS)
- Database EUROMACS Registry for Mechanical Circulatory Support
- Pediatric Heart Transplant Study (PHTS)
- Database ACTION-HF Registry: Advanced Cardiac Therapies Improving Outcomes Network

Our Center Experience

The process of organ donation and retrieval is complex. Multiple factors affect the time from diagnosis of death to organ assessment and retrieval. The main physiological factors are catecholamine surge, fluid management, central diabetes insipidus, hypothermia, and hormonal replacement therapies. Lack of in-depth knowledge and appropriate resources in most of the centers leads to poor organ donation to utilization ratio. Other main factor affecting retrieval was logistics such as availability of cardioplegia solution, transesophageal probe (in donor centers), traveling of retrieval team to donation site, timing of aortic cross clamp by coordinating with other organ retrieval teams. During the surgical procedure for organ procurement, it is essential to prevent any physical injury to the organ during steps such as cross clamping, division of vessels and the allocation of the left atrial cuff in coordination between the heart and lung retrieval teams.

Heart transplantation is considered the definitive treatment for advanced heart failure, offering high survival rates. Traditionally, most centers view patients with high pulmonary vascular resistance (>3 wood units) as unsuitable candidates for transplantation, citing it as an absolute contraindication. However, at our center, successful heart transplants have been performed in patients with high pulmonary vascular resistance, yielding favorable outcomes. The main postoperative challenge in these cases involves managing right ventricular dysfunction, which often requires mechanical circulatory support.

After surgery, patients are assessed based on their hemodynamic status to determine whether they require supports such as VA-ECMO or RVAD. Most patients initially receive VA-ECMO, with a transition to RVAD typically occurring in the second postoperative week. Current guidelines classify age over 70 years as a class 2b recommendation for heart transplantation. Notably, our center successfully completed a heart transplant in a 79-year-old gentleman, demonstrating positive results beyond guideline limitations.

India's first HeartMate-2 device was implanted at our center, achieving the country's longest reported survival of up to 10 years. Additionally, one of our patients successfully underwent heart transplantation at our center after receiving LVAD therapy, which was required due to aortic regurgitation following LVAD implantation.

CONCLUSION

The contemporary management of advanced heart failure through transplantation and LVAD therapy represents one of the most remarkable success stories in modern cardiovascular medicine. This review has examined the current landscape across multiple dimensions, highlighting significant advances while acknowledging persistent challenges and opportunities for further improvement.

REFERENCES

1. Peled Y, Ducharme A, Kittleson M, et al. International Society for Heart and Lung Transplantation Guidelines for the Evaluation and Care of Cardiac Transplant Candidates—2024. J Heart Lung Transplant. 2024;43(10):1529-628.e54.
2. Heidenreich PA, Bozkurt B, Aguilar D, et al. 2022 AHA/ACC/HFSA Guideline for the Management of Heart Failure: A Report of the American College of Cardiology/American Heart Association Joint Committee on Clinical Practice Guidelines. Circulation [Internet]. 2022;145(18).
3. TRANSTAN. (2025). Transplant Authority Government Of Tamil Nadu [Internet]. [online] Available from https://transtan.tn.gov.in/ [Last accessed Nov., 2025].
4. Nesseler N, Mansour A, Cholley B, et al. Perioperative Management of Heart Transplantation: A Clinical Review. Anesthesiology. 2023;139(4):493-510.
5. Kidney Disease: Improving Global Outcomes (KDIGO) CKD Work Group. KDIGO 2024 Clinical Practice Guideline for the Evaluation and Management of Chronic Kidney Disease. Kidney Int. 2024;105(4S):S117-S314.
6. Fried J, Sayer G, Naka Y, et al. State of the Art Review: Evolution and Ongoing Challenges of Left Ventricular Assist Device Therapy. Struct Heart. 2018;2(4):262-73.
7. Kittleson MM, Kobashigawa JA. Cardiac Transplantation: Current Outcomes and Contemporary Controversies. JACC Heart Fail. 2017;5(12):857-68.
8. Spertus JA, Jones PG, Sandhu AT, et al. Interpreting the Kansas City Cardiomyopathy Questionnaire in Clinical Trials and Clinical Care: JACC State-of-the-Art Review. J Am Coll Cardiol. 2020;76(20):2379-90.
9. Bilbao A, Escobar A, García-Perez L, et al. The Minnesota living with heart failure questionnaire: comparison of different factor structures. Health Qual Life Outcomes. 2016;14(1):23.
10. Cyrille-Superville N, Rao SD, et al. PREDICT HF: Risk stratification in advanced heart failure using novel hemodynamic parameters. Clin Cardiol. 2024;47(6):e24277.
11. Lai WT, Yu HP, Lin CC, et al. Right Ventricular Pump Efficiency in Secundum-Type Atrial Septal Defect. Acta Cardiol Sin. 2022;38(1):47-55.

Step-by-Step Coiling in Coronary Tree: Why and How

Atul Kaushik, Ashutosh Marwah

INTRODUCTION

Gianturco coils[1] were first introduced in 1975, and have become standard practice for embolization of vascular structures. Coil closure of patent arterial duct using coil was first described by Cambier et al. in 1992.[2] Since then the role of coils has expanded rapidly, and coils have often been used to close both venous and arterial channels. In pediatric cardiology, the coils have been used to close patent arterial duct, aortopulmonary collaterals in cyanotic patients, and feeder vessels of pulmonary arteriovenous malformations. The coils have also been used to close the venovenous collaterals, decompressing veins in patients with univentricular physiology.[3-5]

In coronary circuit, indications of use of coils could be acute or elective.

COIL CLOSURE OF CORONARY ARTERIOVENOUS FISTULAE

Closure of coronary artery AV fistulas remains the single most elective procedure. Coronary artery fistulae are rare, approximately 0.1% of all congenital abnormalities.[6] The fistula may open into any of the cardiac chambers, coronary sinus, the superior vena cava, or pulmonary artery. The distal opening is most common in pulmonary artery (37%), right atrium (24%), left ventricle (15%) followed by left atrium (9%).[7] Main indications for closure are clinical symptoms and myocardial ischemia. In asymptomatic patients closure is indicated if Qp:Qs > 1.5:1.[8] Coronary fistula rarely become symptomatic and often present with murmur over the precordium. Symptoms in childhood are due to myocardial ischemia/CHF because of high flow state. In adulthood, they may cause heart failure, myocardial ischemia, endocarditis, arrhythmias, and rarely emergency situation due to rupture.[9-11] Surgical clipping of AV fistula is safe and effective with good results. Catheter-based interventional closure has emerged as safe and effective procedure and is acceptable alternative to surgery.[9]

Coil closure has high success rates, 91% having complete closure at follow-up and 93% remaining symptom-free, even when complete closure could not be achieved. Chances of successful closure were higher in patients fulfilling the following criteria:

1. Absence of multiple coronary AV fistulae
2. Absence of multiple large branches
3. Absence of extreme vessel tortuosity
4. Safe accessibility to coronary artery.

A variety of material can be used for embolization of AV fistulae including latex balloons, Gianturco coils, platinum coils, and vascular plugs have been used for closing larger fistulae.

Risks and complications: As with any coronary artery procedure risk of vessel trauma or dissection, rupture, and vessel spasm have been reported. Device embolization may happen in case of larger fistulae. Myocardial infarction can happen in the aneurysmal proximal artery because of stagnant flow after the closure. In series of 76 patients who were managed medically or underwent surgical/transcatheter closure myocardial infarction occurred in 15%.

Drainage into coronary sinus was predictor for long-term ischemic events. Precise placement of device >1 cm away from the origin could reduce the risk of thrombus propagation and future coronary embolization.[10]

COIL CLOSURE OF CORONARY ARTERY PERFORATION

It is single most acute indication for use of coils in coronary artery circuit. Coronary artery perforation occurs as a complication of percutaneous coronary artery intervention for recanalization. Incidence of coronary artery perforation is about 4% of all percutaneous coronary artery interventions even in hands of trained operators.[11] Coronary artery perforations have traditionally been classified into five types (Ellis classification).[12]

1. *Type I:* Focal extraluminal crater without extravasation
2. *Type II:* Pericardial or myocardial blushing without jet extravasation
3. *Type III:* Active jet extravasation
4. *Type IV:* Cavity spilling
5. *Type V:* Distal perforation

Large-vessel perforations can be managed by implantation of covered stents at the site of perforation.[13] However, in case of small-vessel perforation or significant side branch perforation stent implantation may not be possible. In such cases, coil embolization may be a feasible and effective treatment option.

Distal perforations can occur in vessels with chronic total occlusions and even in vessels without occlusion. They are often caused as a result of using a polymer jacket wire or tapered highly penetrative wire. Most cases of coronary artery perforation can be managed with prolonged balloon inflation and reversal of anticoagulation. In some cases microcatheters can be used and the perforation sealed using blood clot or fatty tissue.[14,15] However, occlusion of the vessel using coils is a more definitive treatment, and prevents recanalization and future risk of tamponade. Microspheres should be avoided in coronary tree as they may migrate and cause occlusion of other vessels, which may have catastrophic consequences. Fat embolization should be used only in emergency situations, in case the coils are not available, due to lack of accuracy during embolization procedure. The techniques of coil embolization has been described by Garbo et al.[16]

Trapping technique: Coil embolization with this method is possible if the offending wire is still in position. A microcatheter is advanced at the site of perforation; the position is verified by an injection through the microcatheter. Once in position a suitable coil is then delivered through the microcatheter. A repeat injection is made through the microcatheter and additional coils delivered if necessary **(Figs. 1 to 3)**.

Block and deliver technique (BAD): A balloon is advanced proximal to the site of perforation, the balloon is inflated to stop bleeding, and an microcatheter is then advanced through the same guide catheter using "buddy wire" technique. The microcatheter is advanced near the site of

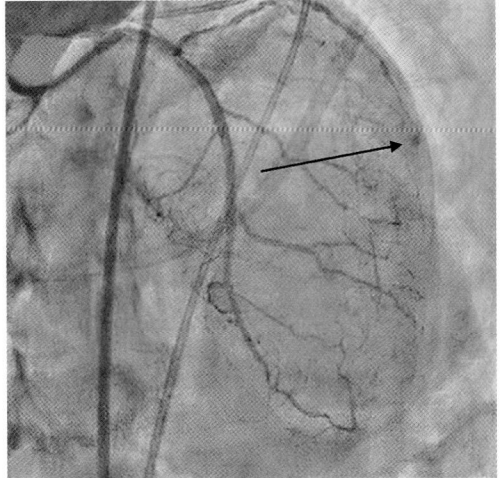

Fig. 1: Coronary artery angiogram showing perforation in a coronary artery branch.

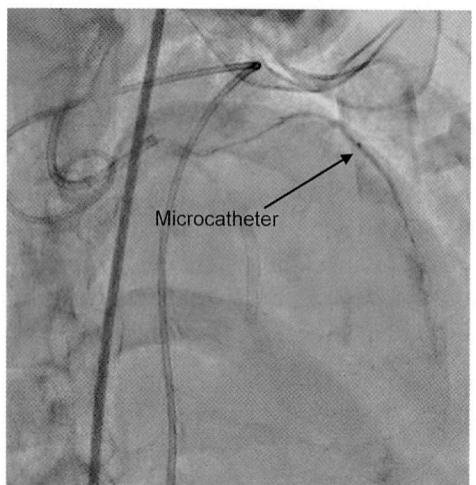

Fig. 2: Selective coronary artery angiogram using a microcatheter (arrow points the tip of catheter).

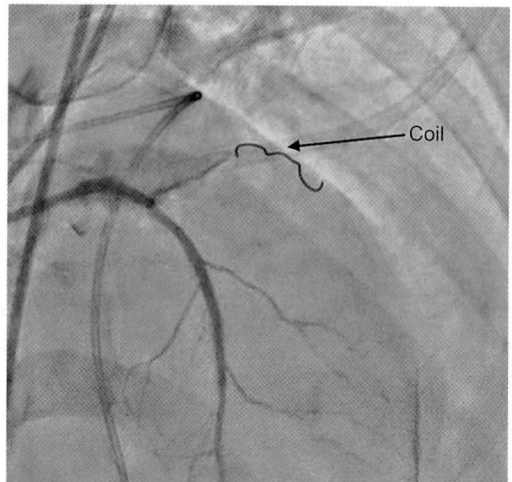

Fig. 3: The coil inside the coronary artery, with complete occlusion of distal segment.

perforation, the balloon needs to be deflated to allow the microcatheter to pass distally. The balloon is reinflated, a test injection is then given through the microcatheter to localize the site correctly. The coil is then inserted into the microcatheter using a delivery wire. The coil is gently advanced to the tip of catheter and deployed just proximal to the site of perforation. A repeat injection from microcatheter is made to see if any residual leak is present, if present, additional coils may be deployed. The BAD technique allows verification of complete hemostasis before removal of catheters and wires. It is considered safe and effective, with a high rate of successful sealing in both non-CTO and CTO PCI.[17]

Complications: The BAD technique is generally safe, distal migration of coil may occur if the size of coil is too small for the vessel diameter. Ventricular arrhythmia has been reported in some cases, immediately after deployment.

CONCLUSION

Coils can be used effectively and safely in coronary circuit. Though the use remains limited to two main indications: Coronary AV fistulae and inadvertent perforations. In both the settings coils provide good long-term resolution.

REFERENCES

1. Gianturco C, Anderson J, Wallace D. Mechanical devices for arterial occlusion. Am J Roentgenol Radium Ther Nucl Med. 1975;124(3):428-35.
2. Cambier P, Kirby W, Wortham D, et al. Percutaneous closure of small (less than 2.5 mm) patent ductus arteriosus using coil embolization. Am J Cardiol. 1992;69(8):815-6.
3. Perry SB, Radtke W, Fellows KE, et al. Coil embolization to occlude aortopulmonary collateral vessels and shunts in patients with congenital heart disease. J Am Coll Cardiol. 1989;13(1):100-8.
4. Ali YA, Nour El-Deen NS, Elshahed GS. Management of collaterals after Glenn procedure and its impact on patient with single ventricle: A single center study. REC Interv Cardiol. 2024;6(4):296-304.
5. Moore JW, Berdjis F. Coil occlusion of congenital vascular malformations and surgical shunts. Prog Pedia Cardiol. 1996;6(2):149-59.
6. Gillebert C, Van Hoof R, Van de Werf F, et al. Coronary artery fistulas in an adult population. Eur Heart J. 1986;7:437-43.

7. Yun G, Nam TH, Chun EJ. Coronary Artery Fistulas: Pathophysiology, Imaging Findings, and Management. Radiographics. 2018;38(3):688-703.
8. Shyamsunder KR, Tharakan JA, Titus T, et al. Coronary artery fistula in children and adults: a review of 25 cases with long-term observation. Int J Cardiol. 1997;58(1):47-53.
9. Armsby LR, Keane JF, Sherwood MC, et al. Management of coronary artery fistulae. Patient selection and results of transcatheter closure. J Am Coll Cardiol. 2002;39:1026-32.
10. Stout KK, Daniels CJ, Aboulhosn JA, et al. 2018 AHA/ACC guideline for the management of adults with congenital heart disease: a report of the American College of Cardiology/American Heart Association Task Force on Clinical Practice Guidelines. J Am Coll Cardiol. 2019;73:e81-e192.
11. Nathan A, Hashemzadeh M, Movahed MR. Percutaneous coronary intervention of chronic total occlusion associated with higher inpatient mortality and complications compared with non-CTO lesions. Am J Med. 2023;136(10):994-9.
12. Gunning MG, Williams IL, Jewitt DE, et al. Coronary artery perforation during percutaneous intervention: incidence and outcome. Heart. 2002;88:495-8.
13. Lemmert ME, van Bommel RJ, Diletti R, et al. Clinical characteristics and management of coronary artery perforations: a single-center 11-year experience and practical overview. J Am Heart Assoc. 2017;6(9):e007049.
14. Dixon SR, Webster MM, Ormiston JA, et al. Gelfoam embolization of a distal coronary artery guidewire perforation. Catheter Cardiovasc Interv. 2000;49(2):214-7.
15. Ajluni SC, Glazier S, Blankenship L, et al. Perforations after percutaneous coronary interventions: clinical, angiographic, and therapeutic observations. Cathet Cardiovasc Diagn. 1994;32(3):206-12.
16. Garbo R, Oreglia JA, Gasparini GL. The balloon-microcatheter technique for treatment of coronary artery perforations. Catheter Cardiovasc Interv. 2017;89:E75-E83.
17. Sanchez JS, Garbo R, Gagnor A, et al. Management and outcomes of coronary artery perforations treated with the block and deliver technique. Catheter Cardiovasc Interv. 2021;98(2):238-45.

CHAPTER 24

Clipping Valves for Regurgitation in 2025

Deepti Yadav, Siddarth Varshney, Nagendra Chouhan, Praveen Chandra

■ INTRODUCTION

Mitral regurgitation (MR) results from anatomical or functional changes in the mitral valve apparatus and affects ~10% of individuals aged ≥75 years.[1] It contributes to left ventricular dysfunction, heart failure (HF), and increased mortality.[2] For high-risk or inoperable patients, *transcatheter edge-to-edge repair (TEER)* offers a less invasive alternative.

Transcatheter edge-to-edge repair mimics the surgical *Alfieri stitch*,[3] using a *clip with grasping arms* (commonly at A2–P2 scallops) to approximate the mitral leaflets, creating a *double-orifice* to reduce MR.

Timeline of TEER milestones:
- *2003:* First-in-human MitraClip procedure[4]
- *2008:* CE mark approval (Europe)
- *2013:* FDA approval for *primary MR* (EVEREST II trial)
- *2016:* First PASCAL device use
- *2019:* FDA approval for *secondary MR* (COAPT trial):
  - TEER proven effective in:
    - Atrial functional MR
    - Severe MAC
    - Post-annuloplasty ring MR
    - Commissural MR
- *2022:* FDA approval for PASCAL

Key trials:
COAPT trial: (COAPT AND EVEREST BOTH REFERENCE 4)
- *Patients:* Symptomatic HF, secondary mitral regurgitation (SMR), LVEF 20–50%, on guideline directed medical therapy.
- *24 months:*
  - *HF hospitalizations:* Reduced from 67.9 to 35.8% ($p < 0.001$)
  - *Mortality:* Reduced from 46.1 to 29.1% ($p < 0.001$)
- *5 years:*
  - *Mortality:* 57.3% (device) versus 67.2% (control), CI: 0.58–0.89
  - *Device-related complications:* 1.4%

EVEREST II trial:[4]
- Compared MitraClip to surgery in degenerative MR
- *1 year:* Less MR reduction with TEER, but better safety and similar outcomes
- *2 years:* No device failures
- *5 years:* MR ≤2+ in 75%; stable safety profile

guidelines for TEER

AHA/ACC valve guidelines 2020:[5] Class IIa recommendation for patients with *high or prohibitive surgical risk*, favorable anatomy for transcatheter repair, and life expectancy >1 year, for both *primary (PMR) and SMR*.

ESC valve guidelines 2021:
- *Primary MR: Class IIb* for symptomatic, inoperable or high-risk patients meeting echocardiographic eligibility and deemed nonfutile by heart team
- *Secondary MR:*
  - *Class IIa* for symptomatic patients unsuitable for surgery with or without coronary artery disease (CAD)
  - *Class IIb* for high-risk symptomatic patients ineligible for surgery without criteria suggesting high TEER response

PROCEDURAL CONSIDERATIONS

Baseline Evaluation

- *Transthoracic echocardiography (TTE):* Initial assessment for MR diagnosis, severity, mechanism, valve area, pulmonary vein flow, septal morphology, presence of clot in left atrium (LA) and left atrial appendage (LAA), pulmonary artery pressure, associated valvular lesions, and left ventricular (LV) and right ventricular (RV) function
- *Transesophageal echocardiography (TEE)* (mandatory for M-TEER candidates):
  - Assess leaflet targets and major MR jets
  - Guide septal puncture and steerable guide catheter navigation
  - Ensure proper clip alignment and confirm leaflet capture
  - Evaluate MR reduction post-clip deployment
  - Exclude significant mitral stenosis and assess residual atrial septal defect (ASD)

M-TEER Systems

Devices available: **Figure 1** shows the comparison between two types of m-TEER devices.
- *MitraClip (Abbott)*
- *MYCLIP (Meril Lifesciences)*
- *PASCAL (Edwards Lifesciences)*

MitraClip System (Fourth Generation G4)

- *Sizes:* NT and XT [4 mm width; 9 mm (NT) and 12 mm (XT) arm lengths], NTW and XTW [6 mm width; 9 mm (NTW) and 12 mm (XTW)] **(Fig. 2)**
- *Features:*
  - Two cobalt-chromium rigid arms with flexible nitinol grippers having longitudinal frictional hooks
  - Longer arms (XT/XTW) for larger coaptation and flail gaps
  - 50% wider grasping area with independent controlled gripper actuation (CGA)
  - Continuous left atrial pressure monitoring
  - Optimized for complex anatomies, reducing clip numbers and leaflet stress

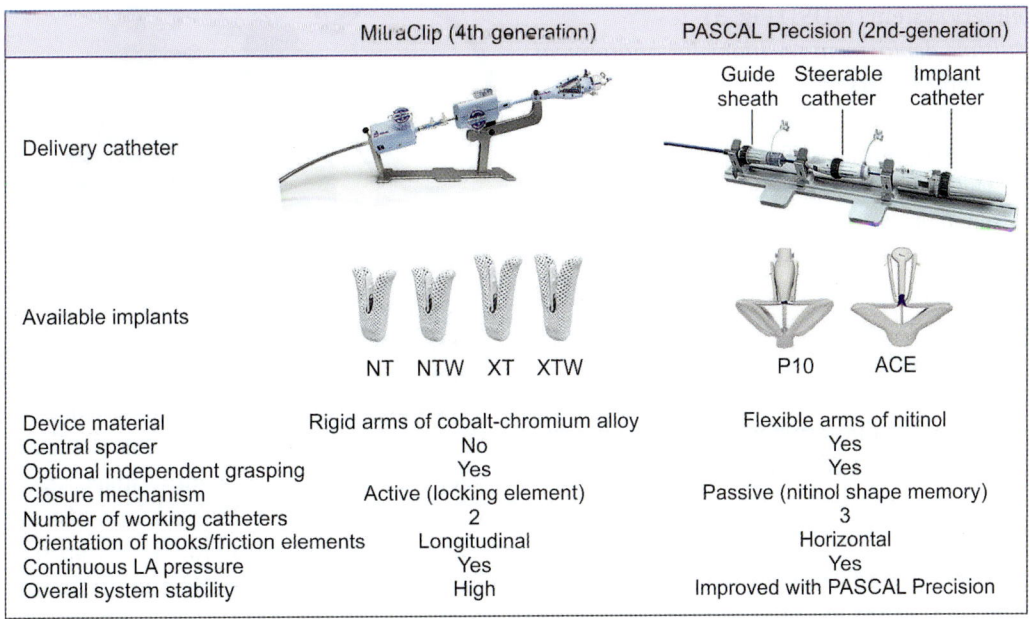

Fig. 1: Comparison of MitraClip and PASCAL device.

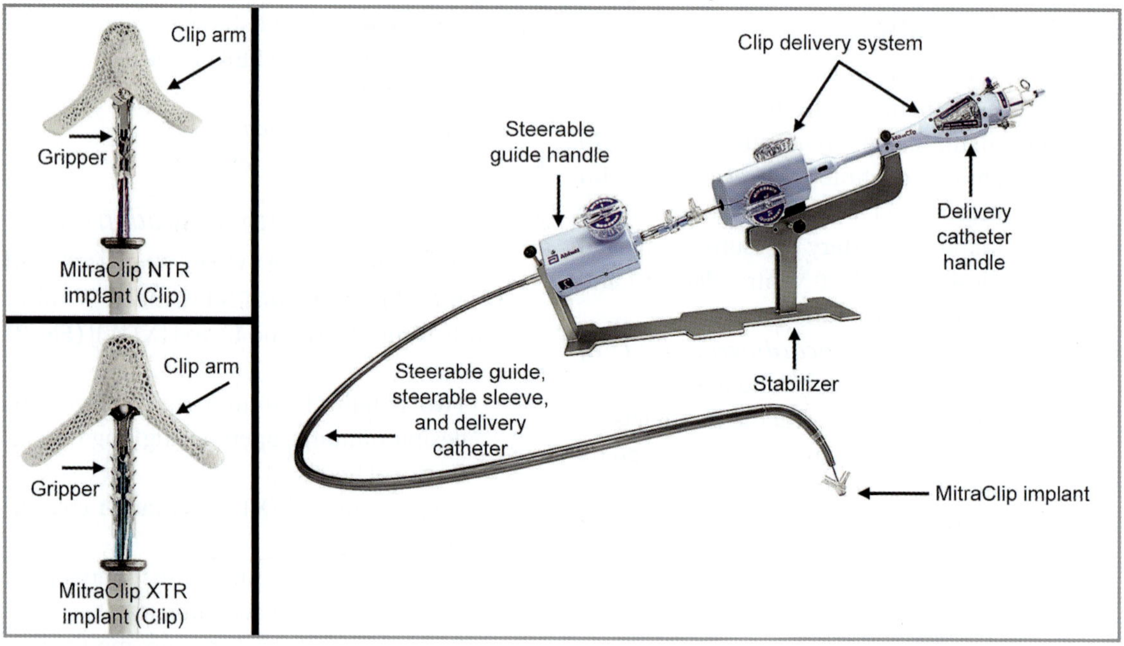

Fig. 2: MitraClip system.

MyClip System (Meril Life Sciences)

- *Components:* Guide catheter (MGC) and clip delivery system (MDS) **(Fig. 3)**
- *Multiple deployment positions for anatomical flexibility* **(Fig. 4)**:
  - *MyClip 60°:* Perpendicular to coaptation line for optimal leaflet grasp
  - *MyClip 120°:* Enables deeper LV access and clip locking
  - *MyClip 180°:* Allows clip inversion in narrow anatomies
  - *MyClip reversed:* Safe transition from LV to LA, reducing leaflet/chordal injury
  - *MyClip closed:* Facilitates insertion through guide catheter and precise micro-adjustments before deployment

PASCAL System (Fourth Generation G4)

- The second-generation PASCAL system **(Figs. 5A to D)** includes a 22-Fr steerable guide sheath, catheter, and an implant catheter for high maneuverability in the left atrium. The nitinol-based PASCAL P10 features two spring-loaded curved paddles (26 mm grasping length) and two individually controlled 10 mm clasps for independent leaflet capture, plus a central spacer to reduce leaflet stress. The PASCAL Ace has similar grasping width with smaller 6 mm paddles for smaller anatomies and multiple implant strategies. The PASCAL Precision platform enhances catheter stability and steerability.

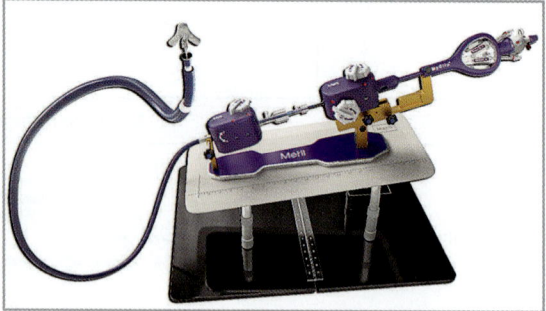

Fig. 3: MyClip delivery system.

- *Anatomical suitability for m-TEER:* Optimal candidates for functional MR meet EVEREST criteria:
  - Mitral valve area (MVA) >4 cm²
  - Minimal leaflet calcification in the grasping area
  - Coaptation length >2 mm
  - Coaptation depth <11 mm
- *For primary MR:* Flail gap should be <10 mm and width <15 mm[6]

- *Complex anatomies include:*
  - Wide coaptation gaps (≥15 mm)
  - Large flail gaps (≥10 mm)
  - Leaflet calcification in the grasping area
  - Transmitral gradient >5 mm Hg
  - Jets outside A2/P2 scallops
  - MVA <4 cm²—factors linked to increased post-procedure gradients[7,8]
  - Severe calcification, active endocarditis, and significant mitral stenosis are contraindications for m-TEER.

Procedure:
- *Trans-septal puncture (Fig. 6):* The ideal puncture site is the posterosuperior fossa ovalis, 4–5 cm above the mitral annulus. Higher punctures suit medial pathologies and primary MR. The septal superior and inferior aspects are identified in the bicaval view; the anterior septum lies closest to the aortic valve on the short-axis view. Biplane imaging confirms a superior-posterior puncture location.

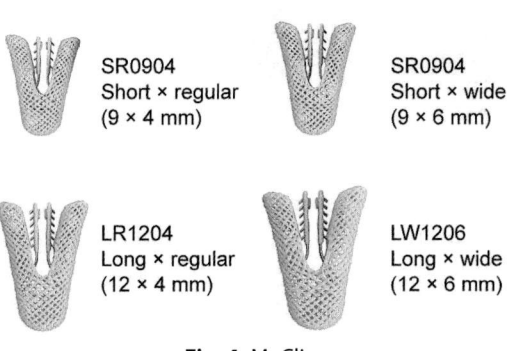

Fig. 4: MyClip.

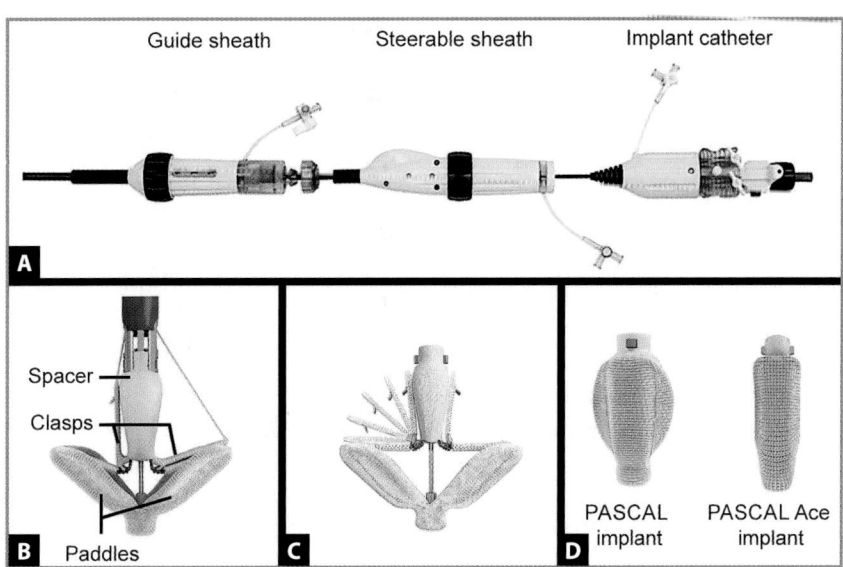

Figs. 5A to D: (A) Components of PASCAL system; (B) PASCAL implant; (C) Independent leaflet capture; (D) PASCAL and PASCAL Ace implant.

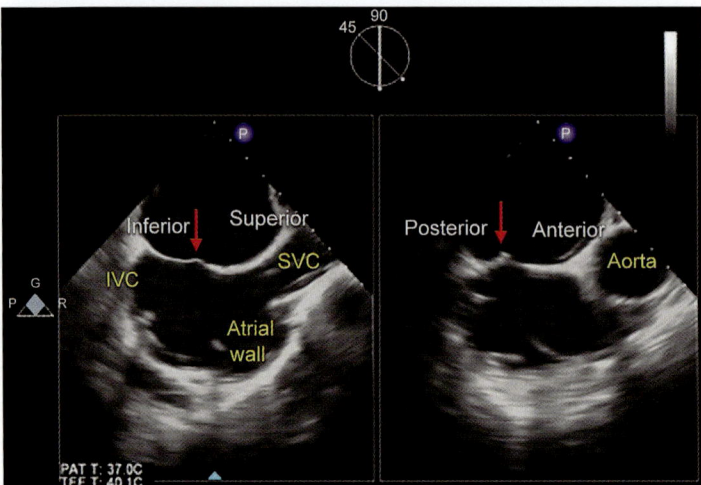

Fig. 6: TEE-guided trans-septal puncture.

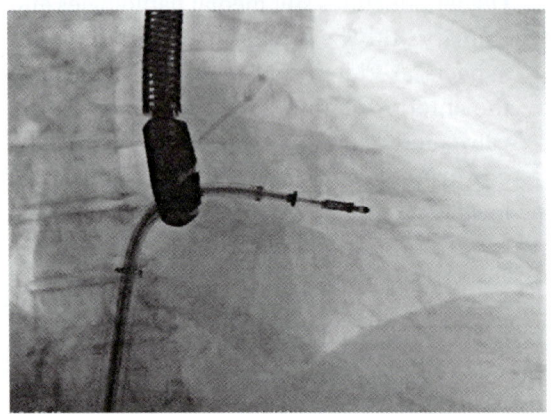

Fig. 7: Steerable guide catheter advancement.

- For distorted fossa ovalis anatomy, needle bending or straightening aids crossing. Thickened or floppy septa may require electrocautery on the needle or using the stiff end of a PCI wire to cross.
- *Advancement of the steerable guide catheter:* A curved-tip stiff wire is passed through the septum into the left upper pulmonary vein, followed by septal dilation. The steerable guide catheter (SGC) is then advanced into the left atrium under 2D and 3D TEE guidance to avoid contact with the left pulmonary vein and left atrial appendage **(Fig. 7)**.

- *Device positioning:* Simultaneous visualization in the intercommissural (50–70°) and LVOT (140–160°) views guides catheter trajectory to optimize leaflet grasping and prevent valve distortion **(Fig. 8)**. Clip arms are oriented perpendicular to the coaptation line **(Fig. 9)**. Manipulations include pushing/pulling to move medially/laterally, clockwise rotation for posterior movement, counterclockwise for anterior, flexing to lower height, and posterior rotation to gain height.
- *Leaflet grasping:* Once device position and trajectory in the left atrium are confirmed, it is advanced into the left ventricle. Clear leaflet visualization ensures adequate tissue grasping **(Fig. 10)**. Leaflet insertion is carefully assessed and quantified before device release.
- *Hemodynamic assessment:* Residual MR is evaluated by regurgitant jet size, pulmonary vein flow **(Fig. 11)**, and left atrial pressure. Significant residual MR warrants device repositioning or adding a second device, provided no mitral stenosis is present. When using multiple clips, the first device is typically placed more medially.

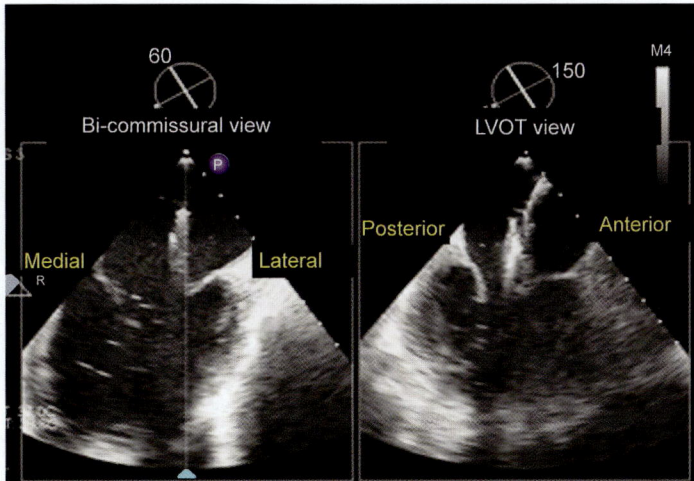

Fig. 8: Device positioning.

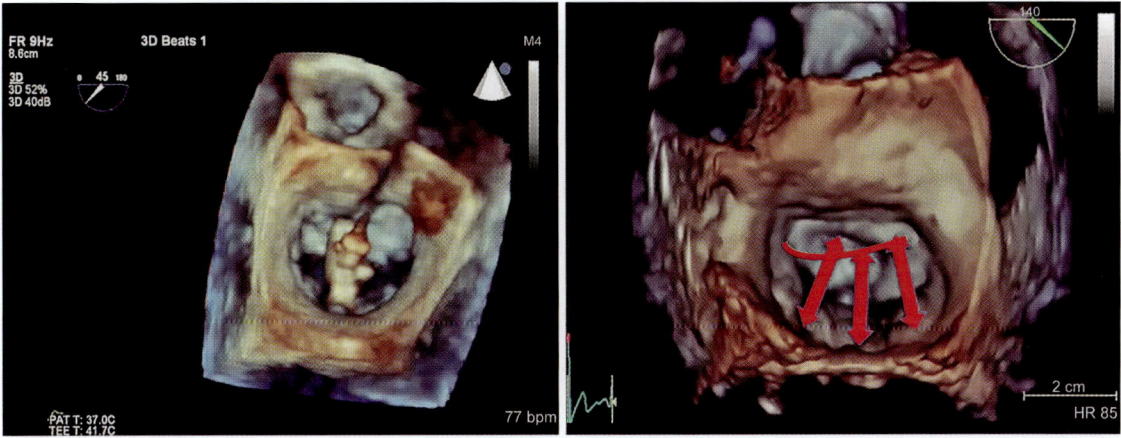

Fig. 9: Clip orientation perpendicular to coaptation line.

Complications:
- *Device-related:*
  - *Residual MR:* Treated with Amplatzer vascular plug or double-disk occluder for significant interclip/paraclip leaks[9,10]
  - *Single leaflet detachment (SLD):* Occurs in 2–5%, caused by leaflet disengagement; prevented by good leaflet grasp and managed with additional clips if possible.
  - *Clip embolization:* Rare (<1%); requires surgical removal if embolized to distal arteries
  - *Leaflet perforation, tear, and chordal rupture*
- *Trans-septal puncture complications:* More common in large/thick septa or prior surgery; includes iatrogenic ASD, tamponade, pericardial effusion, aortic perforation.
- *Other risks:* Infective endocarditis, stroke, vascular dissection, thrombosis, pseudoaneurysm, and bleeding
- *Follow-up:* TTE on post-procedure day 1, at 30 days, and 6–12 months to assess MR and complications.

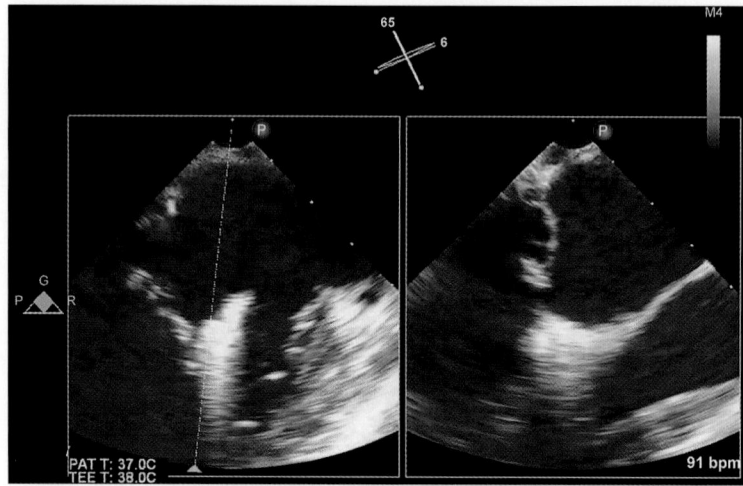

Fig. 10: Adequate leaflet grasping.

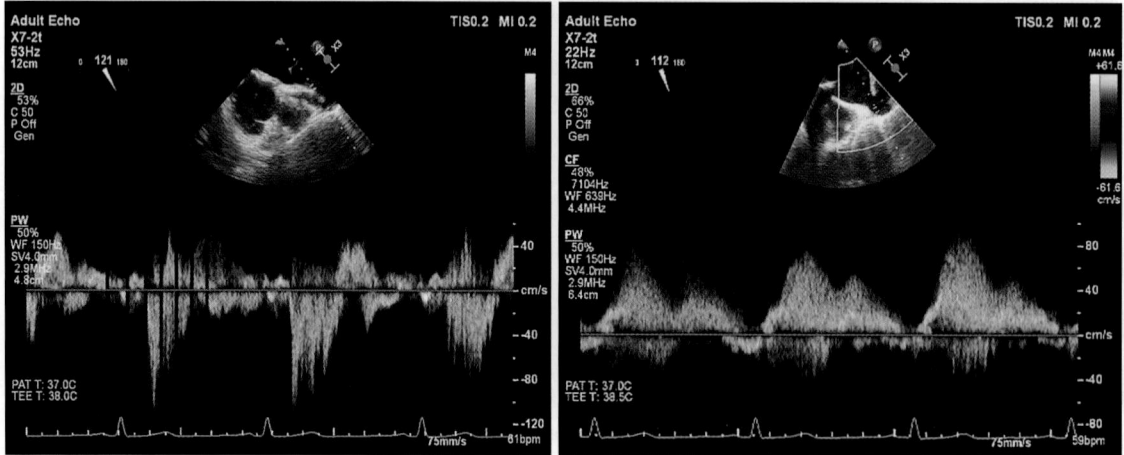

Fig. 11: Pulmonary vein flow before and after m-TEER device.

TRICUSPID REGURGITATION OVERVIEW (TABLE 1)

- Tricuspid regurgitation (TR) affects over two-thirds of the population; significant TR occurs in ~1.5% of men and 5.6% of women over 70.
- Present in nearly one-third of patients undergoing left-sided heart surgery, especially mitral valve procedures[11]

- *Primary TR:* Caused by intrinsic leaflet abnormalities (e.g., carcinoid, endocarditis, trauma, radiotherapy, myxomatous, and congenital)
- *Secondary (functional) TR:* Due to RA or RV enlargement from pulmonary hypertension, left heart disease, atrial fibrillation, or device lead impingement[12]

TABLE 1: Tricuspid regurgitation (primary and secondary).

Recommendations	Class	Level
Recommendations on primary tricuspid regurgitation:		
Surgery is recommended in patients with severe primary tricuspid regurgitation undergoing left-sided valve surgery	I	C
Surgery is recommended in symptomatic patients with isolated severe primary tricuspid regurgitation without severe RV dysfunction	I	C
Surgery should be considered in patients with moderate primary tricuspid regurgitation undergoing left-sided valve surgery	IIa	C
Surgery should be considered in asymptomatic or mildly symptomatic patients with isolated severe primary tricuspid regurgitation and RV dilatation who are appropriate for surgery	IIa	C
Recommendations on secondary tricuspid regurgitation:		
Surgery is recommended in patients with severe secondary tricuspid regurgitation undergoing left-sided valve surgery	I	B
Surgery should be considered in patients with mild or moderate secondary tricuspid regurgitation with a dilated annulus ($\geq$40 mm or >21 mm/m^2 by 2D echocardiography) undergoing left-sided valve surgery	IIa	B
Surgery should be considered in patients with severe secondary tricuspid regurgitation (with or without previous left-sided surgery) who are symptomatic or have RV dilatation, in the absence of severe RV or LV dysfunction and severe pulmonary vascular disease/hypertension	IIa	B
Transcatheter treatment of symptomatic secondary severe tricuspid regurgitation may be considered in inoperable patients at a Heart Valve Centre with expertise in the treatment of tricuspid valve disease	IIb	C

(LV: left ventricle; RV: right ventricle)

ESC/EACTS (European)—2021 valvular heart disease guidelines:

Guidelines (ACC/AHA 2020):
- **Class I:** Surgery for severe TR during left-sided valve surgery
- **Class IIa:** Surgery for severe primary TR with right heart failure
- No current recommendations for TTVI (transcatheter tricuspid valve interventions) in American guidelines

Noninvasive evaluation: Echocardiography (TTE): Diagnosis, TR severity, etiology, RV/RA size, annulus dimension

- *Advanced imaging:*
  - 3D echo and RV strain for detailed assessment
  - Cardiac MRI preferred for RV size/function quantification
- *TR severity:* "Massive" and "torrential" TR have prognostic significance

Risk stratification:
- **TRIO score:** Predicts 10-year mortality for moderate or worse TR to guide referral decisions.
- **TRI score:** Estimates in-hospital mortality risk post-surgical or TV TEER interventions; low-intermediate risk benefits from early intervention

TABLE 2: Transcatheter tricuspid valve intervention landscape.

TTVI	Selection	Considerations	Available devices
Leaflet repair Coaptation enhancement	• *Primary TR:* Confined leaflet prolapse or flail • <7 mm coaptation gap • No significant leaflet calcification • Nonobstructing RV lead • Antero- or posterolateral TR jet	• More residual TR • Concerns for TR progression • Guiding imaging modality • Risk of SLDA • Less invasive	• TriClip • MitraClip • PASCAL • Dragonfly • Mitralix
Annuloplasty	• Secondary TR: Right atrial TR • Dilated annulus • Favorable RCA course • Mild valve tethering • Central jet location • Allows for future interventions	• Risk of RCA obstruction • Large coaptation defect >7 mm • Primary RV lead-induced TR • Severe pulmonary hypertension	• Trialign • Cardioband • TriCinch • Millipede • MIA • PASTA • DaVinci • K-Clip System
Orthotopic valve	• Primary TR—rheumatic, severe prolapse • Coaptation gap >7 mm • Heavily calcified/thickened leaflets • Retracted/perforated leaflets • Prior tricuspid replacement	• Bioprosthetic longevity • Anticoagulation needed • Risk of severe RV dysfunction • Pacemaker rate increased • Mortality/bleeding	• Evoque • Intrepid • V-Dyne • Navigate • Trisol • Lux • Topaz

(SLDA: single leaflet device attachment; TR: tricuspid regurgitation; TTVI: transcatheter tricuspid valve intervention)

- Emerging 1-year mortality risk models exist but lack guideline endorsement **(Table 2)**

Main T-TEER Devices

- *TriClip (Abbott):*
  - Only FDA-approved T-TEER device in the US **(Figs. 12A to E)**
  - Multiple clip sizes (NT, NTW, XT, and XTW), independent leaflet grasping, enhanced steering (G4 generation)
  - TRILUMINATE trial showed high safety, quality-of-life improvements, and sustained TR reduction (89% ≤ moderate TR at 1 year)[13,14]
- *PASCAL (Edwards Lifesciences):*
  - Available in Europe, under study in the US (CLASP II TR study); not FDA-approved yet
  - Features central spacer, nitinol construction for less leaflet stress, flexible positioning[13]
  - The repair system features several enhancements including improved steerability in a septolateral range and a shorter curve for easier height adjustment. Expanded size range and controlled gripper actuation provide more treatment options with predictable results.

Patient Selection

- *Indications:* Severe functional (secondary) TR, high surgical risk, persistent symptoms (fatigue and edema)
- *Exclusions:* Massive leaflet tethering, lead interference, heavy calcification, pacemaker in tricuspid position (relative)

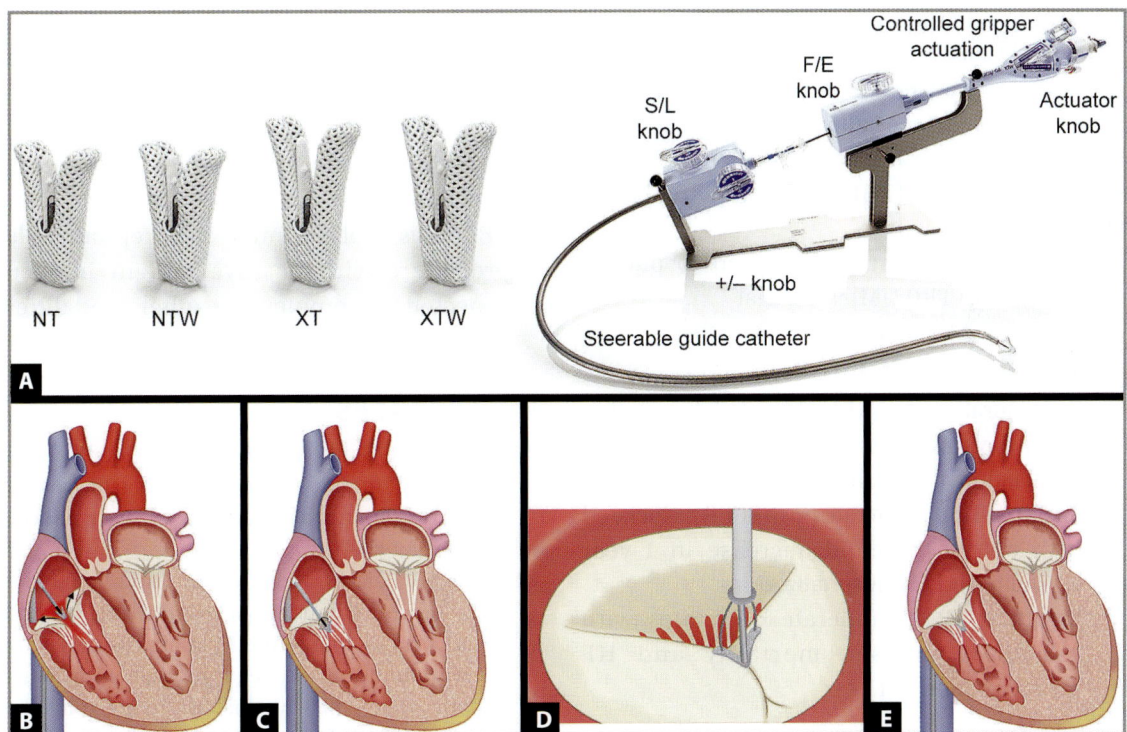

Figs. 12A to E: TriClip G4 transcatheter tricuspid valve repair system. (A) A total of four implants with wider grasping area; (B) The delivery system insertion, positioning and steering in the right atrium; (C and D) Crossing the valve and leaflet grasping; (E) Clip deployment. (F/E: flex/extend; S/L: septal/lateral)

Imaging for Procedural Planning

TEE (2D/3D) and CT to assess leaflet anatomy, coaptation gap (<7 mm ideal), jet location, annulus size, and RV function

Procedure Steps (TriClip)

- Venous access via right femoral vein; 24-F steerable guide catheter advanced to inferior vena cava (IVC)
- Guide catheter navigated to right atrium under fluoroscopy and TEE
- Clip aligned perpendicular to coaptation line using 3D TEE
- Clip advanced across tricuspid valve into RV, then retracted to grasp leaflets (independent grasping available)
- Partial clip closure and TR assessment via TEE; deployed if effective
- Additional clips placed if residual TR persists
- Delivery system withdrawn; femoral access closed

Postprocedure Care

- Monitor for vascular complications, arrhythmias, and pericardial effusion
- Echocardiographic follow-up at discharge, 30 days, 6 months, annually
- Continue guideline-directed medical therapy for RV failure

Complications

- Bleeding (0–11.9%), single leaflet device attachment loss (SLDA, 3.8–13%), device-related surgery (0.2%)[13]
- Tricuspid gradients ≥5 mm Hg in some patients post-procedure[14]

- No significant increase in device-related arrhythmias
- Low major adverse event and mortality rates at 30 days; no mortality benefit over medical therapy beyond 1 year[14,15]
- Stroke (0%), MI (1%), renal failure (5%) post-TEER low[15]
- Favorable early survival linked to patient selection in TRILUMINATE trial[14]

Predictors of Outcome

- Procedural success with ≥1 grade TR reduction at 30 days predicts reduced mortality and heart failure hospitalization[16]
- Residual TR ≤ moderate post-TEER associated with nearly threefold decrease in 1-year mortality and HF hospitalizations[14]
- Residual TR ≥ moderate correlates with 2-3-fold increased mortality and HF hospitalization at 1 year[17]

CONCLUSION AND FUTURE DIRECTIONS

- Positive outcomes from transcatheter TV repair growing; off-label MitraClip use improves quality of life regardless of baseline RA pressure[18]
- BRIGHT trial shows low lead complication rates (~1%) with clipping around cardiac implantable electronic device leads[18]
- Durable TR reduction, few adverse events, and significant clinical benefits support transcatheter treatment of TR.
- Optimal timing critical; late intervention limits benefits due to irreversible ventricular damage.
- T-TEER may not suit all; other transcatheter platforms (annuloplasty, valve replacement) are in development.
- FDA approval in 2024 of TriClip (repair) and Evoque valve (replacement) expected to expand treatment options.
- Advances in imaging, device design, and operator skill improve safety, efficacy, and accessibility.
- Early detection, optimal imaging, and multi-disciplinary care essential for maximizing benefit.
- TEER has evolved into a safe, reproducible procedure with positive patient impact, expected to complement other modalities with ongoing research.

REFERENCES

1. Nkomo VT, Gardin JM, Skelton TN, Gottdiener JS, Scott CG, Enriquez-Sarano M. Burden of valvular heart diseases: a population-based study. Lancet. 2006;368:1005-11.
2. Goel SS, Bajaj N, Aggarwal B, Gupta S, Poddar KL, Ige M, Bdair H, et al. Prevalence and outcomes of unoperated patients with severe symptomatic mitral regurgitation and heart-failure: comprehensive analysis to determine the potential role of MitraClip for this unmet need. J Am Coll Cardiol. 2014;63:185-6.
3. Alfieri O, Maisano F, De Bonis M, Stefano PL, Torracca L, Oppizzi M, et al. The double-orifice technique in mitral valve repair: a simple solution for complex problems. J Thorac Cardiovasc Surg. 2001;122:674-81.
4. Feldman T, Wasserman HS, Herrmann HC, Gray W, Block PC, Whitlow P, et al. Percutaneous mitral valve repair using the edge-to-edge technique: six-month results of the EVEREST Phase I Clinical Trial. J Am Coll Cardiol. 2005;46:2134-40.
5. Otto CM, Nishimura RA, Bonow RO, Carabello BA, Erwin JP 3rd, Gentile F, et al. 2020 ACC/AHA Guideline for the Management of Patients With Valvular Heart Disease: A Report of the American College of Cardiology/American Heart Association Joint Committee on Clinical Practice Guidelines. Circulation. 2021;143(5):e72-e227.
6. Lesevic H, Karl M, Braun D, Barthel P, Orban M, Pache J, et al. Long-Term Outcomes After MitraClip Implantation According to the Presence or Absence of EVEREST Inclusion Criteria. Am J Cardiol. 2017;119:1255-61.

7. Thaden JJ, Malouf JF, Nkomo VT, Pislaru SV, Holmes DR Jr, Reeder GS, et al. Mitral Valve Anatomic Predictors of Hemodynamic Success With Transcatheter Mitral Valve Repair. J Am Heart Assoc. 2018;7:e007315.
8. Oguz D, Padang R, Rashedi N, Pislaru SV, Nkomo VT, Mankad SV, et al. Risk for Increased Mean Diastolic Gradient after Transcatheter Edge-to-Edge Mitral Valve Repair: A Quantitative Three-Dimensional Transesophageal Echocardiographic Analysis. J Am Soc Echocardiogr. 2021;34:595-603.
9. Niikura H, Bae R, Gössl M, Lin D, Jay D, Sorajja P. Transcatheter therapy for residual mitral regurgitation after MitraClip therapy. EuroIntervention. 2019;15:e491-9.
10. Nakajima Y, Kar S. First experience of the usage of a GORE CARDIOFORM Septal Occluder device for treatment of a significant residual commissural mitral regurgitation jet following a MitraClip procedure. Catheter Cardiovasc Interv. 2018;92:607-10.
11. Taramasso M, Vanermen H, Maisano F, Guidotti A, La Canna G, Alfieri O. The growing clinical importance of secondary tricuspid regurgitation. J Am Coll Cardiol. 2012;59:703-10.
12. Song H, Kim MJ, Chung CH, Choo SJ, Song MG, Song JM, et al. Factors associated with development of late significant tricuspid regurgitation after successful left-sided valve surgery. Heart. 2009;95:931-6.
13. Nickenig G, Weber M, Lurz P, von Bardeleben RS, Sitges M, Sorajja P, et al. Transcatheter edge-to-edge repair for reduction of tricuspid regurgitation: 6-month outcomes of the TRILUMINATE single-arm study. Lancet. 2019;394:2002-11.
14. Sorajja P, Whisenant B, Hamid N, Naik H, Makkar R, Tadros P, et al. Transcatheter repair for patients with tricuspid regurgitation. N Engl J Med. 2023; 388:1833-42.
15. Rehan ST, Eqbal F, Ul Hussain H, Ali E, Ali A, Ullah I, et al. Transcatheter edge to-edge repair for tricuspid regurgitation: a systematic review and meta-analysis. Curr Probl Cardiol. 2024;49(1 Pt B): 102055.
16. Besler C, Orban M, Rommel KP, Braun D, Patel M, Hagl C, et al. Predictors of procedural and clinical outcomes in patients with symptomatic tricuspid regurgitation undergoing transcatheter edge-to-edge repair. JACC Cardiovasc Interv. 2018;11:1119-28.
17. Coisne A, Scotti A, Taramasso M, Granada JF, Ludwig S, Rodés-Cabau J, et al. Prognostic value of tricuspid valve gradient after transcatheter edge-to-edge repair: insights from the TriValve registry. JACC Cardiovasc Interv. 2023;16:706-17.
18. Ya'Qoub L, Caughron H, Qasim A, Tolstrop K, Delling FN, Watt C, et al. Clinical improvement with transcatheter edge-to-edge tricuspid repair irrespective of right atrial pressure. JACC Adv. 2024;3:100862.

CHAPTER 25

Weight Reduction by Novel Drugs: What is Their Effect on Cardiovascular Events and Which One to Choose?

Chhavi Agrawal, Shiv Kumar Goel

■ INTRODUCTION

Prevalence of obesity has reached to pandemic proportions. According to a WHO statement, in 2022, 2.5 billion adults were overweight, including 890 million adults living with obesity. In most cases, a multitude of factors contribute to the development of obesity, including genetic, psychosocial factors, and obesogenic environments. According to ICMR–INDIAB study in 2015, the prevalence rate of central obesity varies from 16.9% in women and 36.3% in men.[1] Obesity is a major risk factor for various noncommunicable disease like coronary artery disease, heart failure, T2DM, osteoarthritis, hypertension, ischemic strokes, and certain cancers. The increasing prevalence of obesity and in turn the diseases associated with the same may outweigh the benefits of the advances being seen in management of cardiovascular (CV) diseases.

It is thus essential that weight management should play an integral part of the cardiovascular disease treatment in patients who are overweight and obese. However, cardiologists face a multitude of challenges in managing such cases as one of the most difficult part in managing obesity is to introduce lifestyle measure. It has been shown that efforts to implement dietary and lifestyle changes are difficult and maintaining the weight loss is very challenging. To date, there is no data to support that lifestyle interventions lead to improved CV outcomes.[2] In fact, some of the previous obesity medications like sibutramine and fenfluramine lead to concerns about their effect on CV health due to which they were withdrawn from the market.[3] To ensure the cardio-neutral or cardio-beneficial effects of the antiobesity medications, the Food and Drug Administration (FDA) has mandated that similar to the antidiabetic drugs, antiobesity medications should also undergo cardiovascular outcome trials (CVOTs). Although earlier guidelines did not prioritize obesity pharmacotherapies, ADA 2022 has also advised that weight management should be given priority with focus on GLP1-RAs like semaglutide and dual GLP1-RA/GIP like tirzepatide.

The three different weight loss interventions are:
1. Lifestyle intervention
2. Bariatric surgery
3. Pharmacotherapy

Lifestyle intervention primarily refers to behavioral changes brought about by changes in diet, physical activity, and exercise routine in order to achieve the desired weight loss. Many trials have studied the effect of various lifestyle measures in comparison to usual care in overweight and obese individuals. These trials have shown that lifestyle changes are associated with significantly higher weight loss in comparison to usual care.[4,5] These lifestyle interventions do lead to weight loss but on long-term follow-up, these patients tend to regain the weight. The data does suggest difficulty in maintaining the weight loss due to lack on long-term adherence to the interventions and metabolic adaptations leading to increase in orexigenic hormones like ghrelin.

The Look AHEAD (Action for Health in Diabetes) trial was a randomized controlled trial comparing an Intensive Lifestyle Intervention

(ILI) to a Diabetes Support and Education (DSE) in overweight and obese type 2 diabetes patients to track the development of cardiovascular disease over time. The trial failed to show any CV outcome benefits but was showed weight loss was associated with improvement in sugar and lipid profiles along with blood pressure, lesser sleep apnea, and lower liver fat.[4,6]

■ BARIATRIC SURGERY

Bariatric surgery is a group of surgeries aimed to treat morbidly obese individuals. Commonly performed bariatric procedures include vertical banded gastroplasty or sleeve gastrectomy and Roux-en-Y gastric bypass (RYGB).[7] Studies have shown that weight loss post bariatric surgery is 15–20% over and above the weight loss seen with either medicines or lifestyle interventions. The weight loss attained with the surgeries is usually by 1 year and is sustained up to 5 years, unlike the weight loss associated with lifestyle interventions.[8,9] Though none of the guidelines currently recommend bariatric surgery to support improved CV outcomes with level 1 evidence, European Society of Cardiology's newly issued guidelines for cardiovascular disease prevention, "bariatric surgery for obese high-risk people should be considered when lifestyle adjustment does not result in maintained weight loss," i.e., it is a 2A recommendation. Study by Aminian et al. showed significant improvement in extended MACE (defined as first occurrence of all-cause mortality, coronary events, cerebrovascular events, HF, nephropathy, and atrial fibrillation) in patients who had undergone metabolic surgery, in comparison to patients who did not.[10] The Bariatric Surgery for the Reduction of cArdioVascular Events (BRAVE) Feasibility Trial is an ongoing study in patients with severe obesity [body mass index (BMI) ≥30 kg/m^2] and high-risk cardiovascular disease (CVD), to assess if bariatric surgery compared to medical weight management (MWM) safely reduces the risk of major cardiovascular events.[11] Bariatric surgery is currently indicated for patients with BMI ≥40 or ≥35 with comorbidities,[12] though there are variations among various guidelines.

■ PHARMACOTHERAPY FOR OBESITY

GLP1-RAs have revolutionized the management of obesity. This group of medication primarily acts by mimicking endogenous GLP-1 activity and bind to the GLP-1R in various tissues. GLP1 primarily augments insulin secretion in response to food ingestion **(Table 1)**.

Liraglutide Effect and Action in Diabetes: Evaluation of Cardiovascular Outcome Results (LEADER) trial was among the first trials to show that GLP1 RA use led to a reduction in MACE events.[13] The weight loss efficacy of GLP1 RA is dose dependent, thus the trials have studied different doses for diabetes management and weight loss effect. Liraglutide at a dose of 3 mg is approved for weight loss treatment while

TABLE 1: Various GLP1 RAs and their CVOT outcome data.

Drug	Dose	CVOT	Hazard ratio
Liraglutide	1.8 mg	LEADER	HR 0.87; 95% CI: 0.73–1.00, p = 0.046
Dulaglutide	1.5 mg	REWIND	HR 0.88; 95% CI: 0.79–0.99, p = 0.026
Semaglutide—oral	14 mg	PIONEER 6	HR: 0.79; 95% CI: 0.57–1.11; p < 0.001 for noninferiority
Semaglutide—injection	1 mg	SUSTAIN 6	HR: 0.74, 95% CI: 0.58–0.95, p < 0.001 for noninferiority; p = 0.02 for superiority

(CVOT: cardiovascular outcome trial; GLP1 RA: glucagon-like peptide-1 receptor agonist)

maximum dose of 1.8 mg is recommended for T2DM management. No CVOT data is available for the 3 mg dose, though a post hoc analysis of the SCALE (The Satiety and Clinical Adiposity—Liraglutide Evidence in people with T2D and no diabetes) trial demonstrated that the group of patients that received 3 mg liraglutide had a lesser chance of having CV events.[14]

The Researching Cardiovascular Events with a Weekly Incretin in Diabetes (REWIND) trial was a double blind RCT of weekly dulaglutide that studied more than 9,000 T2DM patients. REWIND trial stands out among the GLP1RA trials due to its long follow-up period of greater than 5 years and 69% of patients did not have history of prior cardiac event. This make it suitable to assess the hypothesis for primary prevention of ASCVD in T2DM patients with dulaglutide. It showed that dulaglutide significantly reduced the composite of primary end point, which was defined as a composite of nonfatal MI, nonfatal stroke, and death from CV or unknown causes.[15]

Subcutaneous semaglutide has been extensively studied in a large population of patients. STEP trials evaluated the effect of 2.4 mg once weekly semaglutide against placebo across varying population groups. The STEP-4 trial was a withdrawal trial that evaluated the effect of continued treatment with semaglutide on weight loss maintenance. Patients who were on weekly 2.4 mg semaglutide for 20 weeks were either continued on the drug or on placebo for the next 48 weeks. Patients on the trial drug maintained the weight loss while those on placebo experienced weight gain. Semaglutide use is associated with reduction in systolic and diastolic blood pressure and favorable changed in lipid parameters across the STEP trials. Semaglutide use showed a tendency to increase heart rate, which was also seen in LEADER trial and could be a class effect[16-19] **(Fig. 1)**.

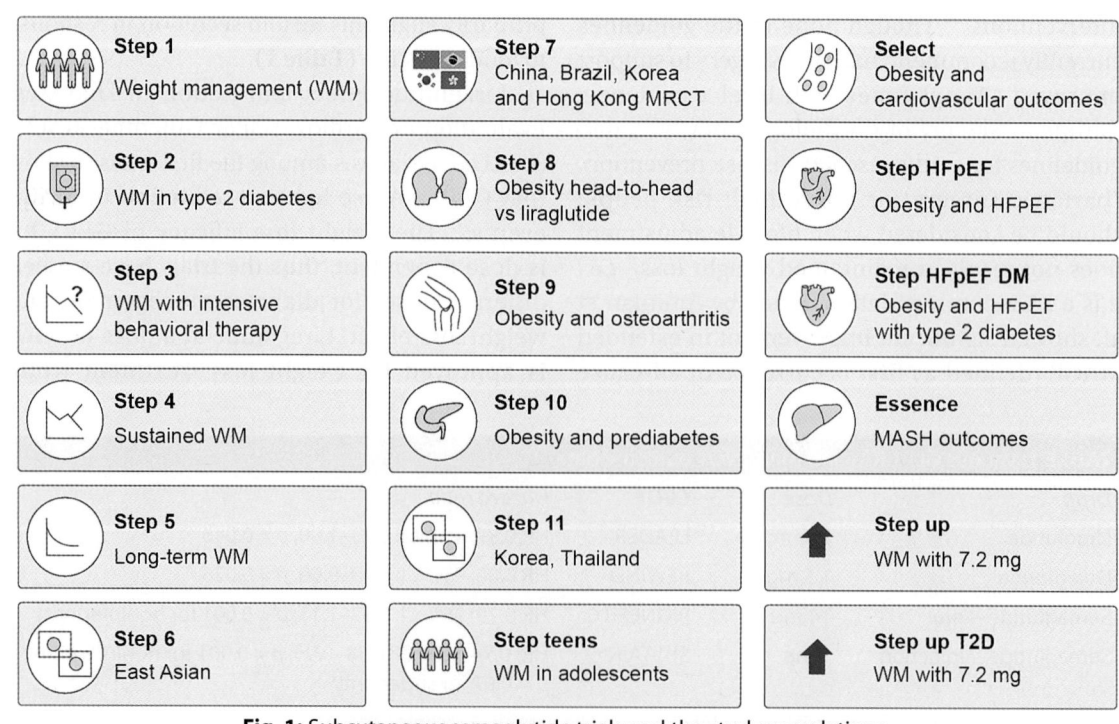

Fig. 1: Subcutaneous semaglutide trials and the study populations.
(HFpEF: heart failure with preserved ejection fraction)

The CVOT trial of semaglutide in patients with T2DM included around 3,300 patients. The Trial to Evaluate Cardiovascular and Other Long-term Outcomes with Semaglutide in Subjects with Type 2 Diabetes (SUSTAIN-6)[20] confirmed noninferiority of semaglutide as compared to placebo. Semaglutide-treated patients had a significantly lower risk of the primary composite outcome of death from cardiovascular causes, nonfatal myocardial infarction, or nonfatal stroke than did those receiving placebo.

SELECT trial was the first CVOT evaluating GLP1 RA in overweight and obese patients without diabetes. It was a superiority trial unlike the SUSTAIN 6 which was a noninferiority trial. More than 17,000 patients were enrolled and the trial demonstrated that overweight or obese patients with pre-existing cardiovascular disease but without diabetes who received 2.4 mg semaglutide had reduced incidence of death from cardiovascular causes, nonfatal myocardial infarction, or nonfatal stroke at a mean follow-up of 39.8 months.[21] This landmark trial leads to important implications in cardiology management as it recommends the drug not only as a weight loss agent but also for secondary prevention of CV disease in obese patients. The STEP-HFpEF (Semaglutide Treatment Effect in People With Obesity and HFpEF) included obese patients with HFpEF who either received semaglutide 2.4 mg once-weekly or placebo. After a follow-up at 1-year, semaglutide significantly improved health-related quality of life, functional status, and CRP levels in addition to the weight reduction in these patients.[22]

Oral semaglutide is the only GLP1 RA which is available in oral formulation. Despite the coformulation with sodium N-(8-(2-hydroxybenzoyl)amino) caprylate (SNAC) to enable gut absorption, bioavailability of the oral formulation remains low, requiring daily ingestion of the medication unlike weekly formulation of injectable semaglutide. The Peptide Innovation for Early Diabetes Treatment (PIONEER) 6 trial[23] was a noninferiority trial in comparison to placebo, which did not any significant difference between the 2 groups though placebo had numerically higher MACE events.

Tirzepatide, also referred to as a "twincretin", because of its dual GLP-1 and GIP receptor efficacy, is approved for glycemic control in diabetes and weight loss in obese patients. Similar to GLP-1, GIP is another incretin hormone released in the gut in response to oral nutrients. Tirzepatide, because of its unique structure, provides additive incretin effect.[24] Administered once weekly, tirzepatide offers dosing flexibility ranging from 2.5 to 15 mg per 0.5 mL injection.[25] SURMOUNT series of trials investigated the efficacy of tirzepatide on primarily weight loss.[26,27] SURMOUNT 1 targeted weight loss in obese patients without diabetes with weekly tirzepatide across doses of 5 mg, 10 mg, and 15 mg. The trial showed weight loss of up to 20.9% after 18 months with 15 mg dose in comparison to 3.1% with placebo while SURMOUNT 2 studied overweight diabetic patients on weekly tirzepatide either 10 mg or 15 mg and patients on 15 mg dose showed 14.7% weight reduction at 18 months.

The SURPASS series of trials[28,29] primarily investigated tirzepatide in participants with T2DM. These trials also showed similar results with weight loss ranging from 5 to 14% across doses of tirzepatide. SURPASS-2 trial compared various doses of tirzepatide to once-weekly subcutaneous semaglutide 1 mg. The trial showed that Tirzepatide at all doses was noninferior and superior to semaglutide. Reductions in body weight were greater with tirzepatide than with semaglutide.[28] A recent meta-analysis of 47 RCTs including more than 17,000 patients found tirzepatide to be the most effective GLP1 RA in weight reduction.[30]

SURPASS-CVOT was a randomized double-blind, active controlled CVOT that compared tirzepatide and dulaglutide in efficacy and safety in adults with type 2 diabetes with established ASCVD. The results found tirzepatide noninferior to dulaglutide (hazard ratio: 0.92; 95.3% CI: 0.83 to 1.01).[31]

Retatrutide is a weekly "triple agonist", acting on glucagon receptors in addition to GLP1 and GIP. In phase 2 study across the doses of 4 mg, 8 mg, and 12 mg, 15% weight reduction was seen in 60%, 75%, and 83% of the study participants respectively. HbA1c reductions of up to 2.2% were seen with the treatment in obese diabetic patients.[32] Initial data from these trials suggest robust weight loss in comparison to the previous drugs available in market; further studies are awaited to understand their impact on CV outcomes and their long-term safety profile.

CONCLUSION

In the last decade, GLP1 RAs have revolutionized the care and management of not only the patients suffering from T2DM but also overweight and obese patients. The focus has shifted from glucocentric management of diabetes primarily targeting the glycemia, to holistic management focusing on drugs targeting the cardiovascular, renal, and hepatic comorbidities. With the availability of CVOT trial data for all new anti-diabetic drugs, individualizing treatment for diabetic patients with ASCVD or heart failure has become the focus of guidelines. CVOT data with newer agents for management of obese patients is awaited. With the advent of new weight loss drugs and trials suggesting that they have beneficial effects on cardiovascular health, cardiologists do need to focus on weight management of patients rather than secondary or tertiary care.

REFERENCES

1. Anjana RM, Deepa M, Pradeepa R, Mahanta J, Narain K, Das HK, et al. Prevalence of diabetes and prediabetes in 15 states of India: results from the ICMR–INDIAB population-based cross-sectional study. Lancet Diabetes Endocrinol. 2017;5(8):585-96.
2. Pi-Sunyer X. The look AHEAD trial: a review and discussion of its outcomes. Curr Nutr Rep. 2014;3:387-91.
3. Müller TD, Blüher M, Tschöp MH, DiMarchi RD. Anti-obesity drug discovery: advances and challenges. Nat Rev Drug Discov. 2022;21:201-23.
4. Look AHEAD Research Group; Wing RR, Bolin P, Brancati FL, Bray GA, Clark JM, et al. Cardiovascular effects of intensive lifestyle intervention in type 2 diabetes. New Engl J Med. 2013;369:145-54.
5. Knowler WC, Barrett-Connor E, Fowler SE, Hamman RF, Lachin JM, Walker EA, et al. Reduction in the incidence of type 2 diabetes with lifestyle intervention or metformin. N Engl J Med 2002;346:393-403.
6. Salvia MG. The Look AHEAD trial: translating lessons learned into clinical practice and further study. Diabetes Spectr. 2017;30:166-70.
7. Arterburn DE, Telem DA, Kushner RF, Courcoulas AP. Benefits and risks of bariatric surgery in adults: a review. JAMA. 2020;324:879-87.
8. Schauer PR, Bhatt DL, Kirwan JP, Wolski K, Aminian A, Brethauer SA, et al. Bariatric surgery versus intensive medical therapy for diabetes—5-year outcomes. New Engl J Med. 2017;376:641-51.
9. Buchwald H, Avidor Y, Braunwald E, Jensen MD, Pories W, Fahrbach K, et al. Bariatric surgery: a systematic review and meta-analysis. JAMA. 2004;292:1724-37.
10. Aminian A, Zajichek A, Arterburn DE, Wolski KE, Brethauer SA, Schauer PR, et al. Association of metabolic surgery with Major adverse cardiovascular outcomes in patients with type 2 diabetes and obesity. JAMA. 2019;322:1271-82.
11. ClinicalTrials.gov. Bariatric Surgery for the Reduction of Cardiovascular Events Feasibility Study (BRAVE). [online] Available from https://clinicaltrials.gov/ct2/show/NCT04226664. [Last accessed November, 2025].
12. Bray GA, Kim KK, Wilding JPH; World Obesity Federation. Obesity: a chronic relapsing progressive disease process. A position statement of the World Obesity Federation. Obes Rev. 2017;18(7):715-23.
13. Marso SP, Daniels GH, Brown-Frandsen K, Kristensen P, Mann JFE, Nauck MA, et al. Liraglutide and Cardiovascular Outcomes in Type 2 Diabetes. N Engl J Med. 2016;375:311-22.

14. Davies MJ, Aronne LJ, Caterson ID, Thomsen AB, Jacobsen PB, Marso SP. Liraglutide and cardiovascular outcomes in adults with overweight or obesity: a post hoc analysis from SCALE randomized controlled trials. Diabetes Obes Metab. 2018;20:734-9.
15. Gerstein HC, Colhoun HM, Dagenais GR, Diaz R, Lakshmanan M, Pais P, et al. Dulaglutide and Cardiovascular Outcomes in Type 2 Diabetes (REWIND): A Double-Blind, Randomised Placebo-Controlled Trial. Lancet. 2019;394:121-30.
16. Wilding JPH, Batterham RL, Calanna S, Davies M, Van Gaal LF, Lingvay I, et al. Once-weekly semaglutide in adults with overweight or obesity. N Engl J Med. 2021;384:989-1002.
17. Davies M, Færch L, Jeppesen OK, Pakseresht A, Pedersen SD, Perreault L, et al. Semaglutide 2.4 mg once a week in adults with overweight or obesity, and type 2 diabetes (STEP 2): a randomised, double-blind, double-dummy, placebo-controlled, phase 3 trial. Lancet. 2021;397:971-84.
18. Wadden TA, Bailey TS, Billings LK, Davies M, Frias JP, Koroleva A, et al. Effect of subcutaneous semaglutide vs placebo as an adjunct to intensive behavioral therapy on body weight in adults with overweight or obesity: the STEP 3 randomized clinical trial. JAMA. 2021;325:1403-13.
19. Rubino D, Abrahamsson N, Davies M, Hesse D, Greenway FL, Jensen C, et al. Effect of continued weekly subcutaneous semaglutide vs placebo on weight loss maintenance in adults with overweight or obesity: the STEP 4 randomized clinical trial. JAMA. 2021;325:1414-25.
20. Marso SP, Bain SC, Consoli A, Eliaschewitz FG, Jódar E, Leiter LA, et al. Semaglutide and Cardiovascular Outcomes in Patients with Type 2 Diabetes. N Engl J Med. 2016;375:1834-44.
21. Lincoff AM, Brown-Frandsen K, Colhoun HM, Deanfield J, Emerson SS, Esbjerg S, et al. Semaglutide and cardiovascular outcomes in obesity without diabetes. N Engl J Med. 2023;389:2221-32.
22. Kosiborod MN, Abildstrøm SZ, Borlaug BA, Butler J, Rasmussen S, Davies M, et al. Semaglutide in patients with heart failure with preserved ejection fraction and obesity. N Engl J Med. 2023;389:1069-84.
23. Husain M, Birkenfeld AL, Donsmark M, Dungan K, Eliaschewitz FG, Franco DR, et al. Oral Semaglutide and Cardiovascular Outcomes in Patients with Type 2 Diabetes. N Engl J Med. 2019;381:841-51.
24. Min T, Bain SC. The role of tirzepatide, dual GIP and GLP-1 receptor agonist, in the management of type 2 diabetes: the SURPASS clinical trials. Diabetes Ther. 2021;12:143-57.
25. Khashayar F, Preeti P. (2024). Tirzepatide. [online] Available from https://www.ncbi.nlm.nih.gov/books/NBK585056/. [Last accessed November, 2025].
26. Jastreboff AM, Aronne LJ, Ahmad NN, Wharton S, Connery L, Alves B, et al. Tirzepatide once weekly for the treatment of obesity. N Engl J Med. 2022;387(3):205-16.
27. Garvey WT, Frias JP, Jastreboff AM, le Roux CW, Sattar N, Aizenberg D, et al. Tirzepatide once weekly for the treatment of obesity in people with type 2 diabetes (SURMOUNT-2): a double-blind, randomised, multicentre, placebo-controlled, phase 3 trial. Lancet. 2023;402(10402):613-26.
28. Frías JP, Davies MJ, Rosenstock J, Pérez Manghi FC, Fernández Landó L, Bergman BK, et al. Tirzepatide versus semaglutide once weekly in patients with type 2 diabetes. N Engl J Med. 2021;385(6):503-15.
29. Rosenstock J, Frías JP, Rodbard HW, Tofé S, Sears E, Huh R, et al. Tirzepatide vs insulin lispro added to basal insulin in type 2 diabetes: the SURPASS-6 randomized clinical trial. JAMA. 2023;330(17):1631-40.
30. Yao H, Zhang A, Li D, Wu Y, Wang CZ, Wan JY, et al. Comparative effectiveness of GLP-1 receptor agonists on glycaemic control, body weight, and lipid profile for type 2 diabetes: systematic review and network meta-analysis. BMJ. 2024;384:e076410.
31. ClinicalTrials.gov. A Study of Tirzepatide (LY3298176) Compared With Dulaglutide on Major Cardiovascular Events in Participants With Type 2 Diabetes (SURPASS-CVOT). [online] Available from https://www.clinicaltrials.gov/study/NCT04255433. [Last accessed November, 2025].
32. Rosenstock J, Frias J, Jastreboff AM, Du Y, Lou J, Gurbuz S, et al. Retatrutide, a GIP, GLP-1 and glucagon receptor agonist, for people with type 2 diabetes: a randomised, double-blind, placebo and active-controlled, parallel-group, phase 2 trial conducted in the USA. Lancet. 2023;402:529-44.

CHAPTER 26

Vegetarian Diet versus Mediterranean Diet: What to Follow? Indian Mediterranean Diet?

Ishi Khosla, Anindita Das

■ INTRODUCTION

Global dietary shifts driven by urbanization and technological changes have caused widespread transition from traditional diets to modern, processed food-heavy patterns.[1] This includes increased consumption of ultra-processed foods high in salt, sugar, and unhealthy fats. These have significantly contributed to the rising global burden of cardiometabolic diseases such as obesity, type 2 diabetes, cardiovascular diseases (CVDs), etc.[2] CVD remains the leading cause of death across the world.[3] Diet, being its modifiable factor, plays a crucial role in its prevention and management.[4] Recently, the emphasis on plant-based and/or plant-forward eating patterns by the American Heart Association and EAT-Lancet Commission have aligned with the core principles of the vegetarian diet (VD) and Mediterranean diet (MD).[5,6] Epidemiological evidence has shown that both these dietary models promise cardioprotective benefits.[7] Although both are predominantly plant-based, they have evolved in different ecological and cultural contexts—one from religious and ethical principles, the other from a traditional cuisine.

The VD primarily restricts or eliminates animal products and have been linked with a 15% relative reduction in CVD incidence and 21% reduced ischemic heart disease risk, apart from improving blood pressure, LDL cholesterol, body weight, and inflammatory markers.[8] MD features a variety of plant foods with olive oil, fish, moderate dairy and wine intake. It has been established as a cardioprotective diet and has been known to reduce all-cause mortality across diverse populations.[9]

Comparing these dietary models is particularly important in dietary management of CVD because, while both diets show robust evidence for cardiovascular benefit, they differ in nutrient profile, adherence, and sustainability considerations. Mechanistically both influence cardiovascular risk through lipid modulation and by improving endothelial function, reducing inflammation, and altering gut microbiota composition.

This chapter reviews the current evidence for these diet models, exploring their nutritional composition, underlying mechanism and clinical outcomes, and highlighting their applicability in real-world clinical practice to inform evidence-based dietary guidance for CVD prevention.

■ IMPACT OF VEGETARIAN DIET ON CARDIOVASCULAR DISEASE RISK FACTORS

The VD excludes animal products such as meat, fish, and poultry and emphasizes on fruits and vegetables, pulses and legumes, nuts and seeds, and whole grains. It has many other forms—lacto-vegetarian (includes dairy only), lacto-ovo vegetarian (includes dairy and eggs), and vegan (excludes all forms of animal-derived foods). A VD typically provides 45–55% of daily energy, though some report higher (~50–60%) from whole grains and legumes.[10] When well planned, it provides around 12–15% of energy from proteins for lacto-ovo vegetarians, but some studies have shown up to 25–30%, especially when emphasizing legumes and soy.[11] VD is naturally rich in dietary fiber (25–40 g/day), unsaturated fatty acids, antioxidants such as vitamin C and E, magnesium, and folate.[12] It is low in cholesterol and saturated fats. All of them are linked to improved cardiometabolic markers and reduced CVD risk.[13,14]

Increased fiber intake slows lipid absorption in the intestine and lowers serum LDL cholesterol, a key contributor to atherosclerosis.[15] Higher soluble fiber and phytosterol intake in the diet facilitates hepatic cholesterol clearance, while antioxidant and polyphenol compounds modulate oxidative pathways that affect vascular tone and insulin signaling.[16,17] Lower saturated fat content reduces LDL oxidation and improves endothelial function, thereby mitigating vascular inflammation and hypertension risk.[18] The combination of high-water content and fiber in plant foods leads to greater satiety, reducing overall energy intake, and supporting healthy weight.[19] Thus, VD help reduce BMI, which decreases cardiometabolic risk through favorable effects on glucose metabolism and inflammatory adipokines.[15,20] VD and plant-based diets are typically lower in branched-chain amino acids and methionine. Lower intake of these amino acids is linked to favorable outcomes on insulin sensitivity and lipid metabolism, both in epidemiological and preclinical studies.[21,22]

The effectiveness of a VD largely depends on its quality. Diets emphasizing whole, minimally processed plant foods differ substantially from those high in refined carbohydrates or fried snacks, despite both qualifying as "vegetarian." A 12-week RCT demonstrated that a whole-food plant-based nutrition program significantly reduced and sustained BMI, blood pressure, total and LDL cholesterol.[23] A 2024 cohort study found that CVD risk was only reduced in those whose plant-based diets prioritized nonultra-processed foods, while diets high in UPFs, even if "meat-free" did not lower and instead may increase the risk of CVD and other metabolic disorders.[24]

A distinguishing feature of VDs is their higher potassium-to-sodium ratio, which supports blood pressure regulation through enhanced natriuresis and vascular relaxation. The higher folate, magnesium, and potassium are attributed to the emphasis on fruits, vegetables, legumes, and whole grains.[12] These micronutrients reduce circulating homocysteine and benefit cardiovascular health.

Recent randomized trials and meta-analyses show that VD are associated with improvement in key CVD risk factors.[8,25] Prospective studies have consistently shown that VD are associated with a lower risk of developing diabetes, CVDs, and certain types of cancers.[20] Cohort studies, particularly the EPIC-Oxford cohort, confirms that those adhered to VD have up to a 32% lower risk of heart disease compared to omnivores.[26] A 2024 umbrella review found that vegan and vegetarian dietary patterns were associated with 15% reduction in CVD incidence and lower concentrations of total and LDL cholesterol, and CRP.[27] RCTs in patients with ischemic heart disease demonstrate that isocaloric VD result in greater reduction of oxidized LDL and total cholesterol, body weight, and favorable shifts in gut microbial composition compared to meat-based diets.[13] The CARDIVEG trial compared a low-calorie VD and MD in patients with ischemic heart disease.[28] Both the diets showed improved weight and fat mass, with VD exhibiting significantly greater LDL reduction. Across studies, the cholesterol-lowering effect is strongest in vegan diets, followed by lacto-ovo vegetarian patterns, indicating a dose-response relationship with the degree of animal product exclusion.[25]

Beyond individual health, vegetarian dietary patterns align with broader sustainability goals, offering lower environmental impact and resource demands compared to meat-based diets.

IMPACT OF MEDITERRANEAN DIET ON CARDIOVASCULAR DISEASE RISK FACTORS

The MD reflects a cultural model emphasizing balance and seasonal variety. Grounded in the traditional eating patterns of countries bordering the Mediterranean Sea, it is characterized by high consumption of whole grains, legumes, fruits, vegetables, nuts, extra virgin olive oil (EVOO), with moderate intake of poultry, fish, dairy and wine, and low consumption of processed and red meats.[29] This diet is rich in monounsaturated fats, mainly derived from EVOO, and omega-3 fats from nuts and fish, alongside abundant dietary fiber, polyphenols, antioxidants, and essential micronutrients.[30] Typically, 35–40% energy is derived from fat, 15–20% from protein, and 40–50% from complex, low-GI carbohydrates.[31,32] Fat quality is prioritized over quantity in a MD.[33]

Consumption of whole grains, fruits, vegetables, and legumes makes the diet rich in dietary fiber, which reduces serum cholesterol, blunts postprandial glycemic spikes, and promotes gut microbiota diversity.[34] Omega-3s lowers triglycerides, reduces platelet aggregation, and stabilizes heart rhythm, thereby providing antiarrhythmic and antithrombotic effects.[35] Moderate red wine intake provides resveratrol, which may further enhance cardioprotective benefits by modulating vascular tone and reducing oxidating milieu.[36] Polyphenols from wine and EVOO increase bioavailability of nitric oxide by modulating endothelial nitric oxide synthase (eNOS). MD involves high intakes of magnesium, potassium, folate, and selenium—all of which are linked to blood pressure regulation, vascular health, and oxidative balance.[34,37] These polyphenols influence transcription factors like peroxisome proliferator-activated receptors (PPARs) and nuclear factor-kappa B (NF-KB), that regulate inflammation and lipid metabolism in the body. It supports higher HDL, lower LDL, improved insulin sensitivity, and reduced inflammatory markers and oxidative stress. The combination of low glycemic load and high MUFA in MD enhances insulin sensitivity and reduces postprandial glucose spikes, contributing to improved metabolic markers.[38]

MD likely reduce the risk of all-cause mortality, cardiovascular mortality, stroke, and nonfatal myocardial infarction compared to minimal interventions.[39] Especially in women, adherence to MD is associated with a 23% lower risk of total mortality and a 24% lower risk of CVD.[40] The PREDIMED trial demonstrates that MD supplemented with either mixed nuts or EVOO relatively reduces major CVD events among high-risk individuals by 30%, compared to a low-fat diet.[30] A long-term review showed that following MD significantly reduces risk of stroke and coronary events, and total and cardiovascular mortality, besides improving endothelial function.[41] MD reduces the incidence of major adverse cardiovascular events (MACE), myocardial infarction, stroke, and CVD-associated death.

DIETARY PATTERNS AND GUT MICROBIOME

Emerging interest of researchers have led to the exploration of how dietary patterns profoundly shape the gut microbiome, which influences cardiovascular health. Higher dietary indices for gut microbiota diversity were strongly and independently associated with reduced CVD risk, partly mediated by improved metabolic parameters and lower BMI.[42] Both VD and MD being rich in plant-based foods and fiber have been associated with a diverse gut microbiome and increased presence of beneficial short-chain fatty acids (SCFAs)-producing bacteria compared to omnivorous or Western-style diets.[43,44] SCFAs bind to G-protein-coupled receptors located in the adipose tissue and colon. When these receptors are activated, they signal anti-inflammatory cascades which suppress insulin signaling in adipose tissue to inhibit fat accumulation, while enhancing systemic insulin sensitivity through lipid and glucose metabolism in liver and muscle.[45] SCFAs production by the gut microbiota reduces inflammation and supports endothelial function, lowering circulating levels of trimethylamine-N-oxide (TMAO).[46] It is a harmful metabolite linked to atherosclerosis.[47] Cross-sectional studies have shown that polyphenol and fiber from a typical MD modulate the gut microbiota and bile acid metabolism, indirectly lowering plasma lipid levels and systemic inflammation.[48]

Interventional study in adults with dysglycemia and obesity showed that switching to a vegan diet lowered plasma TMAO concentration by nearly 50%; the levels rebounded upon returning to an unrestricted diet, confirming diet-dependent effect.[49] This reduction occurred independently of weight loss and was attributed to the elimination of animal-derived TMAO precursors such as choline and L-carnitine, found in eggs, red meat, and fish.

While there is emerging evidence to support the beneficial impact of these diets on both cardiovascular outcomes and microbiome, heterogeneity remains in study results, and the full mechanistic pathways are yet to be completely elucidated. This underscores the need for targeted prospective trials.[41,46]

CLINICAL AND PRACTICAL CONSIDERATIONS

It is important to consider clinical and practical factors while recommending any dietary model to ensure adherence and effectiveness. For VD, ensuring nutrient adequacy is essential, particularly for iron, vitamin B_{12}, and omega-3 fatty acids as these are less abundant in plant-based sources.[50] Nonheme iron in plants is less absorbed in the body compared to heme iron due to inhibition by phytates (found in legumes, whole grains, and nuts) and polyphenols (found in some vegetables, coffee, and tea). These compounds bind iron and reduce its solubility.[51] Similarly, bioavailability of zinc is also reduced by phytic acid in whole grains and legumes which chelate zinc and limits update.[52] Nevertheless, traditional food processing methods such as soaking, germination, and fermentation along with consuming vitamin C-rich foods enhance mineral bioavailability by degrading phytates and promoting absorption. In addition, conversion of plant-derived α-linolenic acid into EPA and DHA is metabolically inefficient. This is why fortified foods and dietary supplementation are often necessary to meet daily requirements, prevent deficiency, and achieve additional protective benefits.[4] Moreover, both VD and MD require attention to calorie control and balanced portion sizes to achieve and maintain healthy weight, which is an important factor in CVD risk reduction.[28]

Strategies such as pairing iron-rich plant foods with vitamin C sources or incorporating sprouted legumes can markedly improve mineral absorption without altering the diet's plant-based nature. Meta-analysis and systematic review support algal oil supplementation for raising plasma and erythrocyte EPA and DHA almost equally to fish oil.[53]

The MD can be adapted globally by replacing Mediterranean staples with culturally relevant, nutritionally equivalent alternatives.[54] For instance, pulses and legumes in India provide fiber and protein analogous to Mediterranean legumes; coastal regions of India have a variety of fishes that can be included in the diet to match the Mediterranean principles. This local tailoring is essential to main the emphasis on whole foods, plant-centered patterns and fat quality, to support both health and cultural acceptance.

CONCLUSION

Individual preferences, cultural background, food availability, and sustainability considerations influence adherence to diet. Both VD and MD have demonstrated flexibility and can be adapted effectively to local cuisines and lifestyles while still providing cardiovascular benefits if appropriately applied.[28] Implementing a hybrid dietary model such as "med-veg" or "plant-forward mediterranean" diet can combine the core principles of both the diets. They unite the strengths of both diets, improving cardiometabolic profiles while maintaining cultural and practical acceptability.[55] All in all whichever diet one follows it must be personalized, gut friendly, and anti-inflammatory.

REFERENCES

1. Ambikapathi R, Schneider KR, Davis B, et al. Global food systems transitions have enabled affordable diets but had less favourable outcomes for nutrition, environmental health, inclusion and equity. Nature Food. 2022;3(9):764-79.
2. Lundberg K, Moragues-Faus A, Thornton L, et al. Paving the way: Urban Health, Food Systems, and the Imperative for Holistic City-Led Action. F1000Research. 2025;14:513-3.
3. Chong B, Jayabaskaran J, Jauhari SM, et al. Global burden of cardiovascular diseases: projections from 2025 to 2050. Eur J Prev Cardiol. 2025;32(11):1001-15.
4. Marques-Vidal P, Tsampasian V, Cassidy A, et al. Diet and nutrition in cardiovascular disease prevention: a scientific statement of the European Association of Preventive Cardiology and the Association of Cardiovascular Nursing & Allied Professions of the European Society of Cardiology. Eur J Prev Cardiol. 2025;32(16):1540-52.
5. American Heart Association. (2025). Plant-based proteins may help lower high blood pressure risk. [Online] Available from https://www.heart.org/en/news/2025/05/15/plant-based-proteins-may-help-lower-high-blood-pressure-risk [Last accessed November, 2025].
6. Commission EL. Eat Lancet's Planetary Health Diets: Plant-based food as part of the solution. [Online] Available from https://www.alprofoundation.org/scientific-updates/eat-lancet-s-planetary-health-diets-plant-based-food-as-part-of-the-solution [Last accessed November, 2025].
7. Dybvik JS, Svendsen M, Aune D. Vegetarian and vegan diets and the risk of cardiovascular disease, ischemic heart disease and stroke: A systematic review and meta-analysis of prospective cohort studies. Eur J Nutr. 2022;62(1):51-69.
8. Wang T, Kroeger CM, Cassidy S, et al. Vegetarian dietary patterns and cardiometabolic risk in people with or at high risk of cardiovascular disease: A systematic review and meta-analysis. JAMA Network Open. 2023;6(7):e2325658.
9. Furbatto M, Lelli D, Antonelli Incalzi R, et al. Mediterranean diet in older adults: Cardiovascular outcomes and mortality from observational and interventional studies—A systematic review and meta-analysis. Nutrients. 2024;16(22):3947.
10. Gomes SC, Pinho JP, Borges C, et al. (2015). Guidelines for a healthy vegetarian diet. National Programme for the Promotion of Healthy Eating - Direção Geral da Saúde. [Online] Available from https://www.researchgate.net/publication/289108166_Guidelines_for_a_healthy_vegetarian_diet [Last accessed November, 2025].
11. Mariotti F, Gardner CD. Dietary protein and amino acids in vegetarian diets-a review. Nutrients. 2019;11(11):E2661.
12. Rizzo NS, Jaceldo-Siegl K, Sabate J, et al. Nutrient profiles of vegetarian and nonvegetarian dietary patterns. J Acad Nutr Diet. 2013;113(12):1610-9.
13. Soo Yong Lee. Vegetarian Diets and Cardiovascular Risk Reduction: Pros. J Lipid Atheroscler. 2023;12(3):315-5.
14. Sung Nim Han. Vegetarian diet for cardiovascular disease risk reduction: Cons. J Lipid Atheroscler. 2023;12(3):323-3.
15. He YM, Chen WL, Kao TW, et al. Association between ideal cardiovascular health and vegetarian dietary patterns among community-dwelling individuals. Front Nutr. 2022;9:761982.
16. Bakr AF, Farag MA. Soluble dietary fibers as antihyperlipidemic agents: A comprehensive

review to maximize their health benefits. ACS Omega. 2023;8(28):24680-94.
17. Feingold KR. The effect of diet on cardiovascular disease and lipid and lipoprotein levels. South Dartmouth (MA): MDText.com, Inc.; 2024.
18. Salehin S, Rasmussen P, Mai S, et al. Plant based diet and its effect on cardiovascular disease. Int J Environ Res Public Health. 2023;20(4):3337.
19. Tan C, Wei H, Zhao X, et al. Effects of dietary fibers with high water-binding capacity and swelling capacity on gastrointestinal functions, food intake and body weight in male rats. Food Nutr Res. 2017;61(1):1308118.
20. Wang T, Masedunskas A, Willett WC, et al. Vegetarian and vegan diets: Benefits and drawbacks. Eur Heart J. 2023;44(36):3423-39.
21. Zheng L, Cai J, Feng Y, et al. The association between dietary branched-chain amino acids and the risk of cardiovascular diseases in Chinese patients with type 2 diabetes: A hospital-based case–control study. Front Nutr. 2022;9:999189.
22. Nguyen DC, Wells CK, Taylor MS, et al. Dietary branched-chain amino acids modify postinfarct cardiac remodeling and function in the murine heart. J Am Heart Assoc. 2025;14(4):e037637.
23. Morin É, Michaud-Létourneau I, Couturier Y, et al. A whole-food, plant-based nutrition program: Evaluation of cardiovascular outcomes and exploration of food choices determinants. Nutrition. 2019;66:54-61.
24. Rauber F, Laura M, Chang K, et al. Implications of food ultra-processing on cardiovascular risk considering plant origin foods: an analysis of the UK Biobank cohort. Lancet Reg Health Eur. 2024;43.100940-0.
25. Koch CA, Kjeldsen EW, Frikke-Schmidt R. Vegetarian or vegan diets and blood lipids: a meta-analysis of randomized trials. Eur Heart J. 2023;44(28):2609-22.
26. Crowe FL, Appleby PN, Travis RC, et al. Risk of hospitalization or death from ischemic heart disease among British vegetarians and nonvegetarians: results from the EPIC-Oxford cohort study. Am J Clin Nutr. 2013;97(3):597-603.
27. Landry MJ, Senkus KE, Mangels AR, et al. Vegetarian dietary patterns and cardiovascular risk factors and disease prevention: An umbrella review of systematic reviews. Am J Prev Cardiol. 2024;20:100868.
28. Sofi F, Dinu M, Pagliai G, et al. Mediterranean versus vegetarian diet for cardiovascular disease prevention (the CARDIVEG study): study protocol for a randomized controlled trial. Trials. 2016;17(1):233.
29. Estruch R, Ros E, Salas-Salvadó J, et al. Primary prevention of cardiovascular disease with a mediterranean diet supplemented with extra-virgin olive oil or nuts. New Engl J Med. 2018;378(25):e34.
30. Miguel A MG, Alfredo G, Miguel RC. The Mediterranean Diet and Cardiovascular Health. Circ Res. 2019;124(5):779-98.
31. Guasch-Ferré M, Merino J, Sun Q, et al. Dietary polyphenols, mediterranean diet, prediabetes, and type 2 diabetes: A narrative review of the evidence. Oxid Med Cell Longev. 2017;2017:1-16.
32. Tosti V, Bertozzi B, Fontana L. Health Benefits of the Mediterranean Diet: Metabolic and Molecular Mechanisms. J Gerontol A Biol Sci Med Sci. 2018;73(3):318-26.
33. Meir AY, Rinott E, Tsaban G, et al. Effect of green-Mediterranean diet on intrahepatic fat: the DIRECT PLUS randomised controlled trial. Gut. 2021;70(11):2085-95.
34. Lu K, Yu T, Cao X, et al. Effect of viscous soluble dietary fiber on glucose and lipid metabolism in patients with type 2 diabetes mellitus: a systematic review and meta-analysis on randomized clinical trials. Front Nutr. 2023;10:1253312.
35. Kaur G, Mason RP, Steg PG, et al. Omega-3 fatty acids for cardiovascular event lowering. Eur J Prev Cardiol. 2024;31(8):1005-14.
36. Ramesh Vidavalur, Otani H, Singal PK, et al. Significance of wine and resveratrol in cardiovascular disease: French paradox revisited. Exp Clin Cardiol. 2024;11(3):217.
37. Davis C, Bryan J, Hodgson J, et al. Definition of the Mediterranean Diet; A Literature Review. Nutrients. 2015;7(11):9139-53.
38. Shannon OM, Stephan BCM, Minihane AM, et al. Nitric Oxide Boosting Effects of the Mediterranean Diet: A Potential Mechanism of Action. J Gerontol A Biol Sci Med Sci. 2018;73(7):902-4.
39. Karam G, Agarwal A, Sadeghirad B, et al. Comparison of seven popular structured dietary programmes and risk of mortality and major cardiovascular events in patients at increased

cardiovascular risk: systematic review and network meta-analysis. BMJ. 2023;380(1):e072003.
40. Pant A, Gribbin Pant A, Gribbin S, et al. Primary prevention of cardiovascular disease in women with a Mediterranean diet: systematic review and meta-analysis. Heart. 2023;109(16).
41. Sebastian SA, Padda I, Johal G. Long-Term Impact of Mediterranean Diet on Cardiovascular Disease Prevention: A Systematic Review and Meta-analysis of Randomized Controlled Trials. Curr Probl Cardiol. 2024;49(5):102509.
42. Luo H, Xia W, Pan L. Association of dietary index for gut microbiota and cardiovascular diseases in American adults: evidence from National Health and Nutrition Examination Survey 1999–2018. Front Nutr. 2025;12:1604891.
43. Fackelmann G, Manghi P, Carlino N, et al. Gut microbiome signatures of vegan, vegetarian and omnivore diets and associated health outcomes across 21,561 individuals. Nat Microbiol. 2025;10(1):41-52.
44. Yu J, Wu Y, Zhu Z, et al. The impact of dietary patterns on gut microbiota for the primary and secondary prevention of cardiovascular disease: a systematic review. Nutr J. 2025;24(1):17.
45. Kimura I, Ozawa K, Inoue D, et al. The gut microbiota suppresses insulin-mediated fat accumulation via the short-chain fatty acid receptor GPR43. Nat Commun. 2013;4(1):1829.
46. Evans M, Dai L, Avesani CM, et al. The dietary source of trimethylamine N-oxide and clinical outcomes: an unexpected liaison. Clin Kidney J. 2023;16(11):1804-12. https://pubmed.ncbi.nlm.nih.gov/37915930/
47. Sidhu SRK, Kok CW, Kunasegaran T, et al. Effect of Plant-Based Diets on Gut Microbiota: A Systematic Review of Interventional Studies. Nutrients. 2023;15(6):1510.
48. Domínguez-López I, Arancibia-Riveros C, Marhuenda-Muñoz M, et al. Association of microbiota polyphenols with cardiovascular health in the context of a Mediterranean diet. Food Res Int. 2023;165:112499.
49. Argyridou S, Davies MJ, Biddle GJH, et al. Evaluation of an 8-Week Vegan Diet on Plasma Trimethylamine-N-Oxide and Postchallenge Glucose in Adults with Dysglycemia or Obesity. J Nutr. 2021;151(7):1844-53.
50. Niklewicz A, Hannibal L, Warren M, et al. A systematic review and meta-analysis of functional vitamin B12 status among adult vegans. Nutr Bull. 2024;49(4):463-79.
51. Neufingerl N, Eilander A. Nutrient intake and status in adults consuming plant-based diets compared to meat-eaters: A systematic review. Nutrients. 2021;14(1):29.
52. Hunt JR. Bioavailability of iron, zinc, and other trace minerals from vegetarian diets. Am J Clin Nutr. 2003;78(3):633S639S.
53. National Institutes of Health. (2023). Omega-3 Fatty Acids. [Online] Available from https://ods.od.nih.gov/factsheets/Omega3FattyAcids-HealthProfessional/ [Last accessed November, 2025].
54. Boujelbane MA, Ammar A, Salem A, et al. Regional variations in Mediterranean diet adherence: a sociodemographic and lifestyle analysis across Mediterranean and non-Mediterranean regions within the MEDIET4ALL project. Front Public Health. 2025;13:1596681.
55. Vij V, Deshmukh K, Vijayageetha M, et al. Effect of predominantly plant-based diets on visceral fat: A systematic review and meta-analysis. J Hum Nutr Diet. 2025;38(2):e70055.

CHAPTER 27

Recent Trials with Clinical Impact: A 360° View

Suman Bhandari, Nilashish Dey

TRANSCATHETER VERSUS SURGICAL AORTIC VALVE REPLACEMENT IN WOMEN: THE RHEIA TRIAL

Tchetche D, Pibarot P, Bax JJ, et al. Transcatheter vs. surgical aortic valve replacement in women: the RHEIA trial. Eur Heart J. 2025;46(22):2079-88.

New Question

Although women with severe symptomatic aortic stenosis have more complications than men when undergoing surgical valve replacement, they are underrepresented in clinical trials. The Randomized researcH in womEn all comers wIth Aortic stenosis (RHEIA) trial investigates the balance of benefits and risks of transcatheter aortic valve implantation (TAVI) versus surgery in women.

Key Findings

At 48 European centers, 443 women underwent randomization, and 420 were treated as randomized. Mean age was 73 years, and the mean estimated surgical risk of death was 2.1% (Society of Thoracic Surgeons risk score). Kaplan–Meier estimates of the primary endpoint event rates at 1 year were 8.9% in the TAVI and 15.6% in the surgery group. This difference of −6.8% with an upper 95% confidence limit of −1.5% demonstrated the noninferiority of TAVI ($p < 0.001$). The two-sided 95% confidence interval of −13.0% to −0.5% further resulted in superiority ($p = 0.034$). The 1-year incidence of the primary endpoint components was: 0.9% with TAVI versus 2.0% with surgery for death from any cause, 3.3% versus 3.0% for stroke, and 5.8% versus 11.4% for rehospitalization (**Fig. 1**).

Clinical Implications and Meaning

Among women with severe aortic stenosis, the incidence of the composite of death, stroke, or rehospitalization at 1 year was lower with TAVI than with surgery.

LONG-TERM OUTCOMES OF PATIENTS REQUIRING PACEMAKER IMPLANTATION AFTER TRANSCATHETER AORTIC VALVE REPLACEMENT: THE SWISS TAVI REGISTRY

Badertscher P, Stortecky S, Serban T, et al. Long-Term Outcomes of Patients Requiring Pacemaker Implantation after Transcatheter Aortic Valve Replacement: The SwissTAVI Registry. 2025;18(9):1163-71.

New Question

To evaluate the all-cause and cardiovascular mortality of patients undergoing pacemaker (PM) implant after transcatheter aortic valve replacement (TAVR).

Key Findings

Among 13,360 patients enrolled [mean age 82 ± 7 years, 47% female, self-expanding valves 48%, median follow-up 889 (365–1765) days], 2028 (15%)

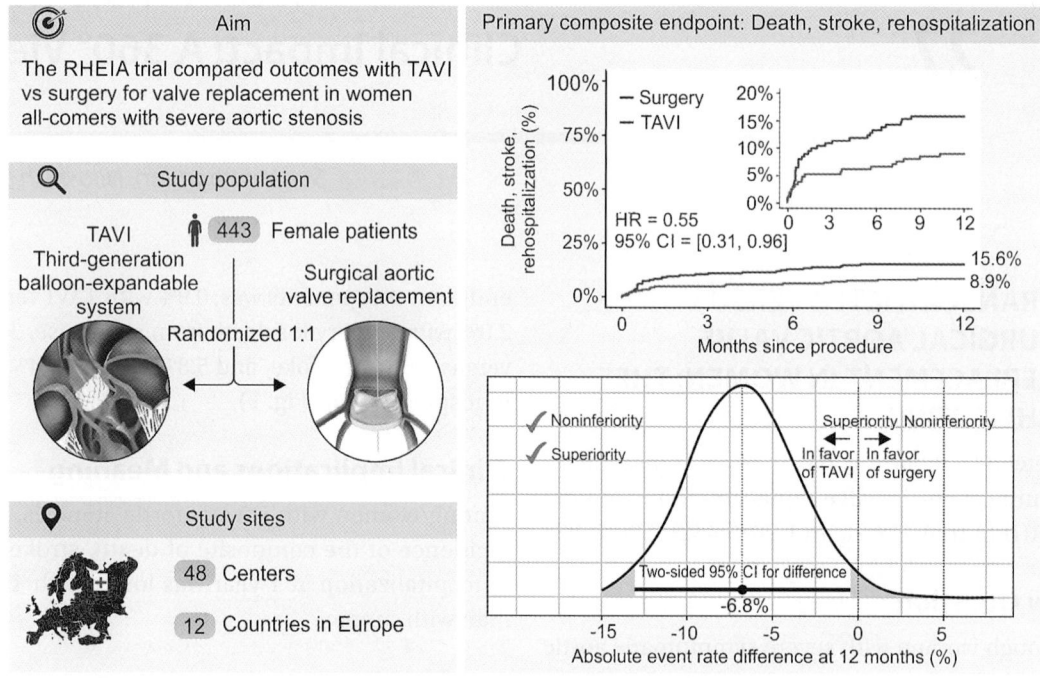

Fig. 1: RHEIA trial: TAVI vs. surgery outcomes.

required PM within 30 days post-TAVR. Patients requiring post-TAVR PM implantation were older (82 ± 6 vs. 81 ± 7 years), predominantly male (58% vs. 50%), and more often had atrial fibrillation (34% vs. 29%). At 1 year follow-up, these patients had higher overall (aHR 1.15, 95% CI 1.05–1.26, $p = 0.002$) and cardiovascular mortality (aHR 1.25, 95% CI 1.06–1.46, $p = 0.006$). These trends persisted at 5- and 10 year follow-up. After multivariable adjustments, significantly higher rates of cardiovascular mortality, LVEF decline ≥10% and NYHA III–IV at 1 year follow-up were observed (aHR 1.44, 95%CI 1.35–1.54, $p < 0.001$), along with higher all-cause and cardiovascular mortality rates at 5- and 10-year follow-up in patients requiring PM implantation following TAVR compared to those not needing a PM **(Fig. 2)**.

Clinical Implications and Meaning

In this large nationwide registry, patients receiving PM implantation within 30 days after TAVR had significantly higher rates of overall and cardiovascular mortality up to 10-years.

ANGIOGRAPHY-DERIVED FRACTIONAL FLOW RESERVE VERSUS INTRAVASCULAR ULTRASOUND TO GUIDE PERCUTANEOUS CORONARY INTERVENTION IN PATIENTS WITH CORONARY ARTERY DISEASE (FLAVOUR II): A MULTICENTER, RANDOMIZED, NONINFERIORITY TRIAL

Hu X, Zhang J, Yang S, et al. Angiography-derived fractional flow reserve versus intravascular

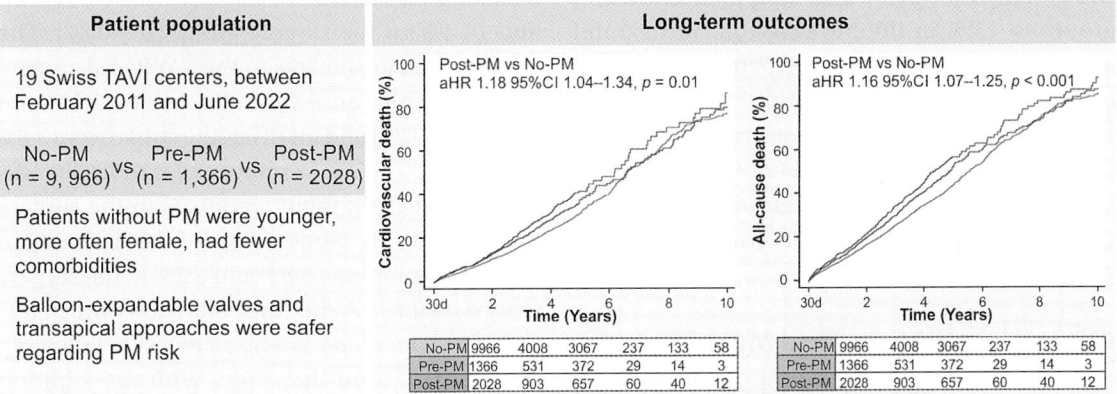

Fig. 2: Long-term outcomes of patients requiring pacemaker implantation after transcatheter aortic valve implantation: The Swiss TAVI registry.

ultrasound to guide percutaneous coronary intervention in patients with coronary artery disease (FLAVOUR II): a multicenter, randomized, non-inferiority trial. Lancet. 2025;405:p1491-504.

New Question

Revascularization decisions based on angiography-derived fractional flow reserve (FFR) or optimization of stent implantation with intravascular ultrasound yield superior clinical outcomes compared with percutaneous coronary intervention (PCI) guided by angiography alone. However, the differences in outcomes when a single approach is used for both purposes remain unclear. We aimed to assess the noninferiority of angiography-derived FFR versus intravascular ultrasound guidance in terms of clinical outcomes at 12 months in patients with angiographically significant stenosis.

Key Findings

Between May 29, 2020, and Sept 20, 2023, 1,872 patients were enrolled. After 33 patients withdrew, 923 patients were randomly assigned to the angiography-derived FFR group and 916 to the intravascular ultrasound group. Median age of the study population was 66.0 years (IQR 58.0–72.0), and 1,248 (67.9%) patients were male and 591 (32.1%) were female. Revascularization was performed in 688 (69.5%) of 990 target vessels in the angiography-derived FFR group and 797 (81.0%) of 984 target vessels in the intravascular ultrasound group. At a median follow-up of 12 months (IQR 12–12), the primary outcome event occurred in 56 patients in the angiography-derived FFR group and 54 patients in the intravascular ultrasound group [6.3% *vs.* 6.0%, absolute difference 0.2 percentage points (upper boundary of one-sided 97·5% CI 2·4),

$p_{non-inferiority}$ = 0.022; hazard ratio 1.04 (95% CI 0.71–1.51)]. Mortality did not differ between the two groups [1.8% in the angiography-derived FFR group vs. 1.3% in the intravascular ultrasound group, absolute difference 0.4 percentage points (95% CI –0.7–1.6)]; [hazard ratio 1.34 (0.63–2.83), p = 0.45]. The incidence of recurrent angina was low in both groups: 26 (2.8%) of 923 patients in the angiography-derived FFR group and 35 (3.8%) of 916 patients in the intravascular ultrasound group.

Clinical Implications and Meaning

The angiography-derived FFR-guided comprehensive PCI strategy, encompassing revascularization decision making and stent optimization, was noninferior to intravascular ultrasound guidance. This finding might have implications for future guidelines on its role and application.

5-YEAR OUTCOMES AFTER TRANSCATHETER OR SURGICAL AORTIC VALVE REPLACEMENT IN LOW-RISK PATIENTS WITH AORTIC STENOSIS

Forrest J, Yakubov S, Deeb G, et al. 5-year outcomes after transcatheter or surgical aortic valve replacement in low-risk patients with aortic stenosis. JACC. 2025;85(15):1523-32.

New Question

This study sought to evaluate 5-year clinical and hemodynamic outcomes with TAVR versus surgery in patients from the Evolut Low Risk trial.

Key Findings

A total of 1,414 patients underwent an attempted implant (n = 730 TAVR, n = 684 surgery). The mean age was 74 years (range 51–88 years), and women accounted for 35% of patients.

At 5 years the Kaplan–Meier estimate for the primary endpoint of all-cause mortality or disabling stroke was 15.5% for the TAVR group and 16.4% for the surgery group (p = 0.47). The Kaplan–Meier estimates in the TAVR and surgery groups for all-cause mortality were 13.5% and 14.9% (p = 0.39) and for disabling stroke were 3.6% and 4.0% (p = 0.57). Cardiovascular mortality was 7.2% in the TAVR group and 9.3% in the surgery group (p = 0.15). Noncardiovascular mortality in the TAVR group was 6.8% and 6.2% in the surgery group (p = 0.73). A site-level vital status sweep was performed for patients who were lost to follow-up or withdrew from the study. With the addition of these patients, the all-cause mortality rate at 5 years for patients undergoing TAVR was 14.7% and for surgery was 15.2% (p = 0.74). Over 5 years, valve reintervention rate was 3.3% for TAVR and 2.5% for surgery (p = 0.44). A sustained improvement in quality of life was observed in both treatment arms with mean Kansas City Cardiomyopathy Questionnaire summary score of 88.3 ± 15.8 in TAVR and 88.5 ± 15.8 in surgery (Fig. 3).

Clinical Implications and Meaning

At 5 years, patients with severe aortic stenosis who were treated with either TAVR or surgery had comparable rates of all-cause mortality or disabling stroke. Valve durability and performance were excellent in both arms.

EARLY EZETIMIBE INITIATION AFTER MYOCARDIAL INFARCTION PROTECTS AGAINST LATER CARDIOVASCULAR OUTCOMES IN THE SWEDEHEART REGISTRY

Leosdottir M, Schubert J, Brandts J, et al. (2025). Early ezetimibe initiation after myocardial infarction protects against later cardiovascular outcomes in the SWEDEHEART registry. J Am Coll Cardiol. 2025;85(15):1550-64.

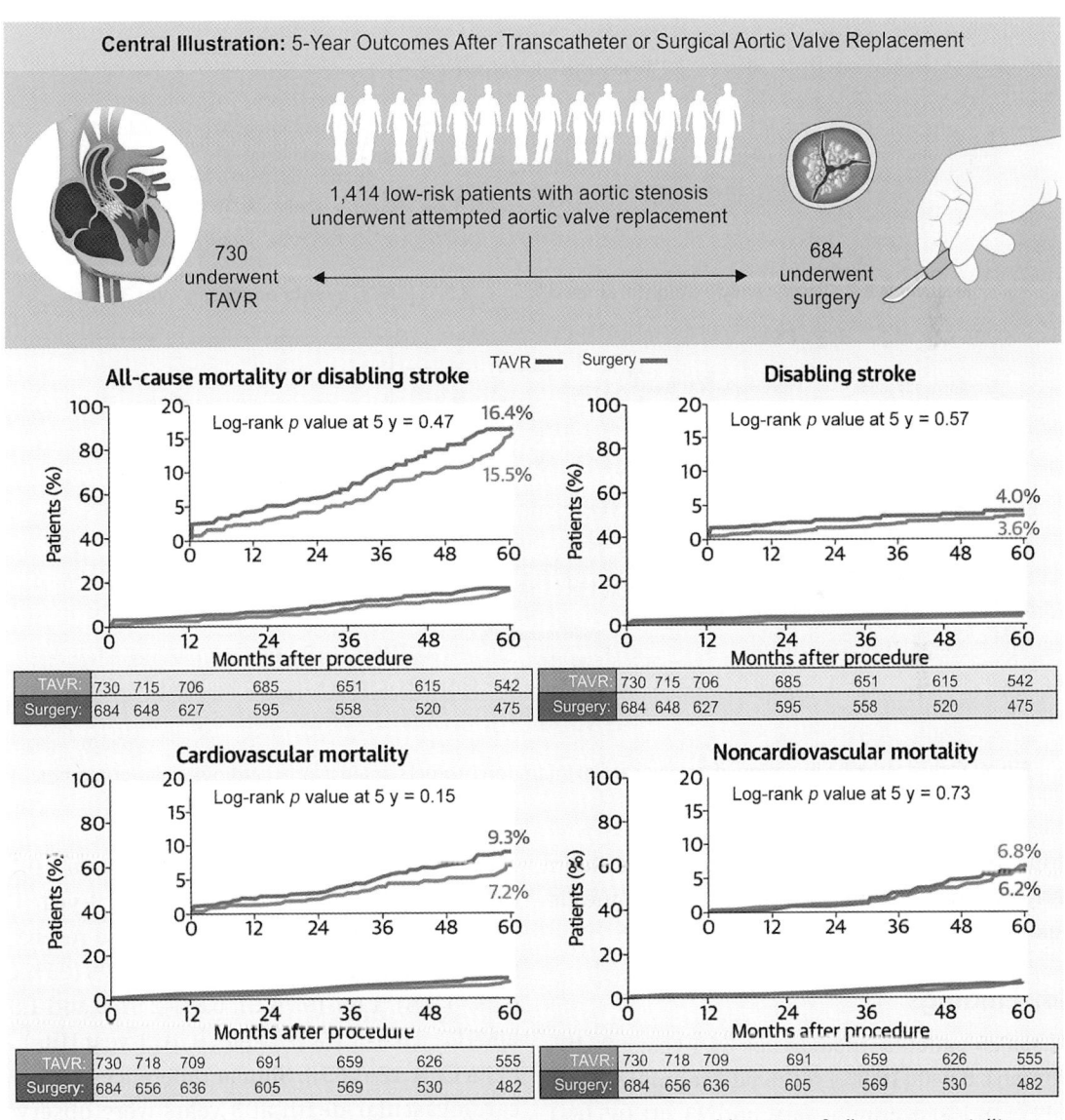

Fig. 3: 5-year outcomes after transcatheter or surgical aortic valve replacement.

New Question

Combination lipid-lowering therapy (LLT) after myocardial infarction (MI) achieves lower low-density lipoprotein cholesterol (LDL-C) levels and better cardiovascular outcomes versus. statin monotherapy. As a result, global guidelines recommend lower LDL-C but, paradoxically, advise treatment through a stepwise approach. Yet the need for combination therapy is inevitable as <20% of patients achieve goals with statins

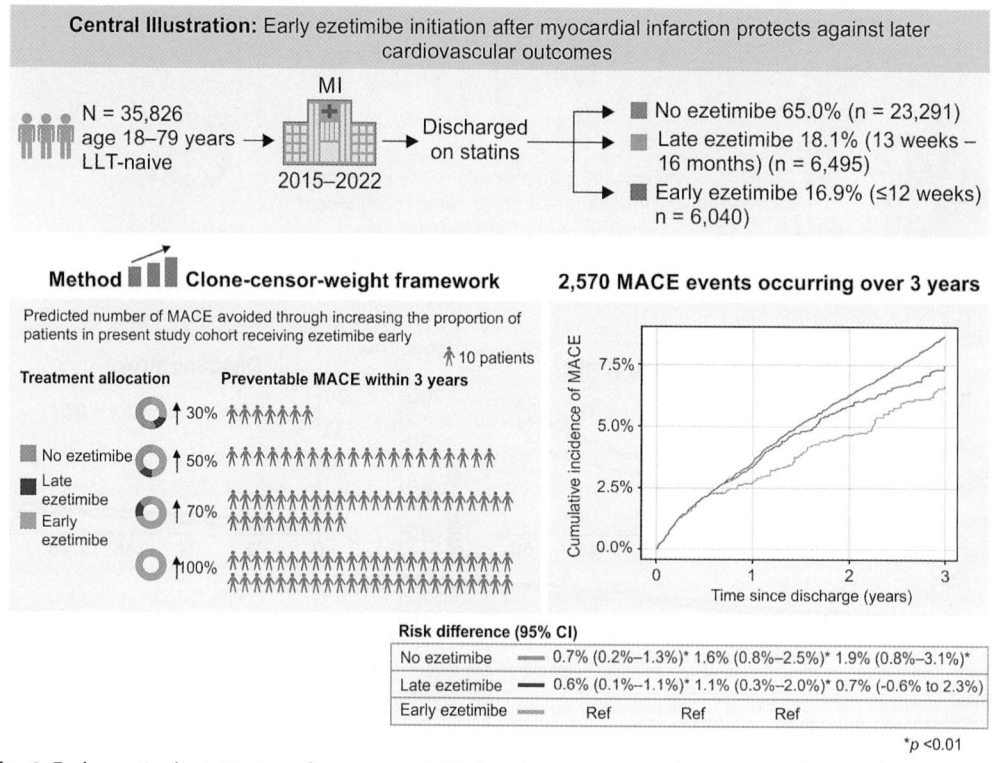

Fig. 4: Early ezetimibe initiation after myocardial infarction protects against later cardiovascular outcomes.

alone. Whether combining ezetimibe with a statin early vs late after MI results in better outcomes is unknown **(Fig. 4)**.

Key Findings

Of 35,826 patients (median age 65.1 years, 26.0% women), 6,040 (16.9%) received ezetimibe early, 6,495 (18.1%) ezetimibe late, and 23,291 (65.0%) received no ezetimibe. High-intensity statin use was ≥ 98% in all groups. Over a median 3.96 years (Q1–Q3: 2.15–5.81 years), 2,570 patients had MACE (440 cardiovascular deaths). 1-year MACE incidences were 1.79 (early), 2.58 (late), and 4.03 (none) per 100 patient-years. Compared with early combination therapy, weighted risk differences in MACE for late combination therapy at 1, 2, and 3 years were 0.6% (95% CI: 0.1%–1.1%; $p < 0.01$), 1.1% (95% CI: 0.3%–2.0%; $p < 0.01$), and 0.7% (95% CI: −0.2%–1.3%; $p = 0.18$), and 3-year HR was 1.14 (95% CI: 0.95–1.41). For those receiving no ezetimibe, risk differences were 0.7% (95% CI: 0.2%–1.3%), 1.6% (95% CI: 0.8%–2.5%), and 1.9% [95% CI: 0.8%–3.1%; p for all < 0.01; 3-year HR: 1.29 (95% CI: 1.12–1.55)]. Similar differences in risk of cardiovascular death at 3 years were observed [HRs vs. early: late: 1.64 (95% CI: 1.15–2.63); none: 1.83 (95% CI: 1.35–2.69)].

Clinical Implications and Meaning

MI care pathways should implement early combination therapy with statins and ezetimibe as standard care, because delaying use of combination LLT or using high-intensity statin monotherapy is associated with avoidable harm.

OUTCOMES OF TRANSCATHETER AORTIC VALVE IMPLANTATION FOR NATIVE AORTIC VALVE REGURGITATION

Ruz RL, Leroux L, Lhermusier T, et al. Outcomes of transcatheter aortic valve implantation for native aortic valve regurgitation. EuroIntervention. 2024;20(17):e1076-85.

New Question

The aim was to report what was the procedural safety and long-term clinical events (CE) in a contemporary cohort of PAVR patients treated with new-generation devices (NGD)?

Key Findings

From 2015-2021, 227 individuals [64.3% males, median age 81.0 (interquartile range {IQR} 73.5-85.0) years, with EuroSCORE II 6.0% (IQR 4.0-10.9)] from 41 centers underwent TAVI with NGD, using either self-expanding (55.1%) or balloon-expandable valves (44.9%; $p = 0.50$). TS was 85.5%, with a nonsignificant trend toward increased TS in high volume activity centers. A second valve implantation (SVI) was needed in 8.8% of patients, independent of valve type ($p = 0.82$). Device size was ≥29 mm in 73.0% of patients, postprocedure grade ≥III residual aortic regurgitation was rare (1.2%), and the permanent pacemaker implantation (PPI) rate was 36.0%. At 30 days, the incidences of mortality and reintervention were 8.4% and 3.5%, respectively. The co-primary endpoint reached 41.6% (IQR 34.4-49.6) at 1 year, increased up to 61.8% (IQR 52.4-71.2) at 4 years, and was independently predicted by TS, with a hazard ratio of 0.45 (95% confidence interval: 0.27-0.76); $p = 0.003$.

Clinical Implications and Relevance

TAVI with NGD in PAVR patients is efficient and reasonably safe. Preventing the need for an SVI embodies the major technical challenge. Larger implanted valves may have limited this complication, outweighing the increased risk of PPI. Despite successful TAVI, PAVR patients experience frequent CE at long-term follow-up.

CARDIAC MYOSIN INHIBITION IN HEART FAILURE WITH NORMAL AND SUPRANORMAL EJECTION FRACTION PRIMARY RESULTS OF THE EMBARK-HFpEF TRIAL

Shah SJ, Rigolli M, Javidialsaadi A, et al. Cardiac myosin inhibition in heart failure with normal and supranormal ejection fraction. JAMA Cardiology. 2025;10(2):170-5.

New Question

What effect does the cardiac myosin inhibitor mavacamten have on cardiac biomarkers in patients with heart failure with preserved ejection fraction (HFpEF) and left ventricular ejection fraction (LVEF) of 60% or greater, and is mavacamten safe in these patients?

Key Findings

A total of 30 patients were enrolled and treated with mavacamten. Median (IQR) patient age was 76 (70-80) years, and 16 patients (53.3%) were female. From baseline to week 26, mavacamten was associated with reductions in NTproBNP (mean reduction, −26%; 95% CI, −44% to −4%; $p = 0.04$), hsTnT (mean reduction, −13%; 95% CI, −23% to −3%; $p = 0.02$), and hsTnI (mean reduction, −20%; 95% CI, −32% to −6%; $p = 0.01$). Cardiac biomarker values returned toward baseline levels 8 weeks after drug discontinuation. NYHA class improved in 10 of 24 patients (41.7%) who had evaluable NYHA class data at the end of treatment, and improvements in echocardiographic markers of LV diastolic function were observed. Mean LVEF decreased by 3.2 absolute percentage points

(95% CI, 1.1–5.4; $p = 0.005$) during treatment. Mavacamten was interrupted in 3 patients (10% of the study population; 95% CI, 2.1%–26.5%) due to protocol prespecified criteria of LVEF < 50% ($n = 2$) or a >20% relative decrease from baseline ($n = 1$; nadir LVEF, 58%), with LVEF recovery observed in all 3 patients. There were no deaths or instances of LVEF <30%; 1 patient had worsening heart failure deemed unrelated to the study drug.

Clinical Implications and Relevance

In an open-label trial in patients with HFpEF with LVEF of 60% or greater, mavacamten was associated with improvements in biomarkers of cardiac wall stress and injury, with no sustained reductions in LVEF observed.

PREHOSPITAL PULSE-DOSE GLUCOCORTICOID IN ST-SEGMENT ELEVATION MYOCARDIAL INFARCTION THE PULSE-MI RANDOMIZED CLINICAL TRIAL

Madsen JM, Engstrøm T, Obling LER, et al. Prehospital Pulse-Dose glucocorticoid in ST-Segment elevation myocardial infarction. JAMA Cardiology. 2024;9(10):882-91.

New Question

Is there any cardioprotective effect of prehospital pulse-dose glucocorticoid in patients with STEMI?

Key Findings

Of 530 included patients [median (IQR) age, 65 (56–75) years; 418 male (78.9%)] with STEMI, 401 (76%) were assessed for the primary outcome, with 198 patients treated with glucocorticoid and 203 with placebo. Median final infarct size was similar in the treatment groups (glucocorticoid, 5%; IQR, 2%–11% vs. placebo, 6%; IQR, 2%–13%; $p = 0.24$). Compared with placebo, the glucocorticoid group had smaller acute infarct size (odds ratio, 0.78; 95% CI, 0.61–1.00), less microvascular obstruction (relative risk ratio, 0.83; 95% CI, 0.71–0.99), and greater acute left ventricular ejection fraction (mean difference, 4.44%; 95% CI, 2.01%–6.87%). Other secondary outcomes were similar in both groups **(Fig. 5)**.

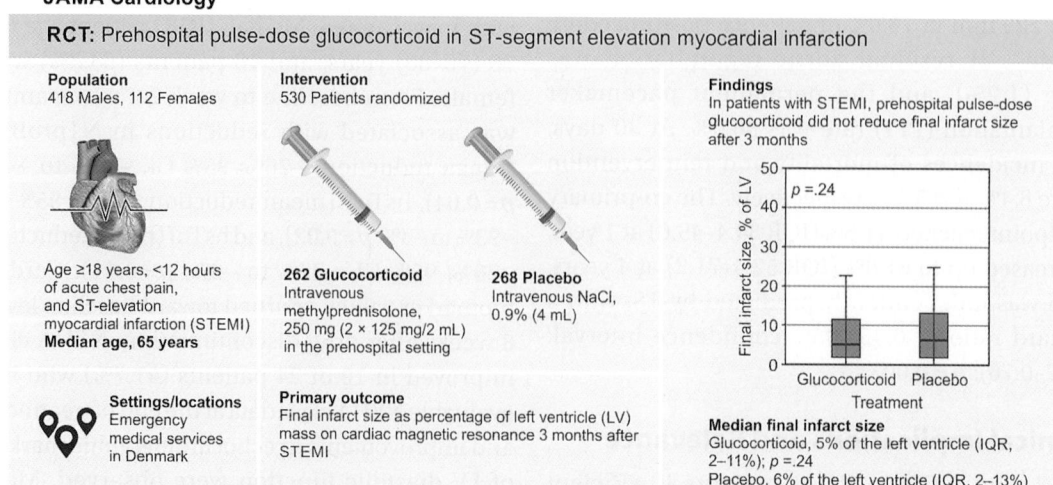

Fig. 5: RCT: prehospital pulse-dose glucocorticoid in ST-segment elevation myocardial infection.

Clinical Implications and Relevance

In patients with STEMI, treatment with prehospital pulse-dose glucocorticoid did not reduce final infarct size after 3 months. However, the trial was likely underpowered as the final infarct size was smaller than anticipated. The glucocorticoid group had improved acute parameters compared with placebo.

EARLY OUTCOMES OF THE NOVEL MYVAL THV SERIES COMPARED TO SAPIEN THV SERIES AND EVOLUT THV SERIES IN INDIVIDUALS WITH SEVERE AORTIC STENOSIS

Van Royen N, Amat-Santos IJ, Hudec M, et al. Early outcomes of the novel Myval THV series compared to SAPIEN THV series and Evolut THV series in individuals with severe aortic stenosis. EuroIntervention, 2025;21(2):e105-18.

New Question

The aim was to evaluate the noninferiority of the balloon-expandable Myval THV series compared to the balloon-expandable SAPIEN THV series or the self-expanding Evolut THV series.

Key Findings

The Myval THV series achieved noninferiority for the primary composite endpoint over the SAPIEN THV series [24.7% vs. 24.1%, risk difference (95% confidence interval {CI}): 0.6% (not applicable {NA} to 8.0); $p = 0.0033$] and the Evolut THV series [24.7% vs. 30.0%, risk difference (95% CI): −5.3% (NA to 2.5); $p < 0.0001$]. The incidences of pacemaker implantation were comparable (Myval THV series: 15.0%, SAPIEN THV series: 17.3%, Evolut THV series: 16.8%). At 30 days, the mean pressure gradient and effective orifice area were significantly better with the Myval THV series compared to the SAPIEN THV series ($p < 0.0001$) and better with the Evolut THV series than with the Myval THV series ($p < 0.0001$). At 30 days, the proportion of moderate-to-severe prosthetic valve regurgitation was numerically higher with the Evolut THV series compared to the Myval THV series (7.4% vs. 3.4%; $p = 0.06$), while not significantly different between the Myval THV series and the SAPIEN THV series (3.4% vs. 1.6%; $p = 0.32$).

Clinical Implications and Relevance

The Myval THV series is noninferior to the SAPIEN THV series and the Evolut THV series in terms of the primary composite endpoint at 30 days. Clinical trial registration: ClinicalTrials.gov: NCT04275726; EudraCT number 2020-000,137-40.

DEVELOPMENT AND VALIDATION OF THE D-PACE SCORING SYSTEM TO PREDICT DELAYED HIGH-GRADE CONDUCTION DISTURBANCES AFTER TRANSCATHETER AORTIC VALVE IMPLANTATION

Bendandi F, Taglieri N, Ciurlanti L, et al. Development and validation of the D-PACE scoring system to predict delayed high-grade conduction disturbances after transcatheter aortic valve implantation. EuroIntervention. 2025;21(2):e119-29.

New Question

This study was designed to identify what were the predictors of high-grade AVB occurring between 24 hours and 30 days after TAVI and to develop and validate a predictive risk score.

Key Findings

Implantation of self-expanding valves, greater implantation depth, longer PR interval in preprocedural electrocardiogram (ECG) and greater increase of PR duration in next-day ECG, preprocedural right bundle branch block (RBBB)

Flowchart 1: Algorithm for delayed high-grade AVB risk stratification. The algorithm should be applied 24 hours after TAVI if there have been no episodes of high-grade AVB in this time interval. Bundle branch blocks are considered persistent if they are present in both postprocedural and next-day (12–24 hours after TAVI) ECGs. Next-day PR variation is the difference in PR interval duration between preprocedural and next-day ECGs.

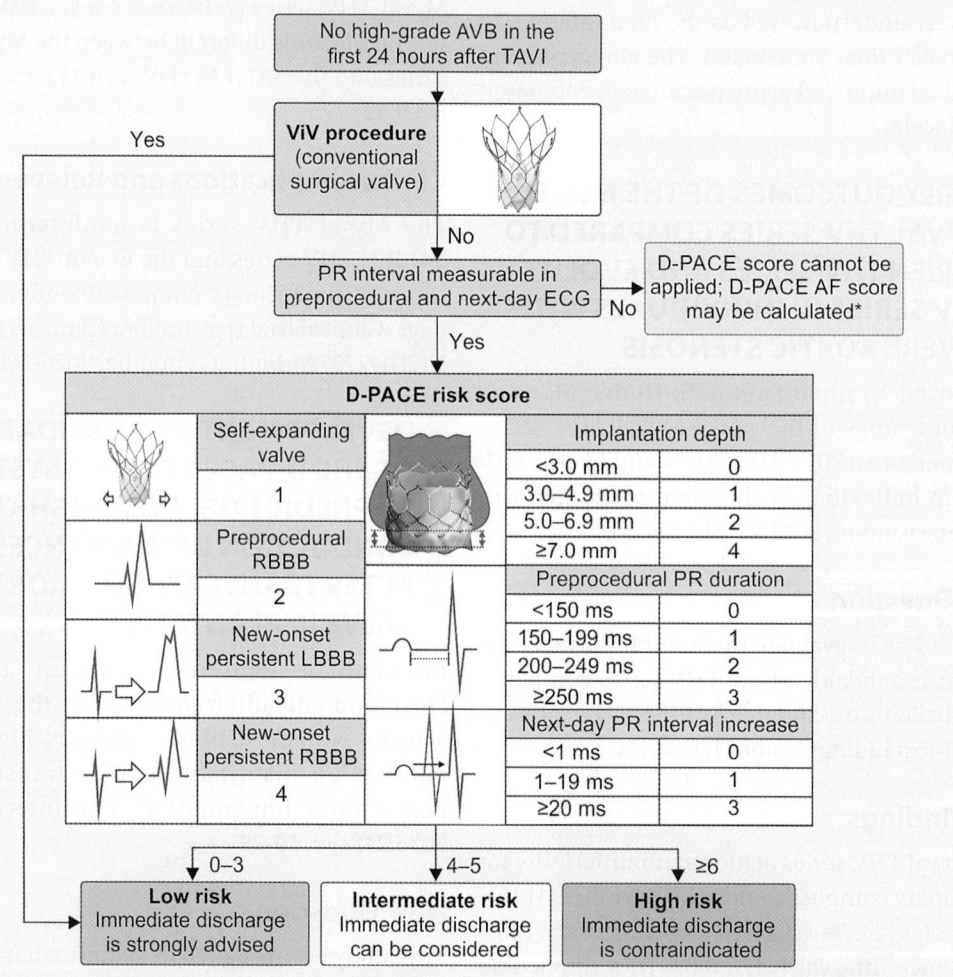

*The D-PACE AF score requires additional validation, and there is no established cutoff for suggesting early discharge. Image adapted from Biorender.com. (AF: atrial fibrillation/flutter: AVB; atrioventricular block; D-PACE: Delayed atrioventricular block Prediction for eArly disChargE: ECG: electrocardiogram: LBBB: left bundle branch block; RBBB: right bundle branch block; TAVI: transcatheter aortic valve implantation; ViV: valve-in-valve)

and new-onset left bundle branch block or RBBB that persisted in next-day ECG were independent predictors of delayed high-grade AVB and were combined to develop the Delayed atrioventricular block Prediction for eArly disChargE (D-PACE) score. The areas under the curve of the score were 0.879 [95% confidence interval (CI): 0.835–0.923] and 0.799 (95% CI: 0.730–0.868) in the derivation and validation cohorts, respectively. Based on the score, patients can be classified into three risk categories; low-risk patients demonstrated an incidence of delayed AVB of <1% and are ideal candidates for next-day discharge **(Fig. 6 and Flowchart 1)**.

Clinical Implications and Relevance

The D-PACE score can be used to stratify TAVI patients according to their risk of delayed high-grade AVB and thereby identify those suitable for next-day discharge.

ABELACIMAB VERSUS RIVAROXABAN IN PATIENTS WITH ATRIAL FIBRILLATION

Ruff CT, Patel SM, Giugliano RP, et al. Abelacimab versus Rivaroxaban in Patients with Atrial Fibrillation. New Engl J Med. 2025;392(4):361-71.

New Question

Abelacimab is a fully human monoclonal antibody that binds to the inactive form of factor XI and blocks its activation. What is the safety of abelacimab as compared with a direct oral anticoagulant in patients with atrial fibrillation?

Key Findings

A total of 1,287 patients underwent randomization; the median age was 74 years, and 44% were women. At 3 months, the median reduction in free factor XI levels with abelacimab at a dose of 150 mg was 99% (interquartile range, 98–99) and with abelacimab at a dose of 90 mg was 97% (interquartile range, 51–99). The trial was stopped early on the recommendation of the independent data monitoring committee because of a greater-than-anticipated reduction in bleeding events with abelacimab. The incidence rate of major or clinically relevant nonmajor bleeding was 3.2 events per 100 person-years with 150-mg abelacimab and 2.6 events per 100 person-years with 90-mg abelacimab, as compared with 8.4 events per 100 person-years with rivaroxaban [hazard ratio for 150-mg abelacimab vs. rivaroxaban, 0.38 (95% confidence interval {CI}, 0.24–0.60); hazard ratio for 90-mg abelacimab vs. rivaroxaban, 0.31 (95% CI, 0.19–0.51); $p < 0.001$ for both comparisons]. The incidence and severity of adverse events appeared to be similar in the three groups **(Fig. 6)**.

Clinical Implications and Relevance

Among patients with atrial fibrillation who were at moderate-to-high risk for stroke, treatment with abelacimab resulted in markedly lower levels of free factor XI and fewer bleeding events than treatment with rivaroxaban.

QUANTITATIVE CORONARY ANGIOGRAPHY VERSUS INTRAVASCULAR ULTRASONOGRAPHY TO GUIDE DRUG-ELUTING STENT IMPLANTATION: A RANDOMIZED CLINICAL TRIAL

Lee PH, Hong SJ, Kim H, et al. Quantitative Coronary Angiography vs Intravascular Ultrasonography to Guide Drug-Eluting Stent Implantation: A Randomized Clinical Trial. JAMA Cardiol. 2024;9(5):428-35.

New Question

Although intravascular ultrasonography (IVUS) guidance promotes favorable outcomes after

The NEW ENGLAND JOURNAL of MEDICINE

Abelacimab versus Rivaroxaban in Atrial Fibrillation
A PLAIN LANGUAGE SUMMARY

Based on the NEJM publication: Abelacimab versus Rivaroxaban in Patients with Atrial Fibrillation by C.T. Ruff et al. (published January 23, 2025)

In this trial, researchers compared the safety of abelacimab—a fully human monoclonal antibody that binds to the inactive form of factor XI and prevents the generation of the activated form (factor XIa)—with that of the direct oral anticoagulant rivaroxaban in patients with atrial fibrillation.

Atrial fibrillation is associated with an increased risk of stroke; consequently, anticoagulation therapy is a cornerstone of treatment.

Why was the trial done?

Guidelines give preference to direct-acting oral anticoagulants (DOACs) over vitamin K antagonists in the treatment of atrial fibrillation because they are at least as effective in reducing ischemic stroke and are much safer with respect to intracranial hemorrhage. However, bleeding, especially gastrointestinal bleeding, remains a major complication of DOAC therapy. Safer anticoagulants are needed.

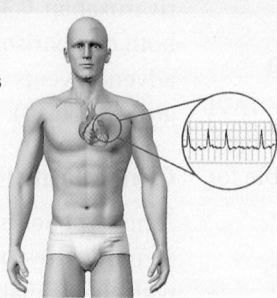

Patients

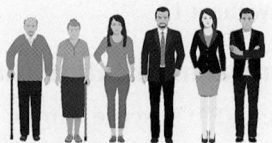

WHO	1287 patients
	55 years of age or older; median, 74 years
	Men: 56%; Women: 44%
	White: 95%; Asian: 5%
Clinical status	History of atrial fibrillation or atrial flutter
	Planned anticoagulation
	Moderate-to-high risk of stroke (CHA_2DSc_2-VASc score ≥4 or a score of 3 with either planned concomitant use of antiplatelet medications or an estimated creatinine clearance ≤50 mL per minute)
Trial design	• Randomized • Active-controlled • Phase 2B • Location: 95 Centers in 7 countries

How was the trial conducted?

Patients with atrial fibrillation and a moderate-to-high risk of stroke were assigned to one of two doses of monthly subcutaneous injections of abelacimab (150 mg or 90 mg) or open-label oral rivaroxaban (20 mg once daily). The primary end point was a composite of major or clinically relevant nonmajor bleeding.

Abelacimab 150 mg	Abelacimab 90 mg	Rivaroxaban
430 Patients	427 Patients	430 Patients

Contd...

Contd...

The NEW ENGLAND JOURNAL of MEDICINE

Results

During a median follow-up of 2.1 years, both abelacimab doses resulted in a lower incidence of major or clinically relevant nonmajor bleeding than rivaroxaban.

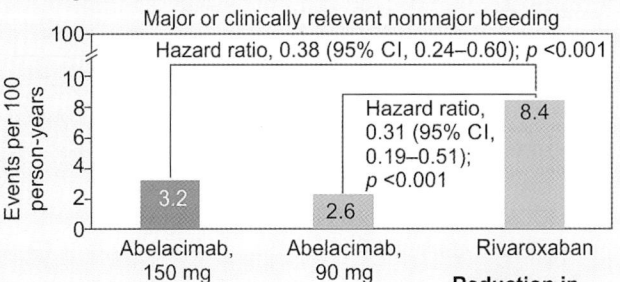

At 3 months, free factor XI levels were reduced by a median of at least 97% among patients who received abelacimab.

The incidence of adverse events, serious adverse events, and adverse events leading to discontinuation of a trial drug appeared to be similar in the three groups.

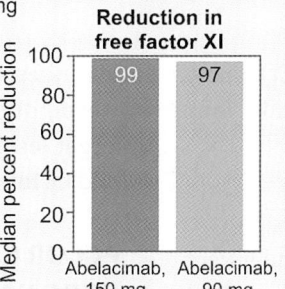

Early termination

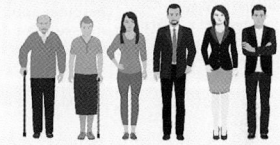

The trial was stopped early at the recommendation of the independent data monitoring committee because of a greater-than-expected reduction in bleeding events observed with both doses of abelacimab relative to rivaroxaban

Limitations and remaining questions

- The relatively small sample size precludes assessment of the clinical efficacy of abelacimab, and larger trials are needed to address this question.
- Most enrolled patients were White, so generalizability to other races is limited.
- Researchers could not make conclusions about how abelacimab would compare with DOACs other than rivaroxaban with respect to bleeding risk.

Links: full article | NEJM quick take| science behind the study

Conclusion

Among patients with atrial fibrillation who were at moderate-to-high risk for stroke, abelacimab resulted in markedly lower levels of free factor XI and fewer bleeding events than rivaroxaban.

Further information

Trial registration: ClinicalTrials.gov number, NCT04755283
Trial funding: Anthos Therapeutics
Full citation: Ruff CT, Patel SM, Giugliano RP, et al. Abelacimab versus rivaroxaban in patients with atrial fibrillation. N Engl J Med 2025;392:361-71. DOI: 10.1056/NEJMoa2405674.
For personal use only. Any commercial reuse of NEJM Group content requires permission. Copyright© 2025 Massachusetts Medical Society.
All rights reserved.

Fig. 6: Abelacimab versus rivaroxaban in atrial fibrillation.

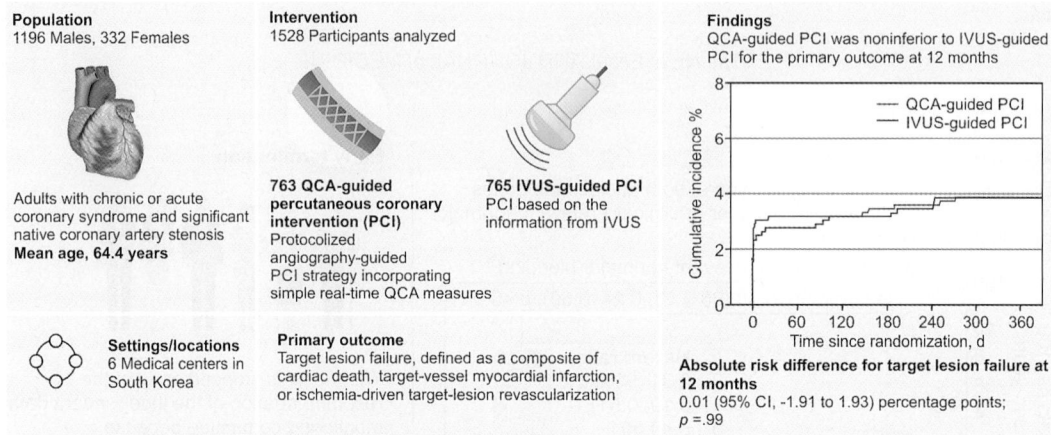

Fig. 7: Quantitative coronary angiography (QCA) vs. intravascular ultrasonography (IVUS) to guide drug-eluting stent implantation.

percutaneous coronary intervention (PCI), many catheterization laboratories worldwide lack access.

Key Findings

The trial included 1,528 patients who underwent PCI with QCA guidance [763; mean (SD) age, 64.1 (9.9) years; 574 males (75.2%)] or IVUS guidance [765; mean (SD) age, 64.6 (9.5) years; 622 males (81.3%)]. The post-PCI mean (SD) minimum lumen diameter was similar between the QCA- and IVUS-guided PCI groups. Target lesion failure at 12 months occurred in 29 of 763 patients (3.81%) in the QCA-guided PCI group and 29 of 765 patients (3.80%) in the IVUS-guided PCI group; hazard ratio. There was no difference in the rates of stent edge dissection, coronary perforation or stent thrombosis between the QCA- and IVUS- guided PCI groups. The risk of the primary end point was consistent regardless of subgroup, with no significant interaction **(Fig. 7)**.

Clinical Implications and Meaning

Findings of this randomized clinical trial indicate that QCA and IVUS guidance during PCI showed similar rates of target lesion failure at 12 months. However, due to the lower-than-expected rates of target lesion failure in this trial, the findings should be interpreted with caution.

PCI OR CABG FOR LEFT MAIN CORONARY ARTERY DISEASE: THE SWEDEHEART REGISTRY

Persson J, Yan J, Angerås O, et al. PCI or CABG for left main coronary artery disease: the SWEDEHEART registry. Eur Heart J. 2023;44(30):2833-42.

New Question

How do the outcomes of coronary artery bypass grafting (CABG) compare to percutaneous coronary intervention (PCI) in an all-comer population with left main coronary artery disease? How can this guide the selection of revascularization strategy to improve patient outcomes?

Key Findings

In this observational study, CABG was associated with lower mortality and fewer major adverse

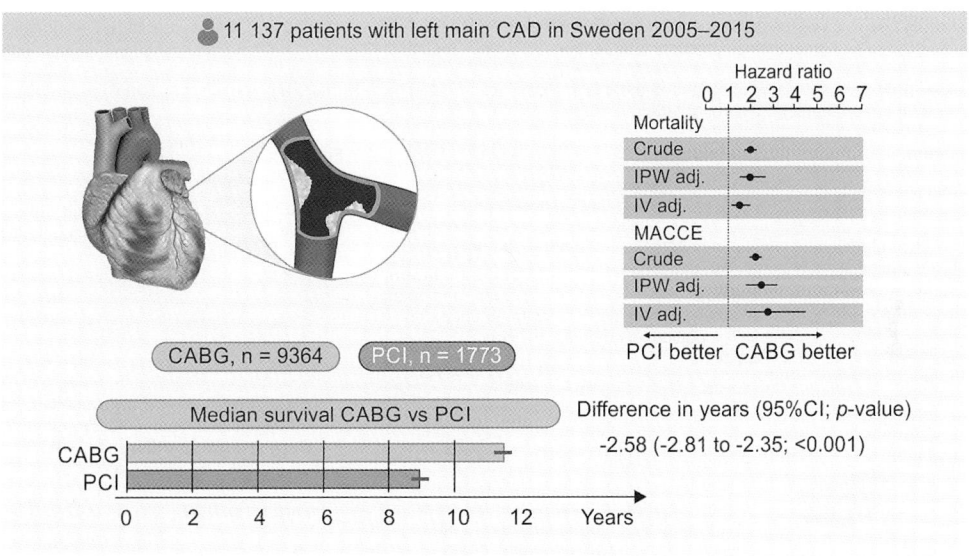

Fig. 8: Results of SWEDEHEART registry. (CABG = coronary artery bypass grafting, CAD = coronary artery disease, CI = confidence interval, PCI = percutaneous coronary intervention, IPW adj. inverse probability weighting adjustment, IV adj. instrumental variable adjusted; MACCE = major adverse cardiovascular and cerebrovascular events)

cardiovascular and cerebrovascular events in patients with left main coronary artery disease compared to PCI after adjustment for confounders during a median follow-up of 4.7 years **(Fig. 8)**.

Clinical Implications and Meaning

This observational study may inform choice between CABG and PCI for left main coronary artery disease, in particular for patients who are not represented in randomized clinical trials.

PACLITAXEL-COATED BALLOON VERSUS UNCOATED BALLOON FOR CORONARY IN-STENT RESTENOSIS THE AGENT IDE RANDOMIZED CLINICAL TRIAL

Yeh RW, Shlofmitz R, Moses J, et al. Paclitaxel-coated balloon vs uncoated balloon for coronary in-stent restenosis: The AGENT IDE randomized clinical trial. JAMA. 2024;331(12):1015-24.

New Question

Is treatment with a coronary paclitaxel-coated balloon superior to an uncoated balloon for 1-year target lesion failure in patients undergoing percutaneous coronary intervention for in-stent restenosis?

Key Findings

In a multicenter randomized trial of 600 patients designed to support US regulatory approval, target lesion failure was significantly lower in the paclitaxel-coated balloon group (17.9%) compared with the uncoated balloon group (28.6%) ($p=0.003$) **(Fig. 6)**. Ischemia-driven target lesion revascularization and target vessel myocardial

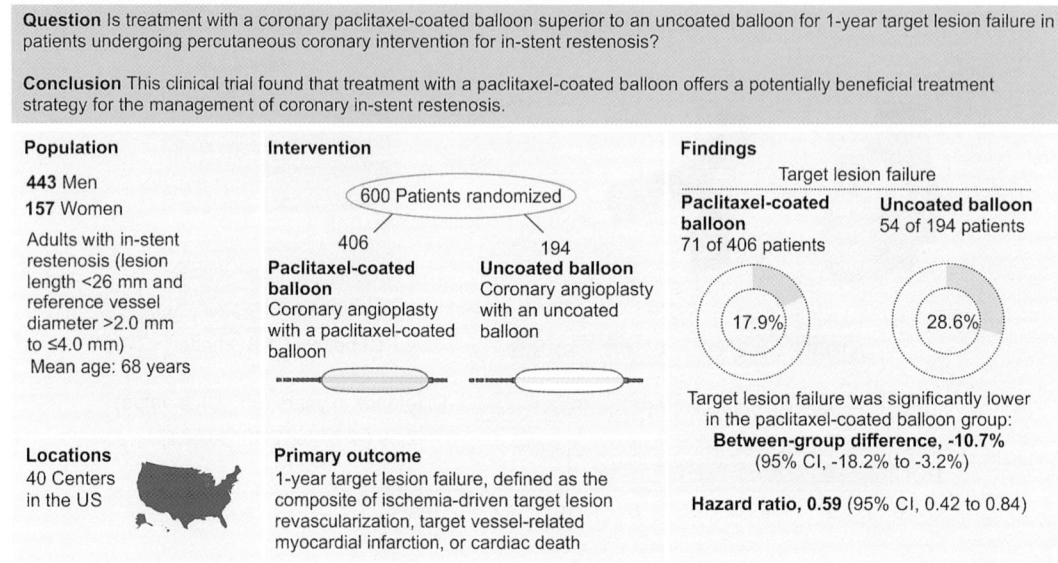

Fig. 9: Summary of AGENT IDE trial.

infarction were also lower after treatment with a paclitaxel-coated balloon **(Fig. 9)**.

Clinical Implications and Meaning

Treatment with a paclitaxel-coated balloon offers an effective treatment strategy for the management of coronary in-stent restenosis.

ROTATIONAL ATHERECTOMY COMBINED WITH CUTTING BALLOON TO OPTIMIZE STENT EXPANSION IN CALCIFIED LESIONS: THE ROTA-CUT RANDOMIZED TRIAL

Sharma SK, Mehran R, Vogel B, et al. Rotational atherectomy combined with cutting balloon to optimise stent expansion in calcified lesions: the ROTA-CUT randomised trial. EuroIntervention. 2024;20(1):75-84.

New Question

We aimed to investigate whether combining rotational atherectomy (RA) with cutting balloon angioplasty (RA + CBA) results in more optimal stent expansion compared with RA followed by noncompliant balloon angioplasty (RA + NCBA).

Key Findings

The mean age was 71.1 ± 9.4 years, and 22% were women. The procedural details of RA were similar between groups, as were procedure duration and contrast use. Minimum stent area was similar with RA + CBA versus RA + NCBA (6.7 ± 1.7 mm^2 vs. 6.9 ± 1.8 mm^2; p = 0.685) **(Fig. 7)**. Furthermore, there were no significant differences regarding the other IVUS and angiographic end points. Procedural complications were rare, and 30-day clinical events included two myocardial infarctions and 1 target vessel revascularization in the RA + CBA

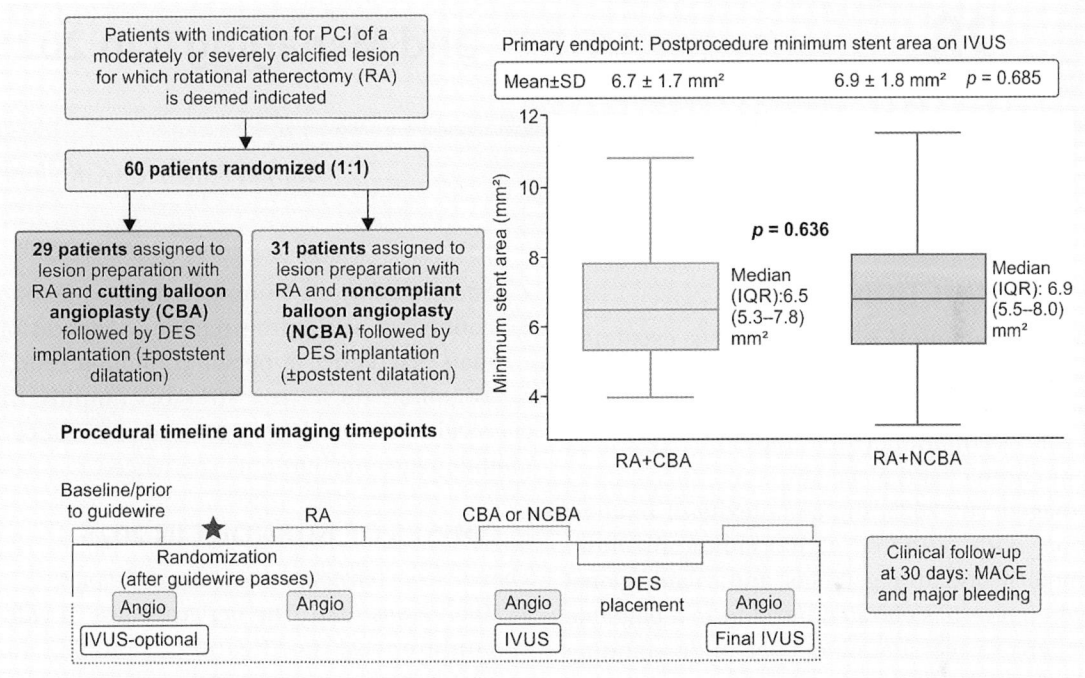

Fig. 10: Design and primary outcome of the ROTA-CUT trial.

group and 1 myocardial infarction in the RA + NCBA group **(Fig. 10)**.

Clinical Implications and Meaning

Combining RA with CBA resulted in a similar minimum stent area compared with RA followed by NCBA in patients undergoing PCI of moderately or severely calcified lesions. RA followed by CBA was safe with rare procedural complications and few clinical adverse events at 30-day.

CHAPTER 28

Burnout: Understanding and Managing it in 2025

Suman Banerjee, GC Khilnani

INTRODUCTION

The phenomenon of burnout has escalated into a global occupational health concern, recognized by the World Health Organization as an "occupational phenomenon" resulting from chronic workplace stress not successfully managed.[1] By 2025, the complexity of modern labor—with saturated digital communication, remote/hybrid arrangements, and volatile global economies—has elevated burnout to a palpable challenge necessitating deeper understanding and proactive strategies.

DEFINING BURNOUT: CLASSICAL AND CONTEMPORARY DIMENSIONS

Originally framed by the Maslach Burnout Inventory, burnout comprises three core dimensions:
1. *Emotional exhaustion:* Persistent feelings of emotional depletion and fatigue[2]
2. *Depersonalization:* Development of cynical or detached attitudes toward work or recipients of one's service[2]
3. *Reduced personal efficacy:* An internal sense of incompetence, decline in productivity, and lack of accomplishment[2]

In 2025, the definition has expanded to integrate contemporary contributors:
- *Digital fatigue:* Exhaustion resulting from continuous screen time, virtual meetings, and email/instant-message overload[3]
- *Cognitive overload:* Deficits in attention and processing capacity due to constant multitasking and information saturation[3]
- *Social isolation:* Diminished interpersonal connection arising from remote and hybrid formats that reduce in-person communication.[3]

Together, these new stressors amplify the classical triad, producing a more pronounced, multidimensional burnout experience.

CAUSES OF BURNOUT IN 2025

The causes of burnout in 2025 are as follows:
- *Digital overload:* The pervasiveness of video conferences, notifications, emails, and instant messaging creates an "always-on" dynamic that affects attention and emotional resources.[3]
- *Work–life boundary erosion:* Hybrid and remote work blur personal–professional distinctions, leading to extended working hours and difficulty disengaging.[3]
- *High performance expectations:* Competitive global markets and productivity paradigms drive pressure for nonstop output and efficiency.[4]
- *Persistent stress in frontline professions:* Healthcare workers and first responders continue to grapple with chronic demands—stemming from postpandemic care backlogs, staffing shortages, and emotional labor.[5]
- *Lack of autonomy:* Excessive micromanagement or curtailed decision-making capacity contributes to feelings of helplessness and disengagement.[4]
- *Cultural and social pressures:* Stigma around mental health, social norms equating worth with productivity, and the "hustle culture"

exacerbate internal stress and reduce help-seeking behavior.[6]

RECOGNIZING BURNOUT: EARLY WARNING SIGNS

Timely recognition is critical.
Common early indicators include:
- Chronic fatigue, energy depletion, and disrupted sleep[7]
- Emotional numbness, apathy, irritability, or mood swings[7]
- Decreased job performance, motivation, or creativity[4]
- Social withdrawal, diminished empathy, and reduced teamwork[7]
- Psychosomatic complaints—tension headaches, GI discomfort, and muscle stiffness.[7]

IMPACT OF BURNOUT

Individuals

Burnout contributes to heightened risk of depression, anxiety disorders, sleep disturbances, substance misuse, and chronic physical ailments (e.g., cardiovascular and musculoskeletal).[5]

Organizations

Organizations suffer from increased attrition, extended absenteeism, reduced productivity, impaired morale, interpersonal conflict, and diminished innovation.[4]

Society

Communities and economies face rising mental healthcare costs, reduced labor force participation, decreased civic engagement, and increasing strain on public health systems.[6]

BURNOUT IN PHYSICIANS IN 2025

Physician burnout on the part of healthcare professionals was at the peak during COVID-19 pandemic. There were long working hours wearing personal protection kits, at times with hot climate, and minimal interaction with colleagues and patients immensely added to frustration and burnout in all healthcare professionals. Lack of gratification due to minimum interaction added to burnout due to seeing extremely sick patients has become one of the most turgent crises in healthcare systems worldwide. Even before the COVID-19 pandemic, studies consistently reported burnout prevalence among physicians ranging from 40 to 60% globally.[8] By 2025, multiple systemic, technological, and cultural pressures have continued to intensify this phenomenon, threatening physician wellbeing, patient safety, and the sustainability of healthcare delivery.

Causes of Physician Burnout in 2025

While physicians share general causes of burnout with other professionals, they also face unique stressors:
- *Excessive workload and staffing shortages:* Persistent postpandemic patient backlogs, combined with physician shortages, have increased working hours and caseloads.[8]
- *Administrative burden:* Electronic Health Records (EHRs), billing codes, and excessive paperwork remain a major source of frustration, often consuming more time than patient care.[9]
- *Digital fatigue:* Constant EHR use, telemedicine consultations, and digital documentation contribute to cognitive overload.[3,9]
- *Emotional burden:* Continuous exposure to suffering, end-of-life care, and ethical dilemmas result in "compassion fatigue," a precursor to burnout.[5]
- *Lack of autonomy:* Physicians often report limited influence over scheduling, treatment decisions, and organizational policy.[4]
- *Work–life conflict:* Night shifts, irregular schedules, and reduced time with family, impair recovery and wellbeing.[6]

- *Stigma in seeking help:* Fear of professional repercussions or licensure consequences often prevents physicians from accessing mental health support.[8]

Warning Signs in Physicians

Burnout in physicians often manifests as:
- Increased irritability or emotional detachment with patients and colleagues[5]
- Reduced empathy and compassion, leading to poorer patient interactions[9]
- Decline in clinical performance, diagnostic errors, and reduced attention to detail[8]
- Somatic complaints such as hypertension, gastrointestinal issues, and sleep disturbances[7]

Impacts of Physician Burnout

Impacts of physician burnout include:
- *On physicians:* Elevated risk of depression, suicidal ideation, substance use disorders, and early retirement[5,8]
- *On patients:* Reduced quality of care, increased risk of medical errors, impaired communication, and lower patient satisfaction[9]
- *On healthcare systems:* Workforce attrition, higher recruitment and training costs, reduced morale, and systemic inefficiencies[6]

STRATEGIES FOR MANAGING BURNOUT IN 2025

Strategies for managing burnout in 2025 are as follows:
- Individual-level interventions
  - *Mindfulness and resilience training:* Structured meditation, breathing techniques, and cognitive strategies to bolster emotional regulation and coping[5]
  - *Digital hygiene:* Defined "tech-free" periods, notification management, and intentional breaks reduce digital fatigue[3]
  - *Work–life integration:* Establishing clear boundaries, honoring rest and leisure, and pursuing nonwork activities[4]
  - *Physical wellbeing:* Prioritizing regular exercise, balanced nutrition, and sufficient restorative sleep[5]
  - *Seeking support:* Engaging counseling services, peer networks, and mental health professionals to strengthen emotional support[6]
- *Organizational approaches:*
  - *Flexible work models:* Hybrid schedules allowing autonomy and accountability, flexible and equitable distribution of shifts and on-call duties help prevent burnout.[4]
  - *Mental health infrastructure:* Easily accessible counseling, employee assistance programs (EAPs), and wellbeing initiatives support proactive care.[6]
  - *Leadership development:* Training leaders to exhibit empathy, transparency, and support fosters psychologically safe environments.[4]
  - *Workload calibration:* Equitable task distribution, realistic targets, recognition of employee efforts, and reward[4]
  - *Smart use of AI and automation:* Employing artificial intelligence (AI) to reduce repetitive tasks, streamline workflows, and support[3]
- *Societal and policy-level measures:*
  - *Regulation of working hours:* Enforcing limits, mandatory rest, and recovery periods to protect against overwork[6]
  - *Mental health literacy campaigns:* Public initiatives aimed at reducing stigma, promoting awareness, and encouraging supportive cultures[6]
  - *Social safety nets:* Policies such as paid leave, subsidized childcare, access to community wellbeing resources, and universal services to relieve stressors[6]
  - *Licensure and credentialing reforms:* Ensuring physicians can seek mental health care without fear of punitive career consequences[8]

- *Investment in workforce expansion:* Training more physicians and allied professionals to reduce workload burdens.[6]

EMERGING TRENDS IN BURNOUT MITIGATION (2025 AND BEYOND)

Emerging trends in burnout mitigation are as follows:

- *Artificial intelligence-driven wellbeing platforms:* Adaptive systems offering personalized stress-management guidance, nudges, and resource recommendations are crucial.[3]
- *Wearable technology:* Devices tracking biomarkers—for example, heart rate variability, electrodermal activity, sleep patterns—can signal early warning flags for burnout onset.[3]
- *Virtual reality (VR) interventions:* Immersive VR experiences can provide guided relaxation, mindfulness, and exposure-based stress relief[5]
- *Predictive organizational analytics:* Data-driven tools to identify patterns suggestive of burnout (absenteeism and interaction decline) and prompt targeted interventions may help.[4]

CONCLUSION

Burnout in 2025 is a complex, multilayered phenomenon shaped by evolving technological, cultural, and occupational landscapes. Its mitigation requires a holistic, integrated approach—empowering individuals, enabling empathetic organizations, and enacting supportive societal policies. Embracing innovation—AI, wearables, VR—alongside mental health advocacy, and sustainable work culture, can transform burnout from a hidden epidemic into an opportunity for resilient, human-centric work ecosystems.

REFERENCES

1. World Health Organization. (2019). Burn-out an "occupational phenomenon": International Classification of Diseases. [online] Available from https://www.who.int/news/item/28-05-2019-burn-out-an-occupational-phenomenon-international-classification-of-diseases [Last accessed November, 2025].
2. Maslach C, Jackson S. The measurement of experienced burnout. J Occup Behav. 1981;2(2): 99-113.
3. Jones A, Patel V, Huang T. Digital fatigue and cognitive overload in hybrid workplaces. J Organ Health. 2024;12(4):210-25.
4. Rivera J. Burnout's organizational toll: Turnover, productivity, and culture. Leadership Quarterly. 2023;24(2):87-100.
5. Smith D, Torres L. Burnout and mental/physical health comorbidity. Occup Med Rev. 2022;15(3): 130-45.
6. Gupta R, Shah S. Societal impacts of professional burnout: Economic and health-system burdens. Glob Public Health. 2024;19(6):900-14.
7. Lee S, Kim H. Psychosomatic manifestations of workplace burnout: A review. Int J Behav Med. 2023;30(1):55-68.
8. Shanafelt T, West CP, Dyrbye LN, et al. Changes in burnout and satisfaction with work-life integration in physicians during the COVID 19 pandemic. Mayo Clin Proc. 2022;97(7):1236-48.
9. Rotenstein L, Torre M, Dudley J. Physician burnout in the digital age: EHR burden, telehealth, and new solutions. NEJM Catalyst Innovations in Care Delivery. 2023;4(2):1-12.

Index

Page numbers followed by *f* refer to figure, *fc* refer to flowchart, and *t* refer to table.

A

Abdominal adiposity 27
Abelacimab 285, 287*f*
Ablation catheter 143
Ablation technique 143*t*
    type of 144*t*
Abluminal wire
    crossing 173
    position 172
Abscesses 123
Academic Research Consortium for High Bleeding Risk 107
Acetylation 55
Acetylcholine infusion 152
Actinobacillus 130
Acute coronary syndrome 98, 99, 107, 114, 116*f*, 171, 202, 209, 212, 219
Acute kidney injury 234, 236
Acute stent thrombosis 189, 191*f*
Adenosine
    infusion 152
    triphosphate 71*f*
Adequate leaflet grasping 256*f*
Adjunctive fibrinolytic therapy 223
Adjunctive therapies 105
Advanced glycation end-products 41
Advanced heart failure 233
    epidemiology of 231
    management of 231
        critical resources for 243
    therapy 243
Advanced intravascular imaging 57
Adventitia 162
Adverse cardiovascular events, increased major 149
AGENT IDE trial 290*f*
Aggregatibacter 130
Air
    bubble artifact 165
    pollution, indoor 28
Airborne nanoplastics 14
Albuminuria 3
    progression of 7

Alfieri stitch 250
Alirocumab 57
Alteplase 220
Altered heart rate 17
Ambulatory blood pressure monitoring 91
Aminoglycoside 125, 129
    resistance, high-level 129
Amoxicillin 128, 131, 137
Amphotericin 132
Ampicillin 130, 131
Amyloid cardiomyopathy 46
Amyloidosis 46, 48*f*
Angina frequency 154
Angiotensin receptor blockers 60, 86
Angiotensin-converting enzyme inhibitors 60, 86
Angiotensin-receptor neprilysin inhibitors 69
Angiovac system 136
Annuloplasty 258
Annulus dimension 257
Antegrade wire crossing 204
Anterior mitral leaflet 197
Anti-adjunctive therapy 183
Antiarrhythmic drug 141
    therapy 141
Antiarrhythmic effects 45
Antibiotic regimen 128*t*
Anticoagulant
    agents 103
    therapy 103
Anticoagulation 219
Antifibrotic effects 43
Antihypertensive 60
    agents, armamentarium of 83
    drug 83
    effect minimally 83
    management 83
    treatment 88, 91
Anti-inflammatory
    cascades, signal 271
    effect 42
    macrophages 56

Anti-ischemic therapy 183
Antiobesity medications 262
Antioxidant
    effect 42
    mimetics 58
Antiphospholipid
    antibodies 123
    syndrome 138
Antiplatelet 52
    activity, mechanisms of 99*f*
    agents 108*f*
    medications 117
    therapy 60, 107, 117
    use of 107, 109*f*
Antisense oligonucleotide 57
Antithrombotic therapy 54, 98
Antithymocyte globulin 235
Aortic dissection 58
Aortic insufficiency 240
Aortic pathology 52
Aortic stenosis 47
    progression 47
    severe 283
Aortic syndromes, medical strategies in 60*t*
Aortopulmonary collaterals 246
Apical dyskinesia 202
Apixaban 116
Apolipoprotein 27
Apoptosis 12, 16, 22
Applanation tonometry 92, 94
Arrhythmia 47*f*
Arrhythmogenic risk 185
Arterial stiffening 150
Arterial tissue concentration 212
Arterial tonometry 92
Arterial wall 54
Arteriolar tone 42
Artifact 163-165
Artificial intelligence
    assisted imaging 228
    driven wellbeing platforms 295
    integration 102
    model 102
Aspergillus 123, 132

Aspiration-based mechanical systems 221
Aspirin 60, 98, 103, 114, 116, 183
Atherectomy 214
Atheroma 19f, 27
  advancing 27
  progression, stage of 27
Atherosclerosis 13, 17, 52, 53f, 55t, 56
  detect subclinical 33
  detection of 31
  early origins of 26f
  impact in 55
  modifying agents 36
  newer concepts 54
  pathobiological determinants of 25
  prevention 37
  risk factors 27
Atherosclerotic
  contemporary management of 57
  coronary plaques 171
  disease 52
  plaque 16, 27, 53
Atherothrombosis 108f
Atherothrombotic events 98
Atrial fibrillation 83, 103, 115, 117f, 141, 287f
  ablation 141
  prevalence of 115, 141
Atrial septal defect 251
Attenuated plaque 163f
Autoimmune disorders 150
Autonomic imbalance 150
Autopsy studies 157
Average peak velocity 152
Azithromycin 137

B

Bactericidal agents 125
Bailout stenting 214
Balance bleeding risk 104
Balancing antiplatelet 103
Ballistocardiography 92
Balloon
  catheter 209
  delivery aids 213
  expansion failure 213
  uncrossable lesions 189, 191
  undilatable lesions 189
Bare metal stents 109, 112f, 114
  development of 209
Bariatric surgery 262, 263
Bartonella 130

Basiliximab 235
Below-knee intervention 196f
Beta-blocker 52, 59, 60, 69, 86, 158,
Beta-hydroxybutyrate 43
Beta-lactam
  allergy 129
  resistance 129
Bifurcation lesions 172, 194f, 210, 211
Bile acid
  secondary 56
  sequestrants 58
Bilirubin 121
Biobeat 92
  monitor 94
Biocompatible polymers 209
Biofilm 125
  sterilization 198
Biofilm-laden leads 196
Bioimpedance 91, 92
Biomarker testing 227
Biomarker-guided intervention 228
Bioresorbable
  scaffolds 103
  stents 103
Bisoprolol 86
Bleeding 259
  higher 104
  risk 104
    assessment 107
    high 99, 107, 111, 114
Bleeding Academic Research Consortium Type 115
Block and deliver technique 247
Blood
  speckles 165
  vessels constrict 181
Blood culture 123
  negative infective endocarditis 123, 130
Blood pressure 30, 88, 218f
  baseline 87
  control 31, 154
    rate 84
  elevated 85
  falls 181
  increasing 181
  lowering, rapid and sustained 84
  measurement method 93
  systolic 83, 234
Blooming 165
Blunt stump 204
Body mass index 3
  higher 236
Bone marrow 55

Bradycardia 154
Brain 41
  arteriovenous malformation 111
Bridging strategy 238
Bridging therapy 103
Brucella 123, 130
Buddy wire
  support 189
  technique 247
Burnout 292
  impact of 293
  mitigation 295

C

Calcific neoatheroma 190
Calcific plaque 162, 163f
Calcification, presence of 205
Calcified lesions 173, 195
Calcified plaque, underlying 170
Calcium
  balance 42
  channel blockers 86, 158
Canakinumab 54
Cap fibroatheroma 171
Capillary density loss 150
Cardiac biomarkers 121
Cardiac computed tomography 123
Cardiac cycle 157
Cardiac dysfunction, evidence of 181
Cardiac hypertrophy 17
Cardiac implantable electronic device infections 135
Cardiac index 234
Cardiac magnetic resonance 203
Cardiac myosin inhibition 281
Cardiac output 181
Cardiac power output 234
Cardiac resynchronization therapy implantation 197
Cardiac surgeons 227
Cardiac tissue 59
Cardiobacterium 130
Cardiogenic shock 65, 180, 184, 187, 232, 234
  latest advances in 184t
  pathophysiology of 180
  pharmacotherapy in 182
  triggers 181
Cardio-kidney-metabolic syndrome 1f
Cardiometabolic diseases 268
Cardiomyocytes 46
Cardiomyopathy 5

Index

Cardioprotection 45
Cardiopulmonary bypass
    management of 239
    time, longer 236
Cardiovascular disease 1, 13, 14t, 27,
            28, 55, 88, 268
    incidence of 29f
    risk factor for 83, 268, 270
Cardiovascular event 24, 262
Cardiovascular implant
            infections 198
Cardiovascular implantable
            electronic devices 137
Cardiovascular outcome trials 262
Cardiovascular protection 7
Cardiovascular risk factors 13t
Cardiovascular system 12
Cardiovascular tissues 16
Cardiovascular toxicity 16
Cardiovascular-kidney-metabolic
            syndrome 1, 2, 9
    pathophysiology of 2, 2f
    spectrum, stages of 4f
    staging of 4
    treatment of 6f
Carotid atherosclerotic plaques 12
Carotid endarterectomy 12
Carotid intima-media thickness 25
Carotid webs 198
Catheter 196
Catheter ablation 141
Catheter-based
    interventional closure 246
    therapeutic interventions 219
Catheter-directed thrombolysis 219
            devices 221f
Catheterization laboratory 176, 181
    access 228
    echo 182
Cavity spilling 247
Cefazolin 128, 135, 137
Ceftaroline 129
Ceftriaxone 130, 131, 137
Celiprolol 59, 60
Central venous
    occlusions 197
    pressures 234
Cephalexin 137
Cerebral abscesses 133
Cerebral oximetry 239
Cerebral venous thrombosis 196
Cerebrovascular accidents 83
Cerebrovascular events 67, 83
Chemotherapy-related subtypes 231

Chest pain 158
Chest X-ray 182
Child health, coordinated
            approach to 30
Chistorical cohort 114
Cholesterol
    crystals 164f
    levels 31
Chronic coronary
            syndrome 98, 99, 107
Chronic inflammatory disease 52, 53f
Chronic kidney disease 1, 7, 33, 43,
            88, 111, 236
Chronic total occlusion 157, 172, 191,
            201, 203, 206
    management 201
    population 203
    score 203, 205
Cilostazol 102
    based triple therapy 102
Ciprofloxacin 136
Circulatory support 236
Clarithromycin 137
Climate change leading to increased
            pollution 14
Clinical data harmonization 36
Clip
    deployment 259f
    embolization 255
Clonal hematopoiesis 55, 58
Clopidogrel 60, 98, 102, 104, 114,
            115, 117
    efficacy 102
    resistance rates, high 105
Clot burden aspirated 222f
Cloxacillin 136
Coagulase-negative staphylococci
            125, 128
Coaptation enhancement 258
Cognitive impairment 83
Coil
    embolization 247
    inside coronary artery 248f
Colchicine 54, 58
Combination pill, low-dose 87
Combination therapy,
            rationale for 83
Community programs 30
Compassion fatigue 293
Conduction disturbances 134
Conductive pathways,
            ablation of 199
Congenital coronary anomaly 157
Congenital heart disease 232, 233

interventions, use in
    pediatric 198
Contemporary cardiac intensive
            care units 180
Continuous noninvasive
            sphygmomanometers 95
Conventional histopathology
            techniques 18
Coronary angiography 157, 161, 170,
            174t, 201, 203
Coronary arteriovenous fistulae, coil
            closure of 246
Coronary artery
    angiogram 247f
    bypass
        grafting 159, 288, 289f
        surgery 12
    calcification, severe 173
    calcium scoring 33
    disease 13, 26, 28, 34, 83, 98, 107,
            201, 213fc, 262, 277, 289f
        left main 172
        nanoplastics in 12
    incidence of 247
    normal 162f
    perforation, coil closure of 247
    spasm, risk of 143
Coronary atheroma 12
    presence of nanoplastics in 18
Coronary atherosclerosis 26, 170
Coronary atherosclerotic
            stenosis 209
Coronary bypass graft surgery 18
Coronary catheterization
            laboratory 161
Coronary computed tomography
            angiography 157
Coronary flow reserve 158
Coronary guidewire 189
Coronary hemodynamics 157
Coronary in-stent restenosis 211
    agent, uncoated balloon for 289
Coronary intervention
            techniques 203
Coronary laser 188
Coronary lesions 175
Coronary microcirculation,
            anatomy of 149
Coronary microvascular dysfunction
    endotypes of 149
    functional 149
    manifestation of 149
    structural 149

Coronary perforation 159
   rates 206
Coronary perfusion 157
Coronary risk factors 12
Coronary tree, step-by-step coiling in 246
Coronary vein occlusion 197
Covered stents 197
Coxiella burnetii 123, 130
Creatinine 121, 182
Cross-boss techniques 206
Cryoablation 142-144
Cryoballoon
   ablation 145*f*
   design 144
Cuffless blood pressure
   devices 91, 93*t*
   measurement devices 91
   technologies 91, 92*t*
Culprit-lesion 185
Cultural pressures 292
Cyclic guanosine monophosphate 71*f*
CYP2C19
   gene 102
   polymorphism 104
   testing common 104
Cytokines 54
   stimulates 53
Cytomegalovirus 236, 237
Cytomembrane destruction 14
Cytotoxicity 14

D

Dalbavancin 132
   role of 132
Dalfopristin 129
Danish-German Cardiogenic Shock 180
Dapagliflozin 6, 44
Dapansutrile 58
Daptomycin 128
Data collection, standard of 36
De novo
   lesions 210, 212
   ostial disease 211
Debulking strategy 172
Defibrillator shocks 233
Degenerative valve disease 137
Delivery system insertion 259*f*
Dendritic cells 54
Depersonalization 292
Dermal contact 16

Device
   positioning 254, 255*f*
   refinement 228
Diabetes mellitus 27, 31, 41, 69, 150
   type 2 268
Diabetes-cardiorenal-metabolic multidisciplinary 8
Diabetic kidney disease 43
Digital fatigue 292, 293
Digital health and remote care 9
Digital hygiene 294
Digital overload 292
Digital subtraction angiography 133
Dilated cardiomyopathy 231, 232
Distal embolization 189
Distal perforation 247
Diuretics 183
Dobutamine 182, 233, 235
   stress echocardiography 203
Donation after circulatory death 243
Donor hearts, shortage of 231
Donor-derived infections 236
Door-to-lactate-free
   metrics 187
   time 180, 181
Door-to-reperfusion targets 185
Door-to-support time 180
Dopamine 233, 235
Dose confusion and polypharmacy 86
Double therapy, duration of 103
Doxycycline 59, 60, 130, 137
Drug delivery facilitation via vascular laser 196
Drug-coated balloon 212
   angioplasty 191*f*
   application 213
   choice of 212
   treatment 190
Drug-coated stent 114, 115
Drug-eluting balloon 209, 212*t*
   evidence for 210
   indications for 211
   limitations of 214
Drug-eluting stent 114
   implantation 285, 288*f*
   trials of 112*f*
Dual antiplatelet therapy 98, 102*t*, 105, 107, 110*f*, 111, 112*f*, 114-116, 183
   duration 99
Dual pathway inhibition 60, 110*f*
Dulaglutide 264
Dural sinus thrombosis 198

Dutch lipid clinic network score 32
Dyslipidemia 27, 29, 31, 150

E

Early atherosclerosis, pathobiology of 25
Early catheter-based interventions, rationale for 219
Early ezetimibe initiation 278
Early stent thrombosis resistant to thrombectomy, LASER to treat 197
Echinocandins, high-dose 132
Echocardiography 123, 202, 219
   parameters 203
Echolucent plaque 163*f*
Ecosystem balance 57
Eculizumab 236
Edoxaban 116
Ehlers-Danlos syndrome, vascular 58
Eikenella 130
Electrical inactivation through tissue heating 142
Electrocardiogram, preprocedural 283
Electrocardiography 91
Electronic health records 36
Electroporation 142, 146
Elevated trimethylamine-noxide promotes 56
Embolic stroke 133
Embolization 107
Emerging pathways 57
Emerging research directions 228
Emotional burden 293
Emotional exhaustion 292
Empagliflozin 6, 44
   effects of 45
Empiric therapy 127
Empirical antibiotic 127
   regimen 128*t*
Encephalopathy 133
Endocarditis 135
Endografts 197
Endoluminal infections, treatment of 196
End-organ dysfunction 233
Endothelial cells 16, 53*f*
Endothelial dysfunction 2, 12, 16, 22, 26, 58, 149
Endothelial muscle cells 16
Endothelial-to-mesenchymal transition 55, 56

Endothelin-1 149
Endothelium 52
Endovascular aortic repair 197
Endovascular procedures 197
Endovascular repair 58
Endovascular system, study of 224
Energy and metabolic efficiency 43
Enterococcal
 endocarditis, treatment of 131t
 infective endocarditis 129
Enterococcus faecalis 125, 127, 128
Environmental exposure models 21
Environmental pollution 12, 14
Epicardial adipose tissues 16
Epicardial fat 43
Epicardial vessels 149
Epigenetic marks 55
Epinephrine 183, 235
Epstein–Barr virus 236
Eradicate atherosclerosis 34, 35t
Eruptive calcified nodule 164f
Erythrocyte sedimentation rate 121
Esophageal fistula, risk of 143
Esophagus 142
Estimated glomerular filtration
 rate 41, 44, 111
Eurointervention 283
Everolimus-eluting stent 114t
Evinacumab 57, 58
Excimer-assisted systems 199
Excimer-laser
 coronary atherectomy 188,
 190, 192
 induced endothelial regeneration,
 research into 198
Exercise 31
Exertional angina 158
Exopolysaccharides 125
Extracardiac emboli 123
Extracellular matrix 54
Extracorporeal membrane
 oxygenation 219, 223
Extracranial bleeding 225
Extra-pulmonary vein lesions,
 ablation of 143
Ezetimibe 54, 60

F

Facilitating valve-in-valve
 procedures 198
Factor XI inhibitors 103
Familial hypercholesterolemia 32
Faster thrombus burden reduction 226

Fatal cardiovascular events 25
Fatty streaks 26
Fenfluramine 262
Fibrin sheaths 196
Fibrinogen 220
Fibrinolysis 223
Fibrinolytic activity 220
 concentrating 220
Fibroatheroma 27
 transform 171
Fibroblast-like phenotype 56
Fibrocalcific lesion, severe 195f
Fibrocalcific plaque 162, 164f
Fibromuscular dysplasia 198
Fibrosis 46
Fibrotic, composition of 162
Fibrous plaque 162, 163f, 164f
Fifth pillar argument 75
First commercial laser 188f
Fistulae 123
Flexible work models 294
Flight mass spectrometry,
 ionization-time of 123
Flowtriever® system 222f
Flucloxacillin 135
Fluconazole 132
Flucytosine 132
Foam cell-like phenotype 56
Focal extraluminal crater 247
Food and water pollutants 14
Fosfomycin 129
Fourier transformed infrared 19f
 spectroscopy 21f
Fractional flow reserve 158
Free entrapped guidewire 198
Fulminant myocarditis 181
Functional cardiomyocytes 16
Fungal endocarditis 132

G

Generate hyperresponsive
 monocytes 55
Generating reactive oxygen
 species 16
Genital infections 48
Genomics 9
Genotype-guided de-escalation 102
Gentamicin 128, 130, 131
Global longitudinal strain 46f
Glomeruli leads 3
Glomerulus 41
Glucagon-like peptide-1 receptor
 agonist 263

Glucose, role of 184
Glycemic control 6, 154
Glycoprotein 107
Glycosuria 6
Glycosuric effects 41
Gripper actuation, controlled 251
Growing public health concern 231
Guanosine triphosphate 71f
Guanylate cyclase 70
Guided subintimal tracking 206
Guideline directed medical
 therapy 7, 69
Guideline endorsements 76
Gut microbiome 56, 270
 targeted therapies 58
Gut microbiota
 composition 268
 diversity 270
 reduces 271

H

Haemophilus 130
Headache 102
Healed plaque 164f
Health workforce strategies 36
Healthcare
 association 122
 systems 9
Healthy diet 30
Heart
 pumping ability drops 181
 rate increases 181
Heart failure 7, 13, 45, 48f, 77, 83,
 122, 232, 250, 262, 281
 management 72
 novel therapies for 71f
 role in 45
 with improved ejection
 fraction 45
 with preserved ejection
 fraction 264f
 with reduced ejection fraction 69
 management 70f
 worsening 70
Heart transplant 231, 240
 candidacy 232
Heart transplantation 233
 number of 232t
 perioperative
 management of 232
 period of 234
Heavy calcification 204
Hematoma 170, 173

Hematopoiesis 57
Hematopoietic stem cells 55
Hemodynamic 183, 220
   assessment 254
   goals 182
   instability 65, 233
   load 60
   mechanisms 2
   monitoring 182
   profiles 234
   stabilization 223
Hemoglobinuria 146
Hemoptysis 218
Hemorrhage 57
   intracranial 111, 224-226
   intraplaque 171
   subarachnoid 133
Hemorrhagic stroke 133
Hemostatic disorders 233
Heparin, unfractionated 219
Hepatic flavin-containing monooxygenase 56
High-density lipoprotein cholesterol, lower 25
Histone methylation 55
Homogenous 162
Homografts 133
Homologous blood pressure 85
Human diseases 14
Hybrid support 187
Hydroxychloroquine 130
Hypercholesterolemia 32
Hyperkalemia 74
   prevention of 44
Hypertension 27-29, 32, 83, 91, 150
   combination therapy for 88, 88t
   epidemic of 69
   management of 84
   mediated organ damage 88
   mild 3
   monotherapy for 84t
   polypills 83
   screening for 31
   stage first 85
Hypertrophic cardiomyopathy 137, 150, 159, 232
Hypokalemia 184
Hypomagnesemia 184
Hypoperfusion, signs of 181
Hypotension 181
   and volume depletion 48
Hypovolemia 240
Hypoxia inducible factor 47f

I

Iatrogenic aortic occlusion 197
Iatrogenic coronary dissection, LASER-assisted management of 197
Immune
   cells, dynamic ecosystem of 54
   dysregulation 57
   mediated microvascular injury 150
   metabolic disease 54
Immunity 54
   metabolic control of 56
   trained 55
Immunohistochemistry, histopathology with 124
Immunometabolism 56
Immunomodulation 58
Immunosuppression 234
   perioperative management of 235
Immunotherapy 35
Impair cardiac contractility 16
Impella 186
Implantable cardiodefibrillator lead extraction 194
Implantable circulatory device 239
Induction therapy 235
Infectious agent 237
Infectious complications 234, 236
Infective endocarditis 121, 122t, 123, 124t, 127t, 128t, 132, 133t, 134, 138
   prevention of 137t, 138
   surgery 133
   surgical management of 132
Inferior vena cava filters, embedded 198
Infiltrative cardiomyopathies 150
Inflammation 12, 16, 22, 52, 58, 171
   chronic 57
Inflammatory hypothesis 54
Inflammatory injury 150
Inflammatory macrophages 57
Inflammatory markers 26
Inflammatory responses, induction of 57
Infrared spectroscopy 12
Ingestion 14
Innate
   cells, memory in 55
   immune cells 55
Innovative financing models 37
Inotropes 182, 185, 187, 233, 236
Inotropic drugs 235
In-stent restenosis 159, 190, 191f, 209, 210

Insulin resistance 29
Integrated care models 8f
Interagency Registry for Mechanically Assisted Circulatory Support 244
Intercellular adhesion molecule 45
Interleukin 59
Intima, disease of 162
Intimal hyperplasia 190
Intra-aortic balloon pump 182, 186
Intracardiac devices 121
Intraglomerular pressure, lowering 42
Intraplaque angiogenesis 57
Intraprocedural fibrinolytic supplementation 224
Intraprocedural hemodynamic assessment 225
Intravascular brachytherapy 197
Intravascular hemolysis 146
Intravascular imaging 161, 163, 167t, 173, 174, 176, 206, 214
   catheters, LASER to facilitate delivery of 197
   systems, technical features of 161
Intravascular lithotripsy 214
Intravascular ultrasonography 285, 288f
Intravascular ultrasound 161, 164t, 165, 172, 175, 190, 206
   guided 288
   plaque characterization 163f
Invasive coronary function testing 152
   protocol 152fc
Inverse probability weighting adjustment 289f
Irbesartan 59, 60
Ischemia 5, 149
   driven target vessel revascularization 115
   long-standing 202
   symptoms of 152
   to atheroma, moving from 24
Ischemic cardiomyopathy 202, 231, 232
Ischemic heart disease, stable 114
Isoechoic 162

K

Kawasaki aneurysm 198
Ketoacidosis 47
   potential for 44

Ketogenesis 43
Kidney
  disease 44
  protection 43
  retain fluid 181
Kingella 130

L

Lampoon 197
Lancet commission 29, 38
  classified 25
Large unruptured aneurysms 134
Large-bore
  aspiration systems 220
  thrombectomy validation 225
Laser
  coronary atherectomy 188
  sheaths 194
Laser-assisted drug delivery 196
Lasing and thrombus aspiration 192*f*
Leadership development 294
Leaflet
  calcification, minimal 253
  capture, independent 253*f*
  grasping 254
  repair 258
Left circumflex arterial territorial
    distribution 202
Left ventricle 234, 257
  dominant shock 234
  primary graft dysfunction,
    classification of 234
Left ventricular 218*f*
  assist device 231, 240
    candidacy 237
    perioperative management
      of 237
    therapy 242
  dysfunction 250
  ejection fraction 45, 203
  hypertrophy 202
Legionella 130
  pneumophila 123
Lepodisiran 58
Lesion
  preparation 172, 213
  severity, assessment of 163
  uncomplicated 213
  uncrossable 189*f*
  undilatable 190*f*
Leukocytosis 121
Leukopenia 121
Levofloxacin 130

Levosimendan 233
Libman-sacks endocarditis 138
Lifestyle 54
  intervention 262
  modification 6
Life-threatening arrhythmia 65
Linezolid 128, 129
Lipid
  lowering 54
  management 7
  metabolism 57
  profiles 30
  storage disorder 52
Lipidic plaque 164*f*
Lipid-rich plaque 164*f*
Lipoprotein 54, 57, 59
  cholesterol, higher low-density 25
  metabolism 57
  modified 52
  reduction, lepodisiran for 57
Liposomal amphotericin 132
Lithotripsy 197, 213
Liver 41
Loeys–Dietz syndrome 58
Losartan 59, 60
Loss-of-function alleles 102
Low blood pressure 233
Low-density lipoprotein 52, 53*f*, 59
  cholesterol 279
Low-dose combination
  advantages of 84
  disadvantages of 84
  therapy, support of 86
Low-thrombogenic stent 108
Lumen
  area stenosis 167
  cross-sectional area 167
Lumenogram 161

M

Machine learning 92
Macroalbuminuria 7
Macrocalcification 57
Macrophages 164*f*
Macrovascular spasm 152
Macula densa 42
Major adverse cardiac events 189, 210
Major adverse cardiovascular event
    45, 67, 206
Maladaptive inflammatory,
    chronic 54
Malapposition 173
  acute 170

Marantic endocarditis 138
Marfan syndrome 58
Maslach burnout inventory 292
Matrix metalloproteinase 45, 46*f*
  inhibition 59
Matrix-assisted laser desorption 123
May-Thurner syndrome 198
Mechanical aspiration
    effectiveness 224
Mechanical atherectomy, excimer
    laser 188
Mechanical circulatory support 180,
    185, 219, 223
  devices 185, 231
    types of 185, 186*f*
Mechanical thrombectomy 220, 222,
    224, 226, 227
  major 221*f*
Mechanical valves 133
Mechanistic novelty 75
Mediterranean diet 268
Meningitis 133
Mental health
  infrastructure 294
  literacy campaigns 294
Merry-go-round effect 165
Metabolic rewiring 55
Metabolizers 102
Metabolomics 9
Metastatic infection 124
Methicillin-resistant *Staphylococcus
    aureus* 120
Microalbuminuria 3
Microbial metabolites 56
Microbial protein fingerprints 123
Microbiome 271
  modulation 57
  targeted interventions 57
Microcalcification 57
Microcatheters 206, 248, 248*f*
  reduce circulating
    homocysteine 269
Microplastics 12
  pathobiology 15*f*
Microvascular angina 149
  pharmacologic options in 153*t*
Microvascular rarefaction 150
Microvascular remodeling and
    fibrosis 150
Microvascular resistance 149
Microvascular spasm 149, 152
Microvasculature 149
Milrinone 233, 235

Mineralocorticoid receptor antagonists 69
Minimum inhibitory concentration data 123
Minimum stent area 191
Mitochondrial damage 42
Mitochondrial dysfunction 12, 16, 22
Mitochondrial health 42
Mitochondrial impairment 14
Mitochondrial lesions 16
MitraClip
  comparison of 251f
  system 251, 252f
Mitral regurgitation, secondary 250
Mitral valve area 253
  suspected 151fc
  treatment strategy for 153fc
Molecular target 59
Monoclonal antibodies 57
Monocytes 55
Monophosphate pathway 69
Monopill low-dose combinations 83
Monotherapy 84, 88, 115
  dose of 84
  group 101
Mortality reduction 65f, 79
Moxifloxacin 128
M-transcatheter edge-to-edge repair systems 251
Mucocutaneous infection 237
Multidisciplinary care 154
Multidisciplinary teams 37
Multifactorial clinical syndrome 180
Multifactorial inflammatory disease 25
Multiorgan failure 181
Multiple chemokines, consequent upregulation of 53
Multispline array 144
Multivessel percutaneous coronary intervention 184
Musculoskeletal manifestations 134
MyClip 253f
  delivery system 252f
  system 252
Mycophenolate mofetil 236
Mycoplasma 130
  pneumoniae 123
Mycotic aneurysms 123, 133
Myocardia 16
Myocardial blushing 247
Myocardial bridging 157
  location of 157
Myocardial fibers 157

Myocardial fibrosis 17
Myocardial infarction 13, 25, 65, 69, 110, 114, 151, 158, 202, 278, 279, 280f
  acute 13, 28, 45
  flow 190
Myocardial perfusion, computed tomography 151
Myocardial salvage 65f
Myocardial tissue 143
Myocardial viability 202
Myocarditis 134

N

Na-hydrogen exchanger 46
Nanoplastic 13, 16, 17
  containing plaques 18
  exposure, chronic 18
  gaining particular attention 13
  quantification of 18
  toxicity 12
  trigger 16
Nanozyme therapy 35
National Pert Consortium 228
Native aortic valve regurgitation 281
Native valve endocarditis 134
Natriuresis, effects on 42
Natriuretic peptides 3, 71f, 121
Neoatherosclerosis 173, 174
Neointimal growth 170
Neointimal hyperplasia 56, 173
Nephrotoxicity, lower risk of 130
Neurohormonal mechanisms 2
Neurohormonal overactivation 69
Neurohumoral activation 217
Neurological complications 134fc
Neurological events 122
New ablation therapies and techniques 142
Next-generation sequencing 124
Nitrates 158
Nitric oxide 69, 71f
Nitroglycerin bolus 152
NLRP3 inflammasome inhibitors 58
Nocturnal hypertension 91
Nonantihypertensive effects 84
Non-bacterial thrombotic endocarditis 138
Noncommunicable diseases 27, 34
Nonculprit
  lesions 185
  territories 184
Noneruptive calcified nodule 164f

Nonheme iron 271
Nonoverlapping safety profile 76
Nonpharmacologic therapy 153
Non-ST-elevation
  acute coronary syndrome 110f
  myocardial infarction 54, 98
Nonsteroidal anti-inflammatory drug 111
Norepinephrine 182, 235
Novel ablation catheters 144t
Novel therapeutic targets 59t
Nuclear factor kappa B 26, 270
Nucleic acid-based therapies 35

O

Obesity 29, 33
  pharmacotherapy for 263
Obesogenic environments 262
Obstructive coronary artery disease 149
Occluded hemodialysis catheters, recanalization of 197
Office-based sphygmomanometers 91
Off-label neurovascular intervention 198
Olpasiran 57, 58
Omecamtiv mecarbil 71f
Omega-3 fats 270
Optical coherence tomography 161, 165
  artifacts 164t
Oral streptococci, treatment of 128
Orbital atherectomy 189, 213
Organ
  damage, target 84
  perfusion markers 183
  sharing, united network for 244
Osteoarthritis 262
Osteogenic phenotype 56
Ostial and bifurcation lesions 193
Ostial lesions 194f, 211
Ostioproximal right coronary artery 172
Outpatient
  antibiotic therapy 131t
  therapy 130
Oxacillin 136
Oxazolidinones 129
Oxidative phosphorylation 55
Oxidative stress 2, 12, 16, 22, 58
  nanoplastics induce 16

Oxidized phospholipids 57
 carriage of 57
Oxygenation impairment 218

P

P value 113, 114
P2Y12 inhibitors 98, 100, 116, 117
Pacemaker 194
 implantation 277f
 lead extraction 195f
Paclitaxel 209
 coated balloon 210, 289
 eluting stents 210
Papillary muscle rupture 181
Paravalvular extension 122
Particulate matter 14
Pascal device 251f
Pascal implant 253f
Pascal system 252
 components of 253f
Patent arterial duct 246
Patent foramen ovale closure 239
Patient's selection 232
Pediatric Heart Transplant Study 244
Pelacarsen 57
Penumbra indigo system 222f
Percutaneous coronary intervention
 65, 98, 107, 109f, 110f, 111,
 117f, 158, 188, 201, 203,
 209, 213, 217, 276, 277, 288,
 289f
 complication 206
 group 288
 recent guidelines for 65t
 roadmap for 161
Percutaneous microaxial flow
 pump 180
Percutaneous transluminal coronary
 angioplasty 188, 209
Perfused boundary region 46f
Pericardial blushing 247
Pericarditis 134
Peripheral artery
 disease 52, 60, 83, 211, 212
Peripheral bypass graft occlusion 198
Peripheral chronic vein occlusion,
 LASER-assisted
 recanalization of 198
Periprocedural myocardial injury 107
Permanent metallic nidus for
 thrombosis 103
Peroxisome proliferator-activated
 receptors 270

Persistent albuminuria, minimal 3
Persistent hyperlactatemia 180
Persistent stress 292
Persistent symptoms despite
 quadruple therapy 75
Pharmacologic therapy 153
Phosphatidylcholine 56
Phosphodiesterase inhibitor 102
Photochemical decomposition 188
Photochemical effect 188
Photomechanical action 188
Photoplethysmography 91, 92
Photothermal effect 188
Phrenic nerve 142
 injury, risk of 143
Physical activity 30, 154
Physical wellbeing 294
Physician burnout
 causes of 293
 impacts of 294
Plaque
 ecosystem 57
 erosion 164f
 fate of 57
 formation 16, 54
  progressive stage of 27
  steps in 52
 mixed 163f
 modification 197
 tools 188
 rupture 107, 164f
Plasminogen 57
 activator 224
Plastic pollution, policies for
 reducing 20
Platelet 198f
 aggregation 149
Pneumocystis jirovecii 237
Point-of-care
 tools, role of 181
 ultrasound 181, 219
Polycystic kidney disease 44
Polymer coated stents,
 modification of 197
Polymer covered stents,
 modification of 197
Polyphenols 270
Polypropylene 19
Polystyrene nanoplastics 16
Population proportionate
 attributable fractions 29f
Positron emission tomography 203
Postcardiopulmonary bypass 239

Postpartum cardiomyopathy 232
Postpercutaneous coronary
 intervention
 complications 169f
Poststent assessment 168
Post-worsening rescue therapy 80
Potassium-to-sodium ratio 269
Practical prescribing 74
Prasugrel 98, 100, 102, 104, 115
Precision medicine 102
Predict stent underexpansion 173
Predictive organizational
 analytics 295
Preshock
 hypotensive normoperfusion 234
 normotensive hypoperfusion 234
Pressure wires 197
Presyncope 158
Primary graft dysfunction 234,
 234t, 235fc
Primary percutaneous coronary
 intervention 192, 192f
Primordial prevention 29
Procalcitonin 121
Programmed cell death 16
Proinflammatory cytokines,
 targeting 58
Proinflammatory endothelial
 activation 158
Proinflammatory macrophages 56
Prolonged dual antiplatelet
 therapy 209
Proprotein convertase subtilisin/
 kexin type 9
 inhibitors 57, 60
Prosthetic material, choice of 133
Prosthetic valve
 endocarditis 125, 134
 infective endocarditis 124
 thrombosis 197
Protein 121
Proteomics 9
Prothrombin time 220
Prothrombotic pathways,
 activation of 17
Protien kinase B 47f
Proton pump inhibitor
 cotherapy 104
Provocative pharmacological
 testing 158
Proximal cap 205
Proximal cap ambiguity 205
Proximal left main branches 172

Proximity artifact 165
Pseudoaneurysms 123
Pseudoresistance 86
Public health
   interventions 20
   response 34
Pulmonary angiography, computed tomography 218
Pulmonary arteriovenous malformations 246
Pulmonary artery 218f
   catheter 239
   chronic thromboembolism, laser in 196
   pulsatility index 234
Pulmonary capillary wedge pressures 234
Pulmonary congestion, use loop diuretics for 183
Pulmonary embolism 217, 223, 229
   massive 224
   pathophysiology 218f
   response teams 226
   submassive 224
   thrombolysis 225
   treatment 221f
Pulmonary valve 136
Pulmonary vascular resistance 233
Pulmonary vasodilators 236
Pulmonary vein
   flow 256f
   isolation 143, 199
   occlusion postablation therapy 198
   stenosis, risk of 143
Pulsatility 240
Pulse
   arrival time 91, 92
   transit time 92
   wave velocity 46f
Pulsed field 143, 144
   ablation 146
      development of 141
Pyrolysis-gas chromatography 18

Q

Q fever 130
Quality of life 241
   impaired 69
Quantitative coronary angiography 285, 288f
Quinupristin 129

R

Radiofrequency ablation 142
Raman spectroscopy 12, 21f
Rapid hemodynamic restoration 219
Recanalized thrombus 164f
Recombinant tissue plasminogen activator 220
Red thrombus 164f
Refractory cardiogenic shock, develop 223
Refractory despite revascularization 184
Reframes vericiguat 78
Regional acute coronary syndrome 228
Regional wall motion abnormality 202, 203
Regulatory measures 20
Remote monitoring 8
Renal dysfunction 74
Renal failure, acute 134
Renal function 72
Renal insufficiency 83
Renal replacement therapy 234
Renin-angiotensin aldosterone system 2, 43
   modulation 43
   system inhibition 69
Reparative macrophages 57
Requires cuff calibration 93
Residual blood artifact 165
Residual lipoprotein risk 52
Restenosis 193f, 211
   high rates of 209
Restrictive cardiomyopathy 232
Retatrutide 266
Retrograde technique 201
Reversible P2Y12 inhibitors 103
Rheia trial 276f
Rheumatic heart disease 137
Rhythm control management 141
Ridaforolimus-eluting stent 114
Rifampicin 125
Rifampin 128, 136
Right atrium 259f
Right bundle branch block 283
Right heart
   catheterization 233
   hemodynamics 236
Right ventricle 4, 234, 257
   dominant shock 234
   primary graft dysfunction, indicators for 234

Right ventricular 218f
   assist devices 223
   dysfunction 218
   failure 240
Ring-down artifact 165
Risk factor control 54
Rivaroxaban 60, 116, 285, 287f
Rotablative techniques 188
Rotational atherectomy 188

S

Saphenous vein graft restenosis 192
Satiety and Clinical Adiposity-Liraglutide Evidence 264
Scanning electron microscopy 12
Seattle angina questionnaire 154
Seeking support 294
Seizures 133
Selective coronary artery angiogram 248f
Semaglutide 265
Septal collateral atherectomy 198
Septic emboli 135
   detecting 124
Serotonin and thromboxane A2 217
Serum lactate 182
Sex-specific strategies 154
Shock team
   integration of 187
   standardization 184
Short dual antiplatelet therapy 109
Short-chain fatty acids 55, 56, 270
Sibutramine 262
Side branch ostium 173
Silent emboli 133
Single leaflet device attachment 258
Single pill 83
Sirolimus-eluting stent 114
Skeletal muscle 41
Skin flora 237
Small-vessel disease 209-211
Smooth muscle hyperreactivity 149
Social pressures 292
Sodium
   handling 42
   hydeogen exchanger 47f
Sodium-glucose
   cotransporter 2 46f
   like transporter 2 inhibitors 48f
Sodium-glucose cotransporter 2 inhibitors 9, 41-44, 42fc, 45-47, 48f, 69, 71f
   mechanisms 47

adverse effects of 47
benefits of 43
mechanisms of action of 41
Soft plaque 163*f*
Solid organ transplant recipients 138
Soluble guanylate cyclase 71*f*
Spiky carina 173
Splenic complications 134
Splenomegaly 122
Spondylodiscitis 124
Spontaneous coronary artery dissection 164*f*
Spotty
   calcification 171
   calcium 164*f*
ST segment-elevation acute coronary syndrome 110*f*
Standard antithrombotic therapy 98
Standard cuff-based brachial 94
Standard techniques fail 191
Standardized detection methods 21
Staphylococcal endocarditis, treatment of 130*t*
Staphylococcus
   aureus 121, 128, 132, 136
   lugdunensis 125
Statins 52, 60, 183
Steerable guide catheter advancement 254, 254*f*
ST-elevated myocardial infarction 46, 54, 98
   reperfusion 206
Stem cell 60
Stent
   edge issues 173
   edge restenosis in bifurcations, treatment of 198
   failure 173
      mechanism of 161
   fracture 159
   implantation 168
   optimization 172
   sizing 166, 168*f*
   strategy 172
   struts 198
      uncovered 173
   thrombosis 98, 107, 159, 189
   underexpanded 193, 194*f*
Stigma 294
Stigmatization 33
Streptococcal endocarditis, treatment of 129*t*
Streptococcus
   gallolyticus 128
   spp. 127, 128, 132

Stress
   cardiac magnetic resonance 151
   electrocardiogram 151
Stroke 13, 25, 114, 115
   acute 196
   response networks 228
ST-segment elevation myocardial infarction 114, 180, 282, 282*f*
Subcutaneous semaglutide 264
   trials 264*f*
Subendocardial hypoperfusion 150
Subendothelial space 52
Suboptimal stent implantation, parameters of 168
Sudden cardiac death 45, 77
Sudden death 25
Sudden-onset dyspnea 218
Supplemental oxygen 182
Surgery
   during index admission 122
   urgency of 133
Surgical aortic valve replacement 275, 279*f*
Surgical embolectomy 219
Surgical management 159
Surgical procedural risk factors 234
Surgical techniques 132
Surveillance systems 36
Swedeheart registry, results of 289*f*
Syncope 158, 218
Systemic fibrinolytic therapy 219
Systemic hypoperfusion 180
Systemic inflammation 150
Systemic ischemic sequelae 117
Systemic lupus erythematosus 138
Systemic thrombolysis 220, 225
Systemic vascular resistance 234

T

Tachycardia 102, 218
Tachypnea 218
Tacrolimus 236
Takayasu aortoarteritis 196*f*
Tamponade 240
Tandem heart 186
Tangential signal dropout 165
Target lesion
   failure 114
   revascularization 114
Telemedicine 8, 228
Temporary mechanical circulatory support 180

Tenecteplase 225
Therapeutic delivery, targeted 219
Thin cap fibroatheroma 164*f*
Thrombectomy, manual 197
Thrombocytopenia 121
Thromboembolic pulmonary hypertension sequelae, chronic 219
Thrombogenesis 12, 17
Thrombolysis 65, 133, 220
   LASER-assisted 196
Thrombosis 192
   beyond platelets 52
Thrombus 193*f*
   aspiration 171
   infected 196
   migration 218*f*
   prolapse 170
Thrombus-Laden vessels 192
Thyroid gland 41
Ticagrelor 98, 100, 102, 104, 114
Tirzepatide 265, 266
   efficacy of 265
Tocilizumab 58
Tolerant bacteria 125
Tonometry 91
Tortuosity, severe 204
Toxoplasma species 236
Training primary care providers 36
Transcatheter 275, 279*f*
   aortic valve implantation 47, 135, 197, 275, 277*f*, 281, 283
   edge-to-edge repair 250
   mitral valve
      repair 233
      replacement 197
   tricuspid valve 258*t*
      intervention 258
Transesophageal
   echocardiography 123, 239, 251
Transformative therapies 72
Transfusion disorders 233
Transient ischemic attacks 133
Translational relevance 55
Translational research 37
   guided transseptal puncture 254*f*
Trans-septal puncture 253
   complications 255
Transthoracic Doppler echocardiography 151
Transthoracic echocardiography 123, 251

Transthyretin amyloid
    cardiomyopathy 48f
Trapping technique 247
Tricuspid
    gradients 259
    regurgitation 256, 257t, 258
Trimethylamine 56
    N-oxide 55, 56, 59, 271
        pathway 56
Tropheryma whipplei 130
Troponins 121
Tubulointerstitial injury 42
Tumor necrosis factor-alpha 53f

U

Ultrasound-accelerated
    catheter-directed
        thrombolysis 220
    thrombolysis 223
Ultrasound-based measurement 92
Unintended stent deformation 168,
    170, 173
Uptitration 83
Urine output 182
Urokinase 220

V

Vacuum thrombectomy, computer-
    assisted 226
Valved conduits 133
Valves most affected 122
Valvular disease, severe 181

Vancomycin 128, 129, 131, 135
Vascular access 182, 197
Vascular cells 54
Vascular damage 25
Vascular endothelial growth factor 43
Vascular extracellular matrix
    remodeling 52
Vascular grafts, testing 197
Vascular inflammation 17
Vascular obstruction 217
Vascular smooth muscle cell 16, 53,
    53f, 55, 56
Vascular surgery 227
Vascular tissue 59
Vascular wall strength 60
Vasoconstriction 149
Vasodilators 183
Vasomotor tone regulation,
    abnormal 149
Vasopressors 182, 187, 235
Vegetarian diet 268
Venoarterial cannulation 223
Venous thromboembolism,
    manifestation of 217
Venous ultrasound 219
Venovenous collaterals 246
Ventricular assist device
    classification of 237, 238f
    system 237
Ventricular septal defects 121
Vericiguat 72, 73
    role of 80
Vertebral osteomyelitis 124
Vicious cycle 181

Viridans streptococci 121
Virtual integrated care program 9
Virtual reality interventions 295
Visi mobile system 94
von Willebrand factor 107
Voriconazole 132
Vulnerable plaque 170
    assessment 170

W

Warfarin 116
Warning signs 294
Wearable technology 295
Weight management 154
White blood cells 46f
White thrombus 164f
Women's Ischemia Syndrome
    Evaluation program 149
Work-life
    boundary erosion 292
    integration 294

X

Xanthomas 32

Z

Zebrafish 17
Zerlasiran 58
Ziltivekimab 35, 57
Zotarolimus-eluting
    endeavor sprint stent 110
    stent 114